AF439742

CHRONIC LYMPHOCYTIC LEUKEMIA

CHRONIC LYMPHOCYTIC LEUKEMIA

Edited by

Susan O'Brien
MD Anderson Cancer Center
Houston, Texas, USA

John G. Gribben
Barts & The London School of Medicine
London, UK

informa
healthcare

New York London

Informa Healthcare USA, Inc.
52 Vanderbilt Avenue
New York, NY 10017

© 2008 by Informa Healthcare USA, Inc.
Informa Healthcare is an Informa business

No claim to original U.S. Government works
Printed in the United States of America on acid-free paper
10 9 8 7 6 5 4 3 2 1

International Standard Book Number-10: 1-4200-6895-4 (Hardcover)
International Standard Book Number-13: 978-1-4200-6895-5 (Hardcover)

This book contains information obtained from authentic and highly regarded sources. Reprinted material is quoted with permission, and sources are indicated. A wide variety of references are listed. Reasonable efforts have been made to publish reliable data and information, but the author and the publisher cannot assume responsibility for the validity of all materials or for the consequence of their use.

No part of this book may be reprinted, reproduced, transmitted, or utilized in any form by any electronic, mechanical, or other means, now known or hereafter invented, including photocopying, microfilming, and recording, or in any information storage or retrieval system, without written permission from the publishers.

For permission to photocopy or use material electronically from this work, please access www.copyright.com (http://www.copyright.com/) or contact the Copyright Clearance Center, Inc. (CCC) 222 Rosewood Drive, Danvers, MA 01923, 978-750-8400. CCC is a not-for-profit organization that provides licenses and registration for a variety of users. For organizations that have been granted a photocopy license by the CCC, a separate system of payment has been arranged.

Trademark Notice: Product or corporate names may be trademarks or registered trademarks, and are used only for identification and explanation without intent to infringe.

Library of Congress Cataloging-in-Publication Data

Chronic lymphocytic leukemia / edited by Susan M. O'Brien, John G. Gribben.
    p. ; cm.
  Includes bibliographical references and index.
  ISBN-13: 978-1-4200-6895-5 (hardcover : alk. paper)
  ISBN-10: 1-4200-6895-4 (hardcover : alk. paper)
  1. Chronic lymphocytic leukemia. I. O'Brien, Susan, 1954- II. Gribben, John.
  [DNLM: 1. Leukemia, Lymphocytic, Chronic, B-Cell—etiology. 2. Leukemia, Lymphocytic, Chronic, B-Cell—therapy. WH 250 C556501 2008]
  RC643.C4842 2008
  616.99′419—dc22

                                          2008030344

For Corporate Sales and Reprint Permissions call 212-520-2700 or write to: Sales Department, 52 Vanderbilt Avenue, 7th floor, New York, NY 10017.

Visit the Informa Web site at
www.informa.com

and the Informa Healthcare Web site at
www.informahealthcare.com

Preface

With this book we have endeavored to develop a comprehensive and up-to-date picture of chronic lymphocytic leukemia. The authors represented herein are some of the leading experts in the field, and the focus is on how new developments in the molecular pathogenesis of this disease impact how we approach and treat patients with CLL. Our introduction to this disease is written by arguably the most famous CLL expert in the United States, Kanti Rai. The initial chapters focus on the origin and nature of the CLL cell and discuss this in relationship to gene expression profiling and molecular abnormalities. Sequencing of immunoglobulin heavy chain genes has shown that patients can be divided into two groups, those with mutated and those with unmutated VH genes (which has significant prognostic import). However, examination of gene expression profiles shows that mutated and unmutated samples are much more similar than different, all having a phenotype of an activated B cell. Thus, these conflicting perspectives on the disease are still being worked out. Another aspect of CLL is the familial clustering that is seen, and the search for genes predisposing to such familial cases is an active area of research. The fascinating finding that a percentage of "normal" people have a small clone of CD5+ B cells provides insight into possible development of the disease, but at the same time raises many questions. Dysregulation of apoptosis is a ubiquitous element in CLL and overexpression of multiple BCL-2 family members can potentially be targeted therapeutically with new molecules that are in clinical trials.

For the past 30 years both the Rai-staging system and the Binet-staging system (which are very similar) have been used to evaluate patients with newly diagnosed CLL. These staging systems are simple, relying only on a physical exam and a complete blood count. Yet they provide significant prognostic information as more advanced stages are associated with shorter survival. However, one limitation of these staging systems is that they are static. That is, in patients presenting with early-stage disease it is difficult to predict which patient is likely to progress and require treatment within a few years and which patient may live 20 years with indolent disease and die of other causes. In the last few years there has been a proliferation of factors, partly derived from research into signaling pathways in CLL, which can provide prognostic information within early-stage disease. Some of these include $\beta 2$ microglobulin, mutation status of the VH gene, presence of CD38 or ZAP70, and molecular abnormalities detected by fluorescent in situ hybridization (FISH). However, this proliferation of important prognostic factors has also raised the question of correlation between factors, and when discordant, which ones are most important. This is an area under active investigation.

Another potential use of these prognostic factors is identifying a subset of patients who might benefit from early treatment. The approach to CLL has always been a watch-and-wait approach based on a number of features, including the fact that patients tend to be older, with an average age of 70 years, may have very indolent disease and be asymptomatic, and the fact that there is no curative therapy for this disease. Thus, the medical axiom "first do no harm" spares patients who are asymptomatic and have indolent disease from the consequences of therapy that may be unnecessary. However, once a patient requires treatment for CLL their median survival averages seven years. Thus, most patients who require treatment for CLL will eventually die of complications of the disease. These patients can be thought of as "ticking time bombs," where the approach of just watching and waiting (or watching and worrying) does not appear very attractive. The presence of these newer prognostic factors can now clearly identify a population of patients who are not going to survive 10 to 20 years without treatment. However, an important question that is not yet answered is: Does early treatment benefit these patients? It is certainly possible that the same factors that predict for more aggressive disease predict for suboptimal response to the current regimens.

Treatment of CLL has evolved significantly over the past 10 years. Historically, chlorambucil, an oral alkylating agent, was the mainstay of therapy and was an effective palliative treatment with an inability to produce complete remission. Fludarabine, a nucleoside analog, proved to be an effective drug for this disease, and in a randomized trial of fludarabine versus chlorambucil it was shown that fludarabine produced higher complete and overall response rates and significantly longer time to progression. However, overall survival was not impacted. There are several potential reasons for this including the crossover design of the trial, the fact that subsequent therapies may also impact survival, and that the complete remission rate with fludarabine was only 20%. Given that this was the most effective single agent and that upfront treatment is the time when the best response is likely to be obtained, the fact that 80% of patients did not achieve a complete remission is certainly one possibility for lack of impact on survival. This has led to the development of new agents as well as combination regimens, which on early analysis appear to be improving survival in this disease, particular combinations including both fludarabine and the monoclonal antibody rituximab. Another monoclonal antibody, alemtuzumab, was approved for the treatment of fludarabine refractory CLL but may, in fact, be better utilized as a consolidation regimen after debulking by chemotherapy, given that it is exquisitely effective in eradicating marrow disease. Combinations of alemtuzumab and fludarabine are also being investigated.

There are a number of exciting agents in clinical trials, including BCL-2 family member inhibitors, new monoclonal antibodies, HSP-90 inhibitors, cyclin D1 inhibitors, and immunomodulatory drugs. Data relevant to all of these are also discussed in chapter 9.

The advent of nonmyeloablative stem cell transplant has made this modality available for the first time to the majority of patients with CLL. The use of myeloablative transplants typically involved high-dose cyclophosphamide and total-body radiation, which were too toxic for older patients, and so most patients with CLL were not candidates for transplant. Recent trials suggest that long-term survival in CLL can be affected in a proportion of patients who undergo stem cell transplant, and improvements in HLA typing also make this feasible for patients without related donors.

The diagnosis of CLL is accompanied by a number of management issues, including the interesting phenomenon of autoimmunity, the potential for development of Richter's transformation to large-cell lymphoma, and treatment of infections related to disease parameters (cytopenias, hypogammaglobulin), as well as parameters induced by treatment including T-cell deficiencies. All of these are discussed and addressed within the textbook.

We hope that readers will find this book enjoyable to read, highly informative, and at the same time clinically relevant in addressing some of the important questions that are being asked by physicians who have the responsibility of taking care of these patients.

Susan M. O'Brien
John G. Gribben

Contents

Preface . . . . *iii*

Contributors . . . . *ix*

Introduction . . . . *xiii*

1. **Origin and Nature of Chronic Lymphocytic Leukemia B Cells** *1*
   Nicholas Chiorazzi and Manlio Ferrarini

2. **Gene Expression Profiling in the Study of Chronic Lymphocytic Leukemia** *19*
   Ulf Klein

3. **Molecular Pathogenesis** *35*
   Arianna Bottoni, Carlo M. Croce, and George A. Calin

4. **Chronic Lymphocytic Leukemia and the B-Cell Receptor** *45*
   Marta Muzio and Federico Caligaris-Cappio

5. **Etiology of CLL: The Role of MBL** *69*
   Paolo Ghia and Andrew C. Rawstron

6. **Apoptosis Dysregulation in CLL** *91*
   Victoria Del Gaizo Moore and Anthony Letai

7. **Differential Diagnosis, Staging, and Prognostic Factors** *103*
   Thorsten Zenz, Hartmut Döhner, and Stephan Stilgenbauer

8. **Frontline Therapy of Chronic Lymphocytic Leukemia** *121*
   Barbara Eichhorst and Michael Hallek

9. **Treatment of Patients with Relapsed or Refractory Chronic Lymphocytic Leukemia** *141*
   Karen W.L. Yee, Michael J. Keating, and Susan M. O'Brien

10. **New Therapies in Chronic Lymphocytic Leukemia** *165*
John C. Byrd, Farrukh Awan, Thomas S. Lin, and Michael R. Grever

11. **Stem Cell Transplantation in CLL** *185*
John G. Gribben

12. **Gene Therapy, Vaccines, and Immune Modulation** *201*
William G. Wierda

13. **Prolymphocytic Leukemias** *217*
Claire E. Dearden

14. **CLL-Specific Complications: Autoimmunity and Richter's Transformation** *231*
Dennis A. Carney and John F. Seymour

15. **Infectious Complications in Patients with Chronic Lymphocytic Leukemia** *261*
Elias Anaissie

Index *293*

Contributors

Elias Anaissie Myeloma Institute for Research and Therapy, University of Arkansas for Medical Sciences, Little Rock, Arkansas, U.S.A.

Farrukh Awan Division of Hematology and Oncology, Department of Internal Medicine and Division of Medicinal Chemistry and Pharmacognosy, College of Pharmacy, The Ohio State University, Columbus, Ohio, U.S.A.

Arianna Bottoni Human Cancer Genetics, Department of Molecular Virology, Immunology, and Medical Genetics, Ohio State University, Columbus, Ohio, U.S.A.

John C. Byrd Division of Hematology and Oncology, Department of Internal Medicine and Division of Medicinal Chemistry and Pharmacognosy, College of Pharmacy, The Ohio State University, Columbus, Ohio, U.S.A.

Federico Caligaris-Cappio Unit and Laboratory of Lymphoid Malignancies, Department of Oncology, Università Vita-Salute San Raffaele and San Raffaele Scientific Institute, Milano, Italy

George A. Calin Departments of Experimental Therapeutics and Cancer Genetics, University of Texas M.D. Anderson Cancer Center, Houston, Texas, U.S.A.

Dennis A. Carney Department of Haematology, Peter MacCallum Cancer Centre, East Melbourne, Victoria, Australia

Nicholas Chiorazzi The Feinstein Institute for Medical Research and the Departments of Medicine and of Cell Biology, North Shore University Hospital and Albert Einstein College of Medicine, Manhasset, New York, U.S.A.

Carlo M. Croce Human Cancer Genetics, Department of Molecular Virology, Immunology, and Medical Genetics, Ohio State University, Columbus, Ohio, U.S.A.

Claire E. Dearden Department of Haemato-Oncology, The Royal Marsden Hospital and Institute of Cancer Research, London, United Kingdom

Victoria Del Gaizo Moore   Medical Oncology, Dana-Farber Cancer Institute, Boston, Massachusetts, U.S.A.

Hartmut Döhner   Department of Internal Medicine III, University of Ulm, Ulm, Germany

Barbara Eichhorst   Klinik I für Innere Medizin, Universität zu Köln, Köln, Germany

Manlio Ferrarini   The Division of Medical Oncology C, Istituto Nazionale per la Ricerca sul Cancro, Dipartmento di Oncologia Clinica e Sperimentale, Universita di Genova, Genova, Italy

Paolo Ghia   Unit and Laboratory of Lymphoid Malignancies, Department of Oncology, Università Vita-Salute San Raffaele and Istituto Scientifico San Raffaele, Milano, Italy

Michael R. Grever   Division of Hematology and Oncology, Department of Internal Medicine and Division of Medicinal Chemistry and Pharmacognosy, College of Pharmacy, The Ohio State University, Columbus, Ohio, U.S.A.

John G. Gribben   St. Bartholomew's Hospital, CRUK Medical Oncology Unit, Barts and The London School of Medicine, London, U.K.

Michael Hallek   Klinik I für Innere Medizin, Universität zu Köln, Köln, Germany

Michael J. Keating   Department of Leukemia, University of Texas M.D. Anderson Cancer Center, Houston, Texas, U.S.A.

Ulf Klein   Institute for Cancer Genetics and Herbert Irving Comprehensive Cancer Center, Columbia University, New York, New York, U.S.A.

Anthony Letai   Medical Oncology, Dana-Farber Cancer Institute, Boston, Massachusetts, U.S.A.

Thomas S. Lin   Division of Hematology and Oncology, Department of Internal Medicine and Division of Medicinal Chemistry and Pharmacognosy, College of Pharmacy, The Ohio State University, Columbus, Ohio, U.S.A.

Marta Muzio   Unit and Laboratory of Lymphoid Malignancies, Department of Oncology, San Raffaele Scientific Institute, Milano, Italy

Susan M. O'Brien   Department of Leukemia, University of Texas M.D. Anderson Cancer Center, Houston, Texas, U.S.A.

Andrew C. Rawstron   Department of Haematology, St. James's Institute of Oncology, HMDS, Leeds Teaching Hospitals, Leeds, U.K.

John F. Seymour   Department of Haematology, Peter MacCallum Cancer Centre, and University of Melbourne, Melbourne, Victoria, Australia

Stephan Stilgenbauer   Department of Internal Medicine III, University of Ulm, Ulm, Germany

William G. Wierda   Department of Leukemia, Division of Cancer Medicine, University of Texas M.D. Anderson Cancer Center, Houston, Texas, U.S.A.

Karen W.L. Yee   Department of Medical Oncology and Hematology, Princess Margaret Hospital, University Health Network, Toronto, Ontario, Canada

Thorsten Zenz   Department of Internal Medicine III, University of Ulm, Ulm, Germany

Introduction

A BRIEF HISTORICAL PERSPECTIVE ON CLL: BENCH VS. BEDSIDE RESEARCH CONTRIBUTIONS

What came first—chicken or the egg? A slight variation of this age-old question can be posed as: Did the progress in our understanding of chronic lymphocytic leukemia (CLL) come first as a result of clinical observations of a few astute physicians or as a result of bench research by a few very smart investigators? Readers might find the chapters that follow in this volume of immense value in answering this question. I would like to start the discussion by citing just a few examples of the dilemma of the primacy issues between bench versus bedside research in this disease.

WHAT IS AT THE CORE OF PATHOPHYSIOLOGY OF CLL? LONG-LIVED LYMPHOCYTES

In the 1960s, Galton (1) and Dameshek (2) came upon their definition of CLL purely by their clinical observations of the natural history of patients with CLL who were under their care. They both suggested that CLL lymphocytes are long lived because they were functionally inert. This was long before the idea of programmed cell death came to the notice of physicians and medical researchers. Even the fact that lymphocytes were broadly classifiable either as B cells or as T cells had not been known when Galton (1) and Dameshek (2) proposed their definition of CLL as a disease of accumulation of long-lived lymphocytes. It took more than a century for basic scientists to find a molecular basis for explaining the longevity of CLL lymphocytes by demonstrating that these cells had altered levels of apoptosis regulating proteins (3) and that these cells had low level expression of miR-15a and miR-16 (4) which, in turn was associated with high levels of bcl-2 (5).

ARE CLL LYMPHOCYTES IMMUNOLOGICALLY NAÏVE?

Until recently, we all believed that CLL lymphocytes are functionally inert and immunologically naïve B cells. This notion was part of the concept of pathogenesis of CLL proposed by Dameshek and Galton. However, recent studies indicate that leukemic lymphocytes in at least half of CLL cases carry mutated IgV_H genes. The process of somatic hypermutation is triggered by a lymphocyte coming in contact with antigen, which turns a naïve B cell—expressing low-affinity surface Ig into a long-lived memory B cell that is a high-affinity antibody producer (6). These observations not only provided us new insights into the nature of the leukemic B cell in patients with CLL but also enabled us to predict clinical behavior and prognosis in this disease based on whether the patients had somatic mutations in IgV_H genes. These observations demonstrated that not all CLL lymphocytes are immunologically naïve. These bench-based findings, in turn, led to numerous additional subsequent studies (covered in the chapters that follow), which all have had important impact on our ability to assign an accurate long-term prognosis for CLL patients. This is an excellent example of clinical medicine benefiting from basic science research.

SMOULDERING CLL: MONOCLONAL B LYMPHOCYTOSIS OF UNKNOWN SIGNIFICANCE

All clinicians who take care of patients with CLL have long recognized that a small subset of early-stage patients, whose disease was diagnosed purely by chance and whose extent of disease barely fulfills the minimum requirements of diagnosis, seem to have what can be termed "smouldering" CLL (7,8). Such patients have a normal life expectancy without ever showing progression. Recently came startling reports that a small minority of healthy, asymptomatic persons, who may or may not be family members of patients with CLL, carry a tiny number of monoclonal B lymphocytes in their blood that have all the phenotypic markers of CLL (9–11). A question legitimately raised is, Whether such persons can be told that they have a preleukemic phase of CLL? Besides the fact that such news is likely to cause psychological havoc for these persons and their families, it also needs to be emphasized that we have little evidence as to whether all such persons or any of them will develop overt CLL in the course of subsequent years or even decades. Thus, it becomes clear that it will be wrong to accept laboratory findings without simultaneously taking into consideration the clinical picture in every case. Who is to determine whether these findings represent a "pre-smouldering" phase of smouldering CLL or a laboratory research–derived genie escaping the bottle and now becoming a monster for society at large?

The chapters that follow in this volume highlight the progresses made at both the basic science level and the clinical level and provide the reader with a balanced picture of CLL as a disease. There should be no primacy in this chicken-and-egg situation, they both are equally important.

Kanti R. Rai

Long Island Jewish Medical Center, New Hyde Park, and Albert Einstein College of Medicine, Bronx, New York, U.S.A.

REFERENCES

1. Galton DAG. The pathogenesis of chronic lymphocytic leukemia. Can Med Assoc J 1966; 94:1005–1010.
2. Dameshek W. Chronic lymphocytic leukemia-accumulative disease of immunologically incompetent lymphocytes. Blood 1967; 29:566–584.

3. Kitada S, Andersen J, Akar S, et al. Expression of apoptosis-regulating proteins in chronic lymphocytic leukemia: correlations with in vitro and in vivo chemoresponses. Blood 1998; 91:3379–3389.

4. Calin GA, Ferracin M, Cimmino A, et al. A unique microRNA signature associated with prognostic factors and disease progression in B cell chronic lymphocytic leukemia. New Engl J Med 2005; 352:1667–1676.

5. Cimmino A, Calin GA, Fabbri M, et al. mlR-15 and miR-16 induce apoptosis by targeting BCL 2. Proc Natl Acad Sci U S A 2005; 102:13944–13949.

6. Wabl M, Cascalho M, Steinberg C. Hypermutation in antibody affinity maturation. Curr Opin Immunol 1999; 11:186–189.

7. Montserrat E, Vinolas N, Reverter JC, et al. Natural history of chronic lymphocytic leukemia: on the progression and prognosis of early clinical stages. Nouvelle Revue Francaise d'Hematologie 1988; 30:359–361.

8. French Cooperative Group on Chronic Lymphocytic Leukaemia. Natural history of stage A chronic lymphocytic leukemia untreated patients. Br J Haematol 1990; 76:45–47.

9. Rawstron AC, Yuille MR, Fuller J, et al. Inherited predisposition of CLL is detectable as subclinical monoclonal B-lymphocyte expansion. Blood 2002; 100:2289–2290.

10. Rawstron AC, Green MJ, Kuzmicki A, et al. Monoclonal B lymphocytes with the characteristics of "indolent" chronic lymphocytic leukemia are present in 3.5% of adults with normal blood counts. Blood 2002; 100:635–639.

11. Rawstron AC, Bennett FL, O'Connor SJ, et al. Monoclonal B-cell lymphocytosis and chronic lymphocytic leukemia. N Engl J Med. 2008; 359(6):575–583.

1
Origin and Nature of Chronic Lymphocytic Leukemia B Cells

Nicholas Chiorazzi
The Feinstein Institute for Medical Research and the Departments of Medicine and of Cell Biology, North Shore University Hospital and Albert Einstein College of Medicine, Manhasset, New York, U.S.A.

Manlio Ferrarini
The Division of Medical Oncology C, Istituto Nazionale per la Ricerca sul Cancro, Dipartmento di Oncologia Clinica e Sperimentale, Universita di Genova, Genova, Italy

INTRODUCTION

In the past, B cells were considered a homogeneous population that gave rise to Ig-secreting cells and memory B cells, following specific antigenic stimulation. In recent years, this view has changed, and B cells are now documented as composed of different subpopulations, each with special functions (Fig. 1). These concepts emerged from observations in both humans and experimental animals suggesting that the B cell–rich zone of peripheral lymphoid tissues segregates into functionally unique areas. For example, B-cell proliferation and selection occur in germinal centers (GCs) of lymphoid follicles during an antigenic response, promoting the specific expansion of the cells equipped with B-cell antigen receptors (BCRs) of the highest affinity for the stimulating antigen. In the mantle of lymphoid follicles, there is an accumulation of "virgin" (foreign antigen inexperienced) cells that may be recruited into GCs by antigen stimulation. In contrast, B cells localized in the splenic marginal zone (MZ) can respond in a T cell–independent fashion by producing IgM antibodies against polysaccharide antigens of encapsulated bacteria. B cells with similar features are detected in subepithelial areas of tonsils, subcapsular areas of lymph nodes, and dome regions of Peyer's patches. Cells of lymphoid follicles and those of the MZ have dissimilar phenotypic and trafficking features, mature by distinct pathways, and respond differently to cytokines and chemokines. This further highlights the diversity of B-cell subsets.

Studies in mice have revealed the existence of specialized subsets of B lymphocytes, categorized by functional rather than anatomic criteria. For example, the peritoneal cavity of mice contains a B-cell subpopulation (B-1) that is capable of

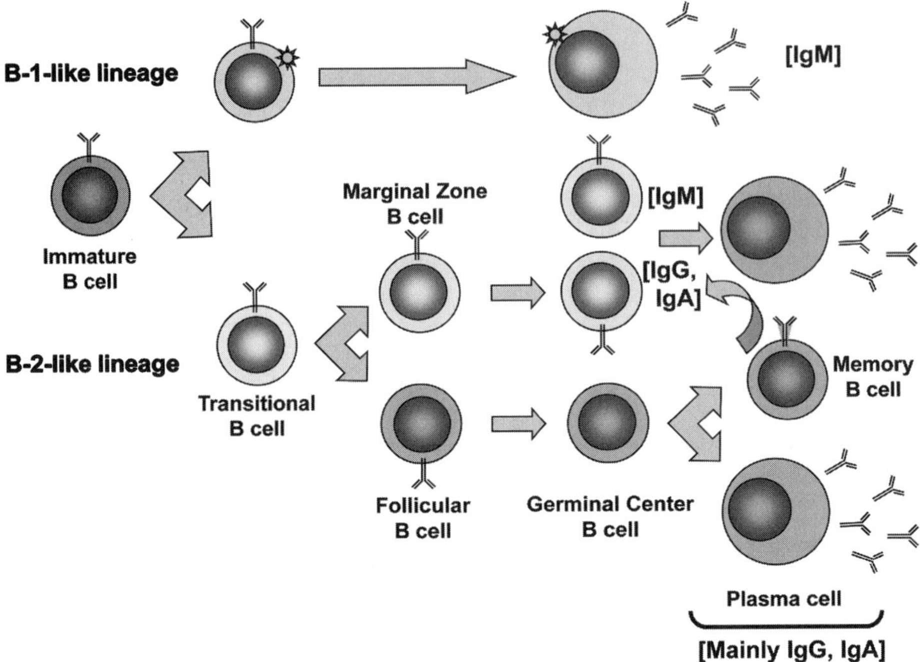

Figure 1 Maturation pathways that normal B lymphocytes follow. This schema is based primarily on studies carried out in mice. The relationship of some of the proposed pathways to human B cells has not been defined (e.g., B-1 cell differentiation pathway) (*See Color Insert*).

self-renewal. These cells produce polyreactive/natural antibodies, mainly of the IgM isotype, reacting with low avidity with a variety of antigens including self- and microbial epitopes. The antigenic determinants recognized by this B-cell subset are frequently nonprotein in nature, consisting of carbohydrates, lipids, and lipoproteins. B-1 cells, which are poorly represented in peripheral lymphoid tissues, are believed to be part of the innate immune system, providing a first line of defense against microbes until an adequate adaptive immune response is achieved. B-1 cells are subdivided into B-1a and B-1b cells on the basis of presence or absence of surface membrane CD5. B-1 cells differ from another functional B-cell subset, B-2 cells, from which high-affinity antibodies and memory B cells specific for stimulating antigens emerge. The phenotypic, trafficking, and maturation features of these B-cell subsets differ markedly.

Human lymphoproliferative disorders, generated by the expansion of a single-cell clone, represent a heterogeneous group of pathological conditions. Part of this heterogeneity is ascribed to their developmental lineages (T cells, B cells, NK cells). The neoplasias emanating from the B-cell lineage are identified on the basis of the B-cell subset of origin. While it has been relatively easy to determine the cell of origin of certain of the B-cell lymphoproliferative disorders (e.g., follicular center cell or MZ lymphomas), for others the cell of origin is still a matter of debate. This is the case for chronic lymphocytic leukemia (CLL), and the issue is especially complicated by the divergent molecular features of cells from patients that differ in clinical course. Although a definite answer to the question of the origin of CLL cells is presently unavailable, we shall review here the principal phenotypic, genetic, structural, and functional features of CLL cells and compare these with those of the major known B-cell subsets.

DISTINGUISHING CHARACTERISTICS OF CLL CELLS THAT COULD PROVIDE CLUES TO THE NORMAL B-CELL EQUIVALENT

As mentioned, B cells are divided into subsets on the basis of several criteria, including expression of cell surface molecules, location in specific geographic regions of lymphoid organs, use of specific genes, and functional properties. Applying these to CLL cells, characteristic patterns emerge.

In this analysis, we shall take into account that there are two major subgroups of CLL, characterized by the use of unmutated versus mutated immunoglobulin heavy chain variable (IgV$_H$) gene segments (1); patients in the former group (U-CLL) have a more aggressive clinical course with shorter survival than patients in the latter group (M-CLL) with a more indolent course and longer life span (2,3). In general, the cells from U-CLL also express ZAP-70 and CD38, while M-CLL cells do not (2,4–8). There are also other distinguishing features between the cells from the two CLL subsets that will be described below.

Surface Membrane Phenotype

CLL cells express surface membrane CD5, along with CD23 and CD27 (9,10). Other distinguishing phenotypic features include diminished levels of surface membrane Ig and CD22. The CD5$^+$CD23$^+$CD27$^+$smIg^{low} phenotype is generally consistent in CLL, although the percentage of cells within a given clone expressing individual molecules can vary. FMC7 and CD10 are usually not displayed on CLL cells, and therefore their expression can be used to distinguish CLL from other types of leukemia should they be present on large numbers of the leukemic clone (e.g., hairy cell leukemia).

Although the expression of a common surface membrane phenotype by CLL cells from multiple patients suggests that the two commonly delineated subgroups of CLL (U-CLL and M-CLL) may derive from the same normal B-cell precursors, the leukemic cells of these two subsets of patients do differ in expression of "activation markers." U-CLL more often than M-CLL express ZAP-70 and CD38 (2,4,5), both activation markers for normal B cells (11–14). In addition, the differential expression of additional molecules upregulated by cell activation (e.g., HLA-DR, CD69, CD71, CD62L, and others) suggests a more marked and recent activation of U-CLL cells (15).

Unfortunately, expression of several of the molecules that define the phenotype of CLL and its subtypes can change at different stages of maturation and activation of normal human B cells (e.g., CD5 and CD38). Furthermore, the defined surface membrane expression pattern of CLL cells does not correlate with a specific normal human B-cell subset. Therefore, the use of surface membrane phenotype alone to assign a CLL cell to a specific normal human B-cell subset can be treacherous.

Anatomic Location and Pattern of Growth

CLL cells circulate throughout the body via blood and lymph vessels, orchestrated by a series of chemokine receptors—CXCR3, CXCR4, CXCR5, and CXCR7—that are functional based on in vitro studies (16). In particular, CXCR4 allows CLL cells to sense a chemokine gradient of its ligand CXCL12/SDF-1, guiding CLL cells to stromal cells producing the ligand (17–19). Upon engagement with CXCL12/SDF-1, CLL cells migrate beneath the stromal cells via a process termed pseudoemperipolesis (17). CXCR3 is also relatively well expressed on CLL cells, in contrast to normal circulating human B cells

(20,21), and interaction with its ligands, IFN-inducible protein 10 (IP-10) and IFN-γ-induced monokine (Mig), leads to migration (21). CLL cells also traffic in response to both of the CXCR7 ligands, CCL19 and CCL21 (16). In normal B cells, CCL21 is secreted by high endothelial venules, inducing adherence to their surfaces, the first step in exiting the vasculature (22,23), from which CCL19 directs the cells into peripheral lymphoid organs (24,25). It has been suggested that CD38 and ZAP-70 regulate trafficking of U-CLL cells in particular, facilitating their tissue invasion (26). This could occur if CD38 interacts with a natural ligand, CD31, on the membrane of endothelial cells, thereby phosphorylating ZAP-70 and making the leukemic cells responsive to CXCL12/SDF-1.

The majority of CLL cells reside in multiple solid lymphoid tissues (bone marrow, lymph nodes, and to a lesser extent spleen) and occasionally in nonlymphoid sites (skin, prostate, others) (27–31). Unlike the characteristic topology and pattern of growth observed for follicular and mantle cell lymphomas, those of CLL can be diverse. Although often diffuse, resembling small lymphocytic lymphoma, other infiltrative patterns can be seen in both lymphoid and nonlymphoid tissues. Thus, histopathology does not help tracing the CLL cell of origin.

Moreover, certain tissue localizations are dictated by cytogenetic lesions and not reflective of normal B-cell biology. For example, patients whose CLL clone has a genomic deletion on the "q" arm of chromosome 11 often show more extensive lymph node involvement than other cases without such a chromosomal abnormality (32). Since this DNA deletion is a somatic event, it does not help in the assignment of a normal precursor.

Functional Responses to Stimulation by Antigens, Other Cells, and Soluble Mediators

Normal B-cell subsets can differ in the types of antigens to which they respond and the nature of the costimulatory interactions they need to carry out these responses. For instance, certain B-cell subsets (e.g., B-1 and MZ B cells) are geared to react with classes of antigenic determinants, proteins versus nonprotein determinants, and do not require T-cell collaboration to promote their activation and maturation. Furthermore, the strength of BCR engagement necessary to yield a response can vary among B-cell subpopulations, as exemplified by the requirement for a much stronger BCR-antigen interaction by B-1 cells than MZ B cells to accomplish cellular activation.

In Vitro Responses Mediated by BCR and TLR Engagement

An analysis of the in vitro responsiveness of CLL cells to specific antigens of different chemical makeup has not been accomplished to date, particularly because information on the antigenic specificity of the BCRs of different leukemic clones has become available only recently (see below). Therefore, a comparison of the response to physiologic ligands of CLL cells with normal B cells has not been made. However, in vitro responses of CLL cells to cross-linking smIgM and smIgD as surrogates for antigen-BCR interaction have been analyzed (33,34). Although these studies are diverse in experimental approach and therefore at times difficult to compare and reconcile, principles have emerged.

CLL cells differ in responsiveness to antibody-mediated BCR cross-linking, both in the ability to transduce a signal through the BCR, as measured by changes in phosphorylation state of intracellular signaling intermediates, as well as by differences in the functional consequences that ensue. Decreased signaling capacity is more often seen in M-CLL than U-CLL, and this has been attributed to anergy (35), potentially due in some instances to retention in the BCR of antigens encountered in vivo (36).

In addition, differences in signal transduction are found when smIgM or smIgD are cross-linked with specific antibodies (33,34). Binding smIgM more often leads to apoptosis, whereas cross-linking smIgD can result in cell survival and plasma cell differentiation.

In vitro induction of apoptosis versus survival can also relate to experimental conditions, such as the use of polyclonal (pAb) versus monoclonal (mAb) antibodies and the use of antibodies that differ in affinity or that are presented in different forms. Recent studies suggest that prolonged BCR engagement through smIgM by antibodies bound to insoluble beads can lead to effective signaling, whereas the same antibodies in soluble form fail to do so or do so at much reduced efficiency (37). In addition, analyses of smIgM cross-linking with mAbs differing in affinity for the Ig target lead to diverse functional outcomes. For instance, cross-linking smIgM with a low-affinity antibody in soluble form can lead to apoptosis of CLL cells, apparently mediated by downregulation of anti-apoptotic molecules such as Mcl-1, whereas the same antibody in multimeric form does not (38).

CLL cells respond well in vitro to nucleic acid ligands that bind to CD180 (39) and to TLR 9 (DNA) and TLR 7 (RNA) (40–42), in particular leukemic cells from patents with U-CLL (40). The proliferation of CLL cells to such stimulation far outstrips that of BCR cross-linking with surrogate antigens (pAbs and mAbs), suggesting that TLR-mediated responses may have special importance in selecting normal B cells for leukemic transformation and expanding CLL cells in vivo. Since some U-CLL BCRs/mAbs can bind apoptotic cells and their products, which often are nucleic acid-protein complexes (43,44), TLR 9 and TLR 7 stimulation might facilitate the clonal evolution of this subset of cases.

T-Cell Dependence of CLL Cell Activation and Maturation

CLL cells do not appear to require T-cell costimulation to avoid apoptosis and proliferate in that phorbol myristate acetate plus ionomycin induces many cases to undergo DNA duplication (45). Furthermore terminal differentiation into Ig-secreting cells can be achieved using mitogenic agents in the absence of T cells (46,47), although the addition of activated T lymphocytes from normal individuals can accomplish this more efficiently (46,48).

T lymphocytes can also block CLL cell apoptosis in vitro thorough signals delivered by physical interactions as well as by soluble mediators. The most well-studied contact signal involves CD40L-CD40 interaction (49). The importance of this interaction has been inferred in vitro by culturing CLL B cells with either soluble CD40L or antibodies to CD40 (50) and documented in vivo by the experiment of nature seen in patients with HyperIgM syndrome due to CD40L structural abnormalities (51,52).

Cytokine and Chemokine Influences

Nonlymphoid cells, such as monocyte-derived nurse-like cells and stromal cell "elements," can block CLL cell spontaneous apoptosis in vitro (53), both by direct contact and by the release of soluble factors. Perhaps the most efficient inhibitors of spontaneous CLL cell apoptosis in vitro are two molecules produced by nurse-like cells and stromal cells that are members of the tumor necrosis factor (TNF) family, "B cell–activating factor belonging to the TNF family"/"B-lymphocyte stimulator"/"TNF and apoptosis ligand-related leukocyte-expressed ligand 1" (BAFF/BLyS/TALL-1) (54–56), and "a proliferation-inducing ligand" (APRIL) (55,57). Like in subsets of normal B cells, these mediators are especially effective in providing survival signals to CLL cells (58–63) via several receptors expressed on CLL cells, BLyS receptor 3 (BR3),

B-cell maturation antigen (BCMA), and transmembrane activator and CAML-interactor (TACI) (64,65).

Furthermore, two cytokines, both members of the IL-2 family, IL-21 and IL-15, influence CLL cells by promoting survival and expansion (IL-15) or by inducing apoptosis (IL-21). Although operating also on untreated cells, the cytokines have their most potent effects on cells activated in vitro via surface membrane CD40 (66–68).

In summary, data on response of CLL to in vitro stimulation suggest that CLL cells respond to BCR cross-linking in the absence of direct T-cell contact, although several cytokines and monokines and even the T cells themselves can modulate this response. The ability to mount a T cell–independent response correlates with the structure of the BCR (i.e., greater response in U-CLL), supporting a link with poor clinical course and outcome. However, the pattern of CLL cell responsiveness is not unique to any of the B-cell subsets so far described.

Gene Expression

CLL cells resemble memory and virgin B cells more than GC cells (69), although their gene expression profile is not especially typical for any of human cell types studied to date (4,69). Furthermore, the genes differentially expressed between U-CLL and M-CLL are remarkably limited (4,69), despite striking differences in IgVH mutations, activation marker expression, and clinical aggressiveness. This finding suggests, but does not prove, derivation of the two types of leukemic cells from a common precursor.

Structure of the BCR

CLL cells display characteristic structural features in the expressed antigen-binding domains of their BCRs, and CLL cases can be split into subgroups on the basis of structural uniqueness (reviewed in Refs. 35, 70–72). This feature may be helpful in extrapolating to a normal B-cell equivalent.

In particular, patients with aggressive U-CLL synthesize BCRs/mAbs that are typically polyreactive, binding multiple foreign as well as autoantigens that do not share apparent structural similarity (73–76). This binding is often of low affinity. In contrast, patients with more indolent M-CLL synthesize BCRs/mAbs that have more restrictive antigen-binding properties.

Of special note is the recent description of polyspecific CLL BCRs/mAbs reactive with structurally conserved epitopes generated during apoptosis and other normal degradative and stress processes (43,44). This specificity resembles closely that of a subset of murine natural antibodies, encoded by IgVH of germline sequence, that react with apoptotic cells (77,78). The targets of these natural autoantibodies are neo-epitopes, conjugated to endogenous proteins, lipoproteins, and lipids, generated by oxidative stress due to mitochondrial dysfunction during the apoptotic process (79) such as malondialdehyde (MDA) and 4-hydroxynonenal (HNE) (80). Strikingly, antibodies reactive with the neo-epitopes also bind determinants on microbes, such as the phosphocholine (PC) head group on *Streptococcus pneumoniae* (81). Of note, the classic murine unmutated T15/S107 mAb (82), which protects against *S. pneumoniae*, reacts effectively with oxidation-specific neo-epitopes (83). In mice, T15$^+$ antibodies are said to be found exclusively among cells of the B-1 compartment (84).

These differences in IgVH mutation status and antigen binding are also reflected at the level of IgV segment use and association (reviewed in Refs. 70–72). The leukemic cells of subsets of CLL patients can express BCRs composed of similar or identical IgVH,

D, and J_H segments with very similar HCDR3 regions (61,85–89). Such rearrangements often pair with the same immunoglobulin light chain variable (IgV_L) gene and even the same J_L gene. These "stereotypic" rearrangements (87) appear to be much enriched in CLL compared with other diseases involving B lymphocytes (e.g., other lymphomas, autoimmunity, allergy) as well as normal human B cells (89). Although stereotypic BCRs can be found among M-CLL clones, they are more often displayed by U-CLL cells. These data strongly suggest antigen selection and drive as a promoting factor in the disease (1,70,72,87,89). It remains unclear if this selection and drive culls susceptible normal B cells from the entire available B-cell repertoire pool or if the selection acts on a subset of cells already skewed in IgV gene use and association (e.g., B-1 and MZ B cells). This uncertainty is in part related to the incomplete characterization of the IgV gene repertoire of different human B-cell subsets.

Composite

On the basis of overall considerations, the normal human B-cell equivalent to a CLL cell likely expresses CD5, constitutively or after stimulation, as well as other markers (CD23 and CD27) indicative of activation in vivo, resides primarily in solid lymphoid tissues, and expresses characteristic BCR structural features, that is, unmutated IgV_H genes coding for polyreactive BCRs/mAbs or somatically mutated IgV_H genes coding for oligo/ monoreactive BCRs/mAbs. In addition, it is likely that selection and drive by either autoantigens or foreign antigens or a combination of both influences the "choice" of which normal B cells or sublineage is promoted into leukemic transformation. This selection and drive is likely made through engagement of structurally restricted BCRs as well as TLRs that bind a limited set of antigenic epitopes including those displayed on apoptotic cells and their products (e.g., DNA in the form of nucleosomes or as nucleic acid-protein complexes). This last set of parameters suggests that the two clinically diverse subgroups of CLL patients (i.e., those with aggressive vs. indolent disease) derive from distinct normal B-cell precursors. However, this conclusion is challenged by the very similar gene expression profiles of U-CLL and M-CLL (4,69).

NORMAL B-CELL SUBSETS IN ANIMALS AND MAN

B-1 Versus B-2 Cells

Using cell surface phenotype, geographic location, functional capabilities, and BCR structure, the most robust B-cell subset categorizations have been made in inbred strains of mice. Of note, in mice two distinct lineages of B cells have been proposed (90–92), although disagreement still exists as to whether these lineages are genetically versus environmentally programmed (93–96). In broad strokes, these two lineages (B-1 vs. B-2) can be distinguished by all four of the above parameters.

Specifically, cells of the B-1 lineage express the CD5 molecule on their surface, whereas cells of the B-2 lineage do not (although a subpopulation of cells within the B-1 cell subset—"B-1b" cells—also may not express CD5) (90). B-1 cells, which have an IgM^{high} IgD^{low} CD23^{low} surface phenotype, are most often found within the peritoneal cavity of mice, in great numerical excess over B-2 cells. Moreover, B-1 cells function uniquely, spontaneously producing IgM antibodies (97,98), without apparent need for the participation of T lymphocytes (99). These antibodies bind multiple antigens, presumably because their IgV segment coding is similar to the murine germline as opposed to having been altered by somatic mutations (100). Furthermore, examples of biased use and association of specific IgV segments is well documented in murine B-1 cells (100–103). These cells and the polyreactive mAbs they produce are currently viewed as making up a B-cell arm of the innate immune system, designed to protect the host against initial infections with various microbes and to cleanse the body of the products of normal cell catabolism and death (104–108).

In contrast, $CD5^-$ B-2 cells are found primarily and in large excess over B-1 cells in solid lymphoid organs such as lymph nodes and spleen. With the cooperation of T lymphocytes and other nonlymphoid cells, B-2 cells produce IgG and IgA antibodies in addition to IgM (109). The antibodies made by B-2 cells bind fewer antigens and with higher affinity than those made by B-1 cells, due to IgV gene changes developed during a GC reaction (110). B-2 cells do not exhibit as biased an IgV repertoire as do B-1 cells. These cells and the oligo/monoreactive antibodies they synthesize comprise the B-cell arm of the adaptive immune system, designed to protect the host against repeated infections. The definition of B-2 cells is based on function rather than phenotype; therefore, B-2 cells may display different phenotypes depending on which stage of B-cell maturation and antibody production is considered.

In humans, this type of lineage discrimination is not as clear as in the mice. For one, human $CD5^-$ B cells can come to express the CD5 molecule after cellular activation in vitro, even in the absence of T cells (111). Therefore, the stability of this marker in vivo has come into question, making it a tenuous indicator of a human B-1-like lineage. The follicular mantle cells from tonsils constitutively express CD5, share many of the feature of virgin B cells, and utilize unmutated IgV_H genes (112). Furthermore, the vast majority of $CD5^+$ B cells from the blood of normal healthy humans, which share the phenotype of follicular mantle cells, utilize unmutated IgV_H region genes and produce IgM molecules that are not polyreactive (76), a cardinal feature of murine B-1 cells. Evidence for marked skewing of IgV segment use and association is not currently available for human $CD5^+$ B cells.

MZ B Cells

The MZ B-cell subpopulation comprises B lymphocytes with a $CD23^-IgM^{high}IgD^{low}$ surface phenotype that use both unmutated and mutated IgV_H segments (113,114). Cells of this compartment serve as a front line of defense against blood-borne microbial infection in both mice and men (83,115–117). Entrance into the MZ compartment is dependent on signaling through the BCR (118), and murine studies suggest that this selection is by autoantigens (115,119,120). The relatively low signaling threshold of MZ B cells (121,122) could support clonal expansion of polyreactive B cells with cross-reactivities with infectious agents, as is seen in CLL (123). Furthermore in mice, anti-carbohydrate antibodies that appear to come from MZ B cells exhibit considerable BCR structural bias (124); this phenomenon has not been documented in man (125).

MZ B cells in both animals and humans, however, do not express CD5 on their surface membranes. However, a recent study described a $CD5^+$ B cell, isolated from activated tonsillar B cells, that expresses a $CD23^-IgM^{high}IgD^{low}$ surface phenotype, responds to T cell–independent type-2 antigens in vitro, and is located in the subepithelial areas of the tonsil, where cells equivalent to the splenic MZ reside (126). Most of these cells utilized unmutated IgV_H genes, although cells with mutated genes could be found in suspensions enriched for $CD27^+$ cells. Common V_HDJ_H gene rearrangements were observed in such cells, suggesting in situ clonal expansion. These $CD5^+$ B cells differ from the majority of tonsil $CD5^+$ B cells, which have the surface phenotype of follicular mantle B cells, lack activation markers, do not respond to T cell–independent antigens, and utilize unmutated IgV$_H$ genes. These cells may represent a link between human MZ B cells and B-1 cells (126).

Circulating IgM$^+$IgD$^+$CD27$^+$ Cells

Human B lymphocytes can be divided into subsets on the basis of expression of IgM, IgD, and CD27 (127). In this way, mature naive B cells (IgD$^+$CD27$^-$) can be distinguished from memory B cells (IgD$^-$CD27$^+$). Another human B-cell subset found in the blood is IgM^{high}, IgD^{low}CD27$^+$ and often displays mutated IgV genes (128). These cells are considered IgM memory B cells that undergo somatic mutation outside of classical GCs and without the need for T-cell help (129,130). This conclusion is supported by the finding that patients with genetic defects in T-B-cell cooperation that prevent formation of classical GCs and IgV gene mutation (e.g., hyperIgM syndrome) still generate mutated IgM$^+$IgD$^+$CD27$^+$ cells (51,52). This subpopulation may be the circulating equivalent of resident MZ B cells (129), based on similarity in surface membrane phenotype (IgM^{high}IgD^{low}CD23$^-$) and the documentation of identical clones circulating in the blood and resident in the spleen.

Transitional B Cells

Finally, there is a B-cell subpopulation that is well characterized in mice and less so in humans termed "transitional" B cells. These cells are immediate descendants of those B cells that have matured in the bone marrow and that are traversing the blood and lymph on their way to solid lymphoid tissues, where they become selected into the long-lived B-cell pool (131–134).

In the mouse, splenic transitional B cells are divided into two or three distinct subpopulations using two cell surface phenotype schemes: transitional type 1, T1 (CD24^{high}CD21^{low}CD23^{low}IgM^{high}IgD^{low}) and transitional type 2, T2 (CD24^{high}CD21^{high}CD23^{high}IgM^{high}IgD^{high}) (132) versus T1 (CD23$^-$IgM^{high}), T2 (CD23$^+$IgM^{high}), and T3 (CD23$^+$IgM^{low}) (131,135), although the existence of the latter subset as a transitional compartment has been challenged (136). BAFF/BLyS/TALL-1 plays an essential role in the maturation from T1 to T2 cells (137,138), and permits maturation to follicular B cells and possibly MZ B cells (138,139). Of note, is the significant responsiveness of murine T2 cells to TLR9 engagement (140), which activates and rapidly matures them to CD27$^+$ IgM-secreting plasma cells producing primarily unmutated mAbs.

In humans, a T1-like subpopulation has been described that has a CD19$^+$CD24^{high}CD38^{high}CD27$^-$ phenotype. These cells also display surface membrane CD5 (133); they also express CD10 normally seen on immature B cells developing in the bone marrow, consistent with their relatively immature state (133). A human T2-equivalent is still in debate. Murine and human transitional B cells use unmutated IgV genes (132,133) and exhibit varying degrees of autoreactivity in mice (141). However, the described human T1-equivalent does not respond well to BAFF/BLyS, although exposure to IL-4 and stromal elements does abort spontaneous apoptosis (133).

MOST LIKELY POSSIBILITIES AS TO THE NORMAL CELLULAR COUNTERPART OF CLL CELLS

As noted above, a number of B-cell subtypes could be progenitors of U-CLL and M-CLL cells. The potential for each of these will be addressed separately in relation to the IgV genotype.

U-CLL Cells

Human Equivalent of the Murine B-1 Cell Subset

CLL cells from patients with aggressive disease closely resemble B-1 cells of mice: they express CD5 (142), do not develop somatic IgV_H mutations (1), and usually produce polyreactive IgM antibodies (76). The dilemma however remains as to what cells constitute the human B-1 cell compartment, should it exist. As mentioned above, circulating human $CD5^+$ cells do not synthesize polyreactive mAbs (76), a cardinal feature of murine B-1 cells. Since the bulk of the human CD5-expressing B-cell population resides in the follicular mantle, $CD5^+$ cells in this anatomic compartment cannot be ruled out. However, unlike murine B-1 cells, human follicular mantle B cells do not respond to T cell–independent stimuli (143). Nevertheless, a B-1 type lineage for CLL cells is an attractive possibility, and efforts are under way to define this subset in man. The cell subpopulation recently described by Dono et al. may represent such a cell, since it expresses CD5, displays unmutated as well as mutated IgV_H, and responds to TI-2 antigens (126).

Transitional B Cells

Although this subset is not as well defined in humans as in mice, such cells could be precursors to CLL cells. The cells express CD5 and CD38 (like U-CLL cells), and they use unmutated IgV genes (133) that can be autoreactive (141). These cells also respond well to TLR stimulation. The major difficulties in assigning transitional B cells as the normal equivalent of CLL cells is the expression of markers not usually seen on CLL cells [e.g., CD10, which is expressed when CLL cells are induced into apoptosis (144)] and the apparent unresponsiveness of these cells to the cytokine BAFF/BLyS/TALL-1 (133), a molecule that supports CLL cell survival very effectively. Moreover, CLL cells are consistently $CD27^+$, while transitional B cells are not. It is conceivable that a yet to be defined human T2-equivalent may have phenotypic and functional characteristics more similar to CLL cells.

Marginal Zone B Cells

In support of this subset as the normal equivalent of CLL cells is the use of unmutated IgV genes (113) to synthesize polyreactive mAbs (115,120). In addition, unlike human $CD5^+$ follicular mantle B cells, human MZ B cells respond to T cell–independent stimuli in vitro (143). An MZ B-cell derivation for CLL cells is also attractive since M-CLL cells could also derive from MZ B cells that have undergone somatic mutation (113). This unified derivation would be consistent with gene expression profiling studies that suggest that U-CLL and M-CLL cells are not distinguished by a large number of differentially express genes (4,69).

M-CLL Cells

Human Equivalent of Murine B-2 Cells

This derivation is the easiest to envision, with one major exception—murine B-2 cells lack CD5 expression, a prerequisite for the diagnosis of CLL (9,10). Nevertheless, the use of somatically mutated IgV_H that code for oligo/monoreactive mAbs (109,110) is consistent with M-CLL. In this scenario, M-CLL cells would derive from post-GC B cells, probably memory cells. A memory cell derivation for M-CLL cells is also supported by gene expression profiling (69). Since chromosomal translocations are rare in

CLL, unlike neoplasias of GC cell origin, M-CLL cells would have transformed after cells exited the GC. A post-GC origin is also somewhat difficult to reconcile because most M-CLL cells express IgM and IgD; although mutated IgM$^+$ B cells exist, post-GC (memory) B cells usually are isotype switched.

Circulating IgM$^+$IgD$^+$CD27$^+$ B Cells and Human Marginal Zone B Cells

These two subpopulations are considered together because IgM$^+$IgD$^+$CD27$^+$ B cells are often viewed as the same population, differing only in location (129). Both of these cell subsets are potential progenitors of M-CLL cells, based primarily on IgV gene and antigen-binding characteristics. Both fall short of a complete match with M-CLL cells because of the lack of CD5 expression. As mentioned above, considering both M-CLL and U-CLL emerging from an MZ population is consistent with gene expression profiling studies that do not find major differences between these two types of CLL (4,69).

OPINION

Figure 2 illustrates the cells most likely to give rise to U-CLL and M-CLL. It is our opinion that U-CLL cells derive either from a heretofore undefined human B-1 cell equivalent or from marginal zone B cells. Furthermore, we propose that M-CLL cells derive either from the human B-2 cell equivalent, through a T cell–dependent GC reaction, or from IgM$^+$IgD$^+$CD27$^+$/MZ B cells, via a T cell–independent mutation mechanism occurring outside of classical GCs.

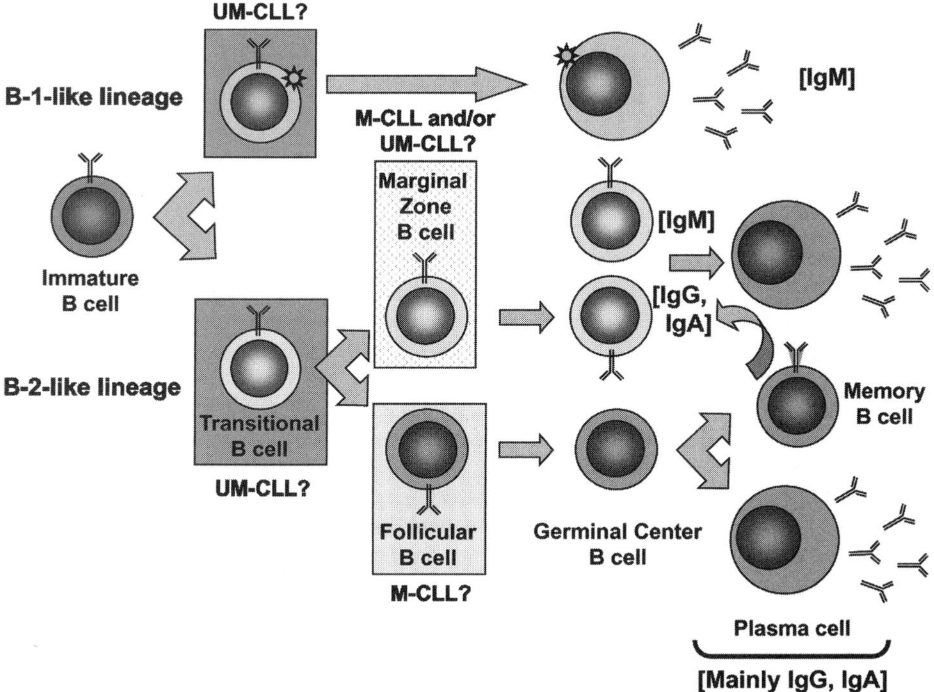

Figure 2 Stages of maturation at which U-CLL and M-CLL cells might emerge (see Figure 1). Boxes indicate potential cell types that could give rise to U-CLL and/or M-CLL. *Abbreviations*: U-CLL, unmutated CLL; M-CLL, mutated CLL (*See Color Insert*).

However, since gene expression profiling suggests that U-CLL cells do not differ from M-CLL cells in a large number of differentially expressed genes, the most parsimonious scenario is that both of these CLL subgroups derive from marginal zone B cells. Nevertheless, if one considers that the similarity between the expression phenotypes of U-CLL and M-CLL could reflect a common transformation process (not a common ancestral lineage), then we would favor the derivation of U-CLL from the human equivalent of B-1 cells and M-CLL from MZ B cells, which could have developed mutations at an extrafollicular site. The possibility that M-CLL derive from follicular B cells that developed IgV$_H$ mutations in classical GCs cannot be excluded, however, especially if such cells subsequently migrated and took up residence in MZ.

ACKNOWLEDGMENTS

We thank the present and past members of the Laboratory of Experimental Immunology, The Feinstein Institute for Medical Research, North Shore-LIJ Health System, of North Shore University Hospital, and of the Division of Medical Oncology C, Istituto Nazionale per la Ricerca sul Cancro for the work that we have discussed in this manuscript.

These studies were supported in part by RO1 grants CA81554 and CA87956 from the National Cancer Institute and an M01 General Clinical Research Center Grant (RR018535) from the National Center for Research Resources, the Associazione Italiana Ricerca sul Cancro (AIRC) and MIUR. The Karches Family Foundation, The Prince Family Foundation, The Marks Family Foundation, The Jean Walton Fund for Lymphoma & Myeloma Research, and The Joseph Eletto Leukemia Research Fund also provided support for these studies.

REFERENCES

1. Fais F, Ghiotto F, Hashimoto S, et al. Chronic lymphocytic leukemia B cells express restricted sets of mutated and unmutated antigen receptors. J Clin Invest 1998; 102:1515–1525.
2. Damle RN, Wasil T, Fais F, et al. Ig V gene mutation status and CD38 expression as novel prognostic indicators in chronic lymphocytic leukemia. Blood 1999; 94:1840–1847.
3. Hamblin TJ, Davis Z, Gardiner A, et al. Unmutated Ig VH genes are associated with a more aggressive form of chronic lymphocytic leukemia. Blood 1999; 94:1848–1854.
4. Rosenwald A, Alizadeh AA, Widhopf G, et al. Relation of gene expression phenotype to immunoglobulin mutation genotype in B cell chronic lymphocytic leukemia. J Exp Med 2001; 194:1639–1647.
5. Wiestner A, Rosenwald A, Barry TS, et al. ZAP-70 expression identifies a chronic lymphocytic leukemia subtype with unmutated immunoglobulin genes, inferior clinical outcome, and distinct gene expression profile. Blood 2003; 101:4944–4951.
6. Hamblin TJ, Orchard JA, Ibbotson RE, et al. CD38 expression and immunoglobulin variable region mutations are independent prognostic variables in chronic lymphocytic leukemia, but CD38 expression may vary during the course of the disease. Blood 2002; 99:1023–1029.
7. Crespo M, Bosch F, Villamor N, et al. ZAP-70 expression as a surrogate for immunoglobulin-variable-region mutations in chronic lymphocytic leukemia. N Engl J Med 2003; 348:1764–1775.
8. Rassenti LZ, Hunynh L, Toy TL, et al. ZAP-70 compared with immunoglobulin heavy-chain genemutation status as a predictor of disease progression in chronic lymphocytic leukemia. N Engl J Med 2004; 351:893–901.
9. Bennett JM, Catovsky D, Daniel MT, et al. Proposals for the classification of chronic (mature) B and T lymphoid leukaemias. French-American-British (FAB) Cooperative Group. J Clin Pathol 1989; 42:567–584.

10. Kuppers R, Klein U, Hansmann ML, et al. Cellular origin of human B-cell lymphomas. N Engl J Med 1999; 341:1520–1529.

11. Nolz JC, Tschumper RC, Pittner BT, et al. ZAP-70 is expressed by a subset of normal human B-lymphocytes displaying an activated phenotype. Leukemia 2005; 19:1018–1024.

12. Cutrona G, Colombo M, Matis S, et al. B lymphocytes in humans express ZAP-70 when activated in vivo. Eur J Immunol 2006; 36:558–569.

13. Scielzo C, Camporeale A, Geuna M, et al. ZAP-70 is expressed by normal and malignant human B-cell subsets of different maturational stage. Leukemia 2006; 20:689–695.

14. Deaglio S, Vaisitti T, Aydin S, et al. In-tandem insight from basic science combined with clinical research: CD38 as both marker and key component of the pathogenetic network underlying chronic lymphocytic leukemia. Blood 2006; 108:1135–1144.

15. Damle RN, Ghiotto F, Valetto A, et al. B-cell chronic lymphocytic leukemia cells express a surface membrane phenotype of activated, antigen-experienced B lymphocytes. Blood 2002; 99:4087–4093.

16. Lopez-Giral S, Quintana NE, Cabrerizo M, et al. Chemokine receptors that mediate B cell homing to secondary lymphoid tissues are highly expressed in B cell chronic lymphocytic leukemia and non-Hodgkin lymphomas with widespread nodular dissemination. J Leukoc Biol 2004; 76:462–471.

17. Burger JA, Burger M, Kipps TJ. Chronic lymphocytic leukemia B cells express functional CXCR4 chemokine receptors that mediate spontaneous migration beneath bone marrow stromal cells. Blood 1999; 94:3658–3667.

18. Burger JA, Kipps TJ. Chemokine receptors and stromal cells in the homing and homeostasis of chronic lymphocytic leukemia B cells. Leuk Lymphoma 2002; 43:461–466.

19. Burger JA, Burkle A. The CXCR4 chemokine receptor in acute and chronic leukaemia: a marrow homing receptor and potential therapeutic target. Br J Haematol 2007; 137:288–296.

20. Ocana E, Delgado-Perez L, Campos-Caro A, et al. The prognostic role of CXCR3 expression by chronic lymphocytic leukemia B cells. Haematologica 2007; 92:349–356.

21. Trentin L, Agostini C, Facco M, et al. The chemokine receptor CXCR3 is expressed on malignant B cells and mediates chemotaxis. J Clin Invest 1999; 104:115–121.

22. Springer T. Traffic signals on endothelium for lymphocyte recirculation and leukocyte emigration. Annu Rev Physiol 1995; 57:827–872.

23. Butcher E, Picker L. Lymphocyte homing and homeostasis. Science 1996; 272:60–66.

24. Ngo VN, Tang HL, Cyster JG. Epstein-Barr virus-induced molecule 1 ligand chemokine is expressed by dendritic cells in lymphoid tissues and strongly attracts naive T cells and activated B cells. J Exp Med 1998; 188:181–191.

25. Reif K, Ekland E, Ohl L, et al. Balanced responsiveness to chemoattractants from adjacent zones determines B-cell position. Nature 2002; 416:94–99.

26. Deaglio S, Vaisitti T, Aydin S, et al. CD38 and ZAP-70 are functionally linked and mark CLL cells with high migratory potential. Blood 2007; 110:4012–4021.

27. Cerroni L, Zenahlik P, Hofler G, et al. Specific cutaneous infiltrates of B-cell chronic lymphocytic leukemia: a clinicopathologic and prognostic study of 42 patients. Am J Surg Pathol 1996; 20:1000–1010.

28. Robak E, Robak T. Skin lesions in chronic lymphocytic leukemia. Leuk Lymphoma 2007; 48:855–865.

29. Bogdan CA, Alexander AA, Gorny MK, et al. Chronic lymphocytic leukemia with prostate infiltration mediated by specific clonal membrane-bound IgM. Cancer Res 2003; 63:2067–2071.

30. Carver JD, Calverley D, Shen P. Chronic lymphocytic leukemia/small lymphocytic lymphoma presenting in urinary bladder without peripheral blood lymphocytosis: case report and literature review. Leuk Lymphoma 2006; 47:1163–1165.

31. Salek J, Sideridis K, White S. Chronic lymphocytic leukemia of the intestinal tract. Gastrointest Endosc 2006; 63:1072–1073.

32. Dohner H, Stilgenbauer S, James MR, et al. 11q deletions identify a new subset of B-cell chronic lymphocytic leukemia characterized by extensive nodal involvement and inferior prognosis. Blood 1997; 89:2516–2522.

33. Zupo S, Massara R, Dono M, et al. Apoptosis or plasma cell differentiation of CD38-positive B-chronic lymphocytic leukemia cells induced by cross-linking of surface IgM or IgD. Blood 2000; 95:1199–1206.

34. Lanham S, Hamblin T, Oscier D, et al. Differential signaling via surface IgM is associated with VH gene mutational status and CD38 expression in chronic lymphocytic leukemia. Blood 2003; 101:1087–1093.

35. Stevenson F, Caligaris-Cappio F. Chronic lymphocytic leukemia: revelations from the B-cell receptor. Blood 2004; 103:4389–4395.

36. Mockridge IC, Potter KN, Wheatley I, et al. Reversible anergy of sIgM-mediated signaling in the two subsets of CLL defined by VH-gene mutational status. Blood 2007; 109:4424–4431.

37. Petlickovski A, Laurenti L, Li X, et al. Sustained signaling through the B-cell receptor induces Mcl-1 and promotes survival of chronic lymphocytic leukemia B cells. Blood 2005; 105: 4820–4827.

38. Paul S, Abu-Helu R, Mongini PKA, et al. Low affinity interactions with CLL B-cell receptors induces apoptosis by down-regulating Mcl-1 and up-regulating Bim. Blood 2007; 110:338a.

39. Porakishvili N, Kulikova N, Jewell AP, et al. Differential expression of CD180 and IgM by B-cell chronic lymphocytic leukaemia cells using mutated and unmutated immunoglobulin VH genes. Br J Haematol 2005; 131:313–319.

40. Longo PG, Laurenti L, Gobessi S, et al. The Akt signaling pathway determines the different proliferative capacity of chronic lymphocytic leukemia B-cells from patients with progressive and stable disease. Leukemia 2007; 21:110–120.

41. Tomic J, White D, Shi Y, et al. Sensitization of IL-2 Signaling through TLR-7 Enhances B Lymphoma Cell Immunogenicity. J Immunol 2006; 176:3830–3839.

42. Spaner DE, Shi Y, White D, et al. Immunomodulatory effects of Toll-like receptor-7 activation on chronic lymphocytic leukemia cells. Leukemia 2006; 20:286–295.

43. Catera R, Hatzi K, Chu CC, et al. Polyreactive monoclonal antibodies synthesized by some B-CLL cells recognize specific antigens on viable and apoptotic T cells. Blood 2006; 108:796a.

44. Catera R, Hatzi K, Seiler T, et al. Binding of CLL B-cell receptors to viable and apoptotic cells offers insights into the role of autoantigens in leukemic transformation. Blood 2007; 110:228a.

45. Tangye SG, Weston KM, Raison RL. Phorbol ester activates CD5+ leukaemic B cells via a T cell-independent mechanism. Immunol Cell Biol 1995; 73:44–51.

46. Fu SM, Chiorazzi N, Kunkel HG, et al. Induction of in vitro differentiation and immunoglobulin synthesis of human leukemic B lymphocytes. J Exp Med 1978; 148:1570–1578.

47. Totterman TH, Nilsson K, Sundstrom C. Phorbol ester-induced differentiation of chronic lymphocytic leukaemia cells. Nature 1980; 288:176–178.

48. Chiorazzi N, Fu S, Montazeri G, et al. T cell helper defect in patients with chronic lymphocytic leukemia. J Immunol 1979; 122:1087–1090.

49. Granziero L, Ghia P, Circosta P, et al. Survivin is expressed on CD40 stimulation and interfaces proliferation and apoptosis in B-cell chronic lymphocytic leukemia. Blood 2001; 97: 2777–2783.

50. Ranheim EA, Kipps TJ. Activated T cells induce expression of B7/BB1 on normal or leukemic B cells through a CD40-dependent signal. J Exp Med 1993; 177:925–935.

51. Agematsu K, Nagumo H, Shinozaki K, et al. Absence of IgD-CD27(+) memory B cell population in X-linked hyper-IgM syndrome. J Clin Invest 1998; 102:853–860.

52. Brezinschek HP, Dorner T, Monson NL, et al. The influence of CD40-CD154 interactions on the expressed human V(H) repertoire: analysis of V(H) genes expressed by individual B cells of a patient with X-linked hyper-IgM syndrome. Int Immunol 2000; 12:767–775.

53. Lagneaux L, Delforge A, De Bruyn C, et al. Adhesion to bone marrow stroma inhibits apoptosis of chronic lymphocytic leukemia cells. Leuk Lymphoma 1999; 35:445–453.

54. Moore PA, Belvedere O, Orr A, et al. BLyS: member of the tumor necrosis factor family and B lymphocyte stimulator. Science 1999; 285:260–263.

55. Schneider P, MacKay F, Steiner V, et al. BAFF, a novel ligand of the tumor necrosis factor family, stimulates B cell growth. J Exp Med 1999; 189:1747–1756.

56. Shu HB, Hu WH, Johnson H. TALL-1 is a novel member of the TNF family that is down-regulated by mitogens. J Leukoc Biol 1999; 65:680–683.
57. Hahne M, Kataoka T, Schroter M, et al. APRIL, a new ligand of the tumor necrosis factor family, stimulates tumor cell growth. J Exp Med 1998; 188:1185–1190.
58. Burger JA, Tsukada N, Burger M, et al. Blood-derived nurse-like cells protect chronic lymphocytic leukemia B cells from spontaneous apoptosis through stromal cell-derived factor-1. Blood 2000; 96:2655–2663.
59. Tsukada N, Burger JA, Zvaifler NJ, et al. Distinctive features of "nurselike" cells that differentiate in the context of chronic lymphocytic leukemia. Blood 2002; 99:1030–1037.
60. Pedersen IM, Kitada S, Leoni LM, et al. Protection of CLL B cells by a follicular dendritic cell line is dependent on induction of Mcl-1. Blood 2002; 100:1795–1801.
61. Widhopf GF 2nd, Rassenti LZ, Toy TL, et al. Chronic lymphocytic leukemia B cells of more than 1% of patients express virtually identical immunoglobulins. Blood 2004; 104:2499–2504.
62. Endo T, Nishio M, Enzler T, et al. BAFF And APRIL support chronic lymphocytic leukemia B cell survival through activation of the canonical NF-{kappa}B pathway. Blood 2007; 109:703–710.
63. Nishio M, Endo T, Tsukada N, et al. Nurselike cells express BAFF and APRIL, which can promote survival of chronic lymphocytic leukemia cells via a paracrine pathway distinct from that of SDF-1alpha. Blood 2005; 106:1012–1020.
64. Gross JA, Johnston J, Mudri S, et al. TACI and BCMA are receptors for a TNF homologue implicated in B-cell autoimmune disease. Nature 2000; 404:995–999.
65. Thompson JS, Bixler SA, Qian F, et al. BAFF-R, a newly identified TNF receptor that specifically interacts with BAFF. Science 2001; 293:2108–2111.
66. de Totero D, Meazza R, Zupo S, et al. Interleukin-21 receptor (IL-21R) is up-regulated by CD40 triggering and mediates proapoptotic signals in chronic lymphocytic leukemia B cells. Blood 2006; 107:3708–3715.
67. de Totero D, Meazza R, Capaia M, et al. The opposite effects of IL-15 and IL-21 on CLL B cells correlate with differential activation of the JAK/STAT and ERK1/2 pathways. Blood 2008; 111:517–524.
68. Gowda A, Roda J, Hussain SR, et al. IL-21 mediates apoptosis through up-regulation of the BH3 family member BIM and enhances both direct and antibody dependent cellular cytotoxicity in primary chronic lymphocytic cells. Blood 2008; 111:4723–4730.
69. Klein U, Tu Y, Stolovitzky GA, et al. Gene expression profiling of B cell chronic lymphocytic leukemia reveals a homogeneous phenotype related to memory B cells. J Exp Med 2001; 194:1625–1638.
70. Chiorazzi N, Ferrarini M. B cell chronic lymphocytic leukemia: lessons learned from studies of the B cell antigen receptor. Ann Rev Immunol 2003; 21:841–894.
71. Ferrarini M, Chiorazzi N. Recent advances in the molecular biology and immunobiology of chronic lymphocytic leukemia. Semin Hematol 2004; 41:207–223.
72. Chiorazzi N, Rai KR, Ferrarini M. Chronic lymphocytic leukemia. N Engl J Med 2005; 352:804–815.
73. Broker BM, Klajman A, Youinou P, ct al. Chronic lymphocytic leukemic cells secrete multispecific autoantibodies. J Autoimmun 1988; 1:469–481.
74. Sthoeger ZM, Wakai M, Tse DB, et al. Production of autoantibodies by CD5-expressing B lymphocytes from patients with chronic lymphocytic leukemia. J Exp Med 1989; 169:255–268.
75. Borche L, Lim A, Binet JL, et al. Evidence that chronic lymphocytic leukemia B lymphocytes are frequently committed to production of natural autoantibodies. Blood 1990; 76:562–569.
76. Herve M, Xu K, Ng Y-S, et al. Unmutated and mutated chronic lymphocytic leukemia derive from common self-reactive B cell precursors despite expressing different antibody reactivity. J Clin Invest 2005; 115:1636–1643.
77. Chang MK, Bergmark C, Laurila A, et al. Monoclonal antibodies against oxidized low-density lipoprotein bind to apoptotic cells and inhibit their phagocytosis by elicited macrophages: evidence that oxidation-specific epitopes mediate macrophage recognition. Proc Natl Acad Sci U S A 1999; 96:6353–6358.

78. Chang MK, Binder CJ, Miller YI, et al. Apoptotic cells with oxidation-specific epitopes are immunogenic and proinflammatory. J Exp Med 2004; 200:1359–1370.
79. Shaw PX, Horkko S, Chang MK, et al. Natural antibodies with the T15 idiotype may act in atherosclerosis, apoptotic clearance, and protective immunity. J Clin Invest 2000; 105: 1731–1740.
80. Esterbauer H, Schaur RJ, Zollner H. Chemistry and biochemistry of 4-hydroxynonenal, malonaldehyde and related aldehydes. Free Radic Biol Med 1991; 11:81–128.
81. Diamond B, Scharff MD. Somatic mutation of the T15 heavy chain gives rise to an antibody with autoantibody specificity. Proc Natl Acad Sci U S A 1984; 81:5841–5844.
82. Crews S, Griffin J, Huang H, et al. A single VH gene segment encodes the immune response to phosphorylcholine: somatic mutation is correlated with the class of the antibody. Cell 1981; 25:59–66.
83. Briles DE, Nahm M, Schroer K, et al. Antiphosphocholine antibodies found in normal mouse serum are protective against intravenous infection with type 3 streptococcus pneumoniae. J Exp Med 1981; 153:694–705.
84. Masmoudi H, Mota-Santos T, Huetz F, et al. All T15 Id-positive antibodies (but not the majority of VHT15+ antibodies) are produced by peritoneal CD5+ B lymphocytes. Int Immunol 1990; 2:515–520.
85. Tobin G, Thunberg U, Johnson A, et al. Chronic lymphocytic leukemias utilizing the VH3-21 gene display highly restricted V{lambda}2-14 gene use and homologous CDR3s: implicating recognition of a common antigen epitope. Blood 2003; 101:4952–4957.
86. Ghiotto F, Fais F, Valetto A, et al. Remarkably similar antigen receptors among a subset of patients with chronic lymphocytic leukemia. J Clin Invest 2004; 113:1008–1016.
87. Messmer BT, Albesiano E, Efremov DG, et al. Multiple distinct sets of stereotyped antigen receptors indicate a key role for antigen in promoting chronic lymphocytic leukemia. J Exp Med 2004; 200:519–525.
88. Tobin G, Thunberg U, Karlsson K, et al. Subsets with restricted immunoglobulin gene rearrangement features indicate a role for antigen selection in the development of chronic lymphocytic leukemia. Blood 2004; 104:2879–2885.
89. Stamatopoulos K, Belessi C, Moreno C, et al. Over 20% of patients with chronic lymphocytic leukemia carry stereotyped receptors: pathogenetic implications and clinical correlations. Blood 2007; 109:259–270.
90. Herzenberg LA, Stall AM, Lalor PA, et al. The Ly-1 B cell lineage. Immunol Rev 1986; 93:81–102.
91. Herzenberg LA, Kantor AB. B-cell lineages exist in the mouse. Immunol Today 1993; 14:79–83.
92. Herzenberg LA. B-1 cells: the lineage question revisited. Immunol Rev 2000; 175:9–22.
93. Wortis H. Surface markers, heavy chain sequences and B cell lineages. Intern Rev Immunol 1992; 8:235–246.
94. Wortis HH, Teutsch M, Higer M, et al. B-cell activation by crosslinking of surface IgM or ligation of CD40 involves alternative signal pathways and results in different B-cell phenotypes. Proc Natl Acad Sci U S A 1995; 92:3348–3352.
95. Wortis HH, Berland R. Cutting edge commentary: origins of B-1 cells. J Immunol 2001; 166:2163–2166.
96. Rothstein T.L. Cutting edge commentary: two B-1 or not to be one. J Immunol 2002; 168:4257–4261.
97. Klinman DM, Holmes KL. Differences in the repertoire expressed by peritoneal and splenic Ly-1 (CD5)+ B cells. J Immunol 1990; 144:4520–4525.
98. Tumang JR, Frances R, Yeo SG, et al. Spontaneously Ig-secreting B-1 cells violate the accepted paradigm for expression of differentiation-associated transcription factors. J Immunol 2005; 174:3173–3177.
99. Hardy RR, Carmack CE, Li YS, et al. Distinctive developmental origins and specificities of murine CD5+ B cells. Immunol Rev 1994; 137:91–118.
100. Hardy RR, Hayakawa K. Developmental origins, specificities and immunoglobulin gene biases of murine Ly-1 B cells. Int Rev Immunol 1992; 8:189–207.

101. Tarlinton D, Stall AM, Herzenberg LA. Repetitive usage of immunoglobulin VH and D gene segments in CD5+ Ly-1 B clones of (NZB × NZW)F1 mice. EMBO J 1988; 7: 3705–3710.
102. Kantor AB, Merrill CE, Herzenberg LA, et al. An unbiased analysis of V(H)-D-J(H) sequences from B-1a, B-1b, and conventional B cells. J Immunol 1997; 158:1175–1186.
103. Seidl KJ, MacKenzie JD, Wang D, et al. Frequent occurrence of identical heavy and light chain Ig rearrangements. Int Immunol 1997; 9:689–702.
104. Herzenberg LA, Herzenberg LA. Toward a layered immune system. Cell 1989; 59:953–954.
105. Fehr T, Naim HY, Bachmann MF, et al. T-cell independent IgM and enduring protective IgG antibodies induced by chimeric measles viruses. Nat Med 1998; 4:945–948.
106. Ochsenbein AF, Fehr T, Lutz C, et al. Control of early viral and bacterial distribution and disease by natural antibodies. Science 1999; 286:2156–2159.
107. Baumgarth N, Herman OC, Jager GC, et al. Innate and acquired humoral immunities to influenza virus are mediated by distinct arms of the immune system. Proc Natl Acad Sci U S A 1999; 96:2250–2255.
108. Haas KM, Poe JC, Steeber DA, et al. B-1a and B-1b cells exhibit distinct developmental requirements and have unique functional roles in innate and adaptive immunity to S. pneumoniae. Immunity 2005; 23:7–18.
109. Rajewsky K. Clonal selection and learning in the antibody system. Nature 1996; 381:751–758.
110. Klein U, Goossens T, Fischer M, et al. Somatic hypermutation in normal and transformed human B cells. Immunol Rev 1998; 162:261–280.
111. Zupo S, Dono M, Massara R, et al. Expression of CD5 and CD38 by human CD5- B cells: requirement for special stimuli. Eur J Immunol 1994; 24:1426–1433.
112. Dono M, Burgio VL, Tacchetti C, et al. Subepithelial B cells in the human palatine tonsil. Morphologic I, cytochemical and phenotypic characterization. Eur J Immunol 1996; 26: 2035–2042.
113. Dono M, Zupo S, Leanza N, et al. Heterogeneity of tonsillar subepithelial B lymphocytes, the splenic marginal zone equivalents. J Immunol 2000; 164:5596–5604.
114. Martin F, Kearney J. Marginal-zone B cells. Nat Rev Immunol 2002; 2:323–335.
115. Chen X, Martin F, Forbush KA, et al. Evidence for selection of a population of multi-reactive B cells into the splenic marginal zone. Int Immunol 1997; 9:27–41.
116. Martin F, Oliver AM, Kearney JF. Marginal zone and B1 B cells unite in the early response against T-independent blood-borne particulate antigens. Immunity 2001; 14:617–629.
117. Martin F, Kearney JF. B-cell subsets and the mature preimmune repertoire. Marginal zone and B1 B cells as part of a "natural immune memory". Immunol Rev 2000; 175:70–79.
118. Martin F, Kearney JF. Positive selection from newly formed to marginal zone B cells depends on the rate of clonal production, CD19, and btk. Immunity 2000; 12:39–49.
119. Li Y, Li H, Weigert M. Autoreactive B cells in the marginal zone that express dual receptors. J Exp Med 2002; 195:181–188.
120. Kanayama N, Cascalho M, Ohmori H. Analysis of marginal zone B cell development in the mouse with limited B cell diversity: role of the antigen receptor signals in the recruitment of B cells to the marginal zone. J Immunol 2005; 174:1438–1445.
121. Watanabe N, Nisitani S, Ikuta K, et al. Expression levels of B cell surface immunoglobulin regulate efficiency of allelic exclusion and size of autoreactive B-1 cell compartment. J Exp Med 1999; 190:461–469.
122. Martin F, Kearney JF. Marginal-zone B cells. Nat Rev Immunol 2002; 2:323–335.
123. Hatzi K, Catera R, Ferrarini M, et al. B-cell chronic lymphocytic leukemia (B-CLL) cells expresss antibodies reactive with antigenic epitopes expressed on the surface of common bacteria. Blood 2006; 108:12a.
124. Casadevall A, Scharff MD. The mouse antibody response to infection with Cryptococcus neoformans: VH and VL usage in polysaccharide binding antibodies. J Exp Med 1991; 174:151–160.
125. Insel RA, Adderson EE, Carroll WL. The repertoire of human antibody to the Haemophilus influenzae type b capsular polysaccharide. Int Rev Immunol 1992; 9:25–43.

126. Dono M, Burgio VL, Colombo M, et al. CD5(+) B cells with the features of subepithelial B cells found in human tonsils. Eur J Immunol 2007; 37:2138–2147.

127. Agematsu K, Nagumo H, Yang FC, et al. B cell subpopulations separated by CD27 and crucial collaboration of CD27+ B cells and helper T cells in immunoglobulin production. Eur J Immunol 1997; 27:2073–2079.

128. Klein U, Rajewsky K, Kuppers R. Human immunoglobulin (Ig)M+IgD+ peripheral blood B cells expressing the CD27 cell surface antigen carry somatically mutated variable region genes: CD27 as a general marker for somatically mutated (memory) B cells. J Exp Med 1998; 188:1679–1689.

129. Weller S, Braun MC, Tan BK, et al. Human blood IgM "memory" B cells are circulating splenic marginal zone B cells harboring a prediversified immunoglobulin repertoire. Blood 2004; 104:3647–3654.

130. Kruetzmann S, Rosado MM, Weber H, et al. Human immunoglobulin M memory B cells controlling Streptococcus pneumoniae infections are generated in the spleen. J Exp Med 2003; 197:939–945.

131. Rolink AG, Andersson J, Melchers F. Characterization of immature B cells by a novel monoclonal antibody, by turnover and by mitogen reactivity. Eur J Immunol 1998; 28: 3738–3748.

132. Loder F, Mutschler B, Ray RJ, et al. B cell development in the spleen takes place in discrete steps and is determined by the quality of B cell receptor-derived signals. J Exp Med 1999; 190:75–89.

133. Sims GP, Ettinger R, Shirota Y, et al. Identification and characterization of circulating human transitional B cells. Blood 2005; 105:4390–4398.

134. Lindsley RC, Thomas M, Srivastava B, et al. Generation of peripheral B cells occurs via two spatially and temporally distinct pathways. Blood 2007; 109:2521–2528.

135. Allman D, Lindsley RC, DeMuth W, et al. Resolution of three nonproliferative immature splenic B cell subsets reveals multiple selection points during peripheral B cell maturation. J Immunol 2001; 167:6834–6840.

136. Cambier JC, Gauld SB, Merrell KT, et al. B-cell anergy: from transgenic models to naturally occurring anergic B cells? Nat Rev Immunol 2007; 7:633–643.

137. Levine MH, Haberman AM, Sant'Angelo DB, et al. A B-cell receptor-specific selection step governs immature to mature B cell differentiation. Proc Natl Acad Sci U S A 2000; 97: 2743–2748.

138. Allman D, Srivastava B, Lindsley RC. Alternative routes to maturity: branch points and pathways for generating follicular and marginal zone B cells. Immunol Rev 2004; 197: 147–160.

139. Tardivel A, Tinel A, Lens S, et al. The anti-apoptotic factor Bcl-2 can functionally substitute for the B cell survival but not for the marginal zone B cell differentiation activity of BAFF. Eur J Immunol 2004; 34:509–518.

140. Capolunghi F, Cascioli S, Giorda E, et al. CpG drives human transitional B cells to terminal differentiation and production of natural antibodies. J Immunol 2008; 180:800–808.

141. Casola S. Control of peripheral B-cell development. Curr Opin Immunol 2007; 19:143–149.

142. Kipps T.J. The CD5 B cell. Adv Immunol 1989; 47:117–185.

143. Dono M, Zupo S, Massara R, et al. In vitro stimulation of human tonsillar subepithelial B cells: requirement for interaction with activated T cells. Eur J Immunol 2001; 31:752–756.

144. Morabito F, Mangiola M, Rapezzi D, et al. Expression of CD10 by B-chronic lymphocytic leukemia cells undergoing apoptosis in vivo and in vitro. Haematologica 2003; 88:864–873.

2

Gene Expression Profiling in the Study of Chronic Lymphocytic Leukemia

Ulf Klein
*Institute for Cancer Genetics and Herbert Irving Comprehensive Cancer Center,
Columbia University, New York, New York, U.S.A.*

INTRODUCTION

B-cell chronic lymphocytic leukemia (CLL) had long been recognized as a morphologically homogeneous disease of mature, resting B lymphocytes. CLL cells are characterized by the expression of the cell surface antigens CD5, CD23, and CD27, and low level of surface immunoglobulin (Ig), a pattern not observed on any normal B cell (1,2). Despite their uniform histological appearance, however, CLL cases turned out to be surprisingly heterogeneous. First, the rearranged Ig variable region (IgV) genes of CLL cases can be either somatically mutated or unmutated (3–5), implying that the corresponding precursor cells may originate from either T cell–dependent or T cell–independent responses. In addition, there is a correlation between the IgV mutational status and clinical course (6,7); thus, somatically mutated CLL cases generally show a better prognosis than unmutated CLL. Second, CLL cases can differ in their immunophenotype, e.g., by their differential expression of the CD38 cell surface antigen (6,8,9). Third, CLL exhibits genetic lesions that are distinct from those observed in other malignancies of mature B cells, such as reciprocal balanced chromosome translocations. CLL show various genomic alterations, mostly chromosomal deletions (10), which are more typical of non-hematological tumors. As yet no common genetic lesion has been identified for CLL. Taken together, the unique phenotypic and genetic characteristics of CLL do not allow a conclusive assignment of this tumor to a particular cell of origin or to understand the mechanisms involved in its pathogenesis.

Global gene expression profiling, made possible by the invention of DNA microarray technology in the late 1990s, allows comparative analysis of a large number of genotypically or otherwise distinct tumor samples by measuring and connecting an enormous number of data points to assess possible relationships between individual samples. Since there were many questions remaining about CLL physiology and pathophysiology, this disease was an especially intriguing target for global gene expression profiling (GEP) analysis. These studies, together with investigations on CLL and normal B lymphocytes performed simultaneously using other methodological approaches, helped gain new insights into phenotype, cell derivation, and pathogenesis of CLL. This chapter summarizes what we have learned so far about CLL from GEP analyses and discusses the surprising observations that emerged from the studies demonstrating that all CLL show a homogeneous expression profile, then explores the identity of the subtler CLL subtypes as well as the relation of the tumor cells to a putative normal counterpart, and attempts to place CLL in the framework of the various B-cell malignancies. The final section is dedicated to the use of global GEP approaches in the quest to identify the in vitro response of CLL cells to activation stimuli and candidate drugs for therapy.

BASICS OF GENE EXPRESSION PROFILE ANALYSIS

Global GEP analysis using DNA microarrays allows the simultaneous screening of thousands of expressed genes in a tissue sample. This not only allowed the number of genes that could be interrogated with this technology to become considerably higher, but its unbiased approach also allowed the identification of genes not previously associated with an expression in the tissue studied. These advances evidently led to progress in the identification of novel tumor (sub)types and the identification of the putative normal cellular counterpart of the tumor, as well as identification of tumor-associated genes or pattern of genes, commonly referred to as *signature*, with potential value for therapy and diagnosis.

In a typical GEP analysis, RNA is isolated from tissue samples of a cohort of normal cell subsets or tumor cases. Labeled probe generated from this RNA is then hybridized to DNA microarrays that contain DNA fragments representing distinct mRNA sequences spotted on silica slides (11,12). Nonbinding probes are washed off, and fluorescent signals emitted by binding probes are measured by a detector. The resulting signals are normalized, and the corresponding gene expression values can be fed into biostatistical analysis platforms to identify specific gene expression patterns.

Two biostatistical analysis methods are employed in the identification of gene expression patterns, namely unsupervised learning and supervised learning (13–15) (Fig. 1). Their use depends on the particular biological question. Unsupervised learning is the method of choice for the identification of novel cell types that have not been classified a priori. Supervised learning, on the other hand, allows identification of genes differentially expressed between samples that were defined a priori on the basis of certain criteria that could be different cell types, genotypic differences among individual cases of a cell type such as the level of IgV somatic hypermutation or genomic alterations, or clinical parameters.

Unsupervised learning, or unsupervised hierarchical cluster analysis, uses algorithms that identify similarities in the gene expression data among a panel of samples (that could be tumor cases), and ranks the samples according to their relatedness to each other (Fig. 1). The output of an unsupervised hierarchical cluster analysis is the dendrogram, in which sample relatedness is visualized by branches. Lower-order branches identify immediate neighbors, higher-order branches identify subgroups of samples. A dendrogram resulting from an unsupervised analysis readily reveals the relationship of all of the samples of a GEP study among each other, and may potentially result in the separation of the samples into subgroups or classes. Thus, this approach is suited for class discovery for identification of subcategories among a group of samples.

Supervised learning, or supervised pattern discovery analysis, is the method of choice for class prediction and for the identification of tissue-specific genes (Fig. 1). The results of a supervised analysis are often represented as a color-coded matrix that

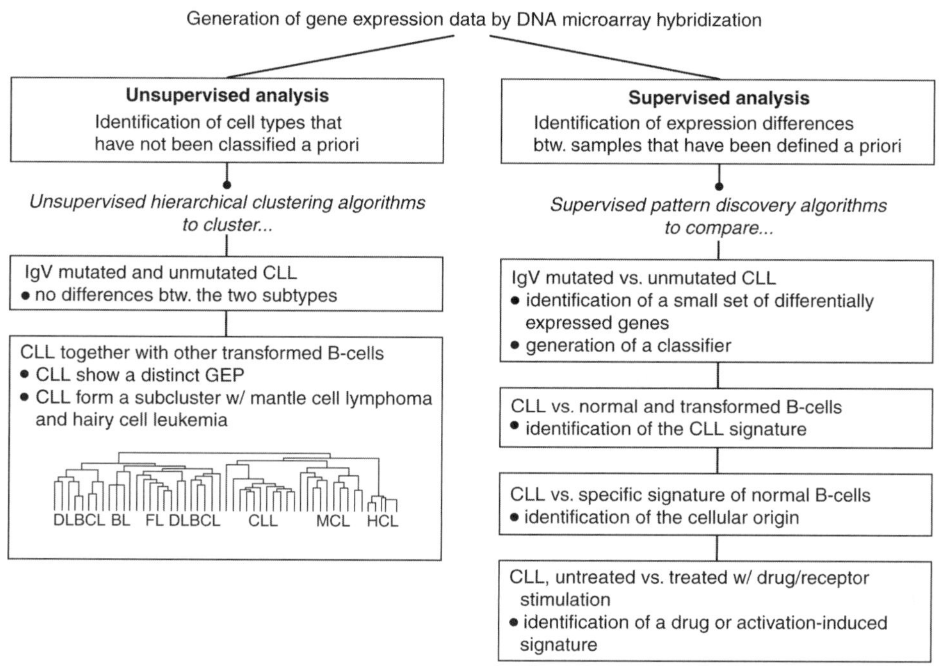

Figure 1 GEP-based strategies for the identification of CLL subtypes and differentially expressed genes between CLL subtypes. Gene expression data generated by DNA microarray hybridization are analyzed by unsupervised or supervised analysis methods, depending on the particular question (indicated in the boxes). The dendrogram resulting from unsupervised hierarchical clustering of samples representing various types of mature B-cell malignancies (*bottom left*). *Abbreviation*: CLL, chronic lymphocytic leukemia (*See Color Insert*).

visualizes the transcript levels of each gene across the samples. Supervised analysis uses algorithms that lead to the identification of a set of genes specifically expressed in a particular tissue subtype. In a classification analysis, this tissue-specific pattern can then identify samples among an independent panel that belong to the particular subtype. Historically, the feasibility of using GEP data for a tumor classification analysis was first demonstrated by the ability to distinguish acute lymphoblastic leukemia (ALL) from acute myeloid leukemia (AML) solely on the basis of their transcriptomes (14). In this analysis, a class predictor was established on a panel of cases that without previous knowledge about the tissue derivation of tumor samples of an independent panel was able to classify these cases into either ALL or AML categories. Classifiers generated by supervised learning have since been successfully employed for tumor class prediction in multiple studies on all different kinds of tissues, and supervised analysis is now widely used for the identification of tumor-associated genes that may lead to improvements in diagnosis, prognosis, and/or therapy.

Over the last several years, various types of lymphoid malignancies and normal lymphocytes have been analyzed by GEP analysis, often leading to new and unexpected insights into the classification and pathogenesis of lymphomas (16,17). One of the first B cell–derived malignancies analyzed by GEP analysis was diffuse large B-cell lymphoma (DLBCL), a non-Hodgkin lymphoma entity of mature B cells with extensive phenotypic and clinical heterogeneity. The initial analysis discovered that a panel of DLBCL can be separated into two subtypes only on the basis of their specific gene expression (18). Moreover, the particular genes expressed in these subtypes suggested a phenotypic relation to particular normal B-cell subpopulations, namely germinal center (GC) B cells and in vitro–activated B cells, respectively. This discovery has given rise to the now generally accepted division of DLBCL into GC-type DLBCL and activated B-cell (ABC)-type DLBCL (18), and, as subsequent studies uncovered, into at least one additional DLBCL category (19,20). The GEP-based finding that DLBCL can be subdivided into biologically distinct subgroups has evidently had a large impact on the development of new concepts about the molecular pathogenesis of this disease. Clearly, the insights gained from GEP analyses on DLBCL provide a classic example for the value of GEP in the study of lymphoid malignancies.

CLL SHOWS A HOMOGENEOUS GENE EXPRESSION PROFILE

GEP analyses performed by independent laboratories have found that all CLLs displayed a common gene expression profile that is independent of the level of IgV somatic hypermutation (21–23) or of the expression of CD38 (24). Only more sensitive analysis methods were able to extract subtle differences in the genotypically defined subsets (see next section). Thus, despite the heterogeneity in IgV mutational status, the expression of certain cell surface markers, and genomic alterations, CLL represents a phenotypically homogeneous disease. The results of the GEP analyses are thus inconsistent with the hypothesis that IgV-unmutated and somatically mutated CLL derive from separate B-cell developmental stages, namely the antigen-inexperienced (naïve) and antigen-experienced (memory) stages. In this regard, CLL is clearly distinct from DLBCL, a tumor entity that is characterized by extensive heterogeneity and distinct cellular derivation (see previous paragraph). Instead, these observations strongly suggest that all CLL originate from a common cellular precursor as a result of a common pathogenetic mechanism (21,22).

In an unsupervised hierarchical cluster analysis, CLL clusters separately from all other B cell–derived malignancies and normal B-cell subpopulations (21,22,25), thus identifying a CLL-specific gene expression signature. Although different DNA micro-array platforms have been employed by the various laboratories that studied CLL by unsupervised and supervised analysis, there is a considerable overlap in the actual genes that are specifically up- or downregulated in CLL compared with other normal and transformed B cells (21–23,26). This circumstance strengthens the validity of a GEP-based approach to gain new insights into CLL biology and pathophysiology. Through these highly specific as well as largely unbiased biostatistical approaches, new CLL-specific genes were identified that are presently being further evaluated for their potential use in diagnosis or treatment. Moreover, the CLL-specific signature revealed that the transcripts encoding proliferation and cell cycle–associated genes were strongly downregulated compared with other normal and transformed B cells, including even mature, resting B cells (naïve and memory B cells) (21). This observation is in agreement with the well-known low proliferation capacity of CLL tumor cells isolated from the peripheral blood. When the expression profile of CLL was specifically compared with that of normal B lymphocytes, it emerged that pro-apoptotic genes were downregulated and anti-apoptotic genes were upregulated in the tumor cells, which is in accordance with the known apoptosis-resistant phenotype of CLL (21–23). Moreover, transcripts encoding certain cytokine and chemokine receptors were found to be specifically upregulated in CLL cells compared with normal B cells, suggesting that the tumor cells may exert abnormal physiological responses to the respective cytokines/chemokines. The GEP data obtained so far not only spurred new investigations into the phenotype of CLL and CLL pathogenesis; since the data are publicly available, they also serve as a valuable repository for research on CLL because it is possible to look up the expression of almost any gene of interest.

The realization that microRNAs convey essential cellular functions raised the question as to whether specific microRNAs are expressed in the CLL tumor cells versus normal B cells. Initial results, using either DNA microarrays (27) or large-scale polymerase chain reaction (PCR) based methods (28), suggested that some microRNAs are indeed specifically overexpressed in CLL samples. When extending the analysis to the various subtypes of B-cell malignancies, it will be interesting to see whether the upregulated expression of several microRNAs, which may include miR-155 and miR-21 (28), is specific for CLL, and what might be the functional consequences. For further reading in this area, see chapter 3 (Calin chapter).

SUBTYPES OF CLL

Several observations suggested the existence of CLL subtypes despite the marked morphological homogeneity of the CLL tumor cells present in peripheral blood. First, the realization in the 1990s that CLL cases can express either somatically mutated or unmutated IgV genes (3–5) suggested the existence of subgroups of CLL that originate from the oncogenic transformation of developmentally distinct precursor cells. Thus, the occurrence of somatic mutations in the rearranged IgV genes of a subset of CLL cases was suggestive of an antigen-experienced, memory B-cell derivation, while the unmutated CLLs were thought to be related to antigen-inexperienced, naïve B cells. Second, the clinical course of CLL can be benign or aggressive, with a strong correlation between the IgV somatic mutation status and clinical prognosis (6,7). Third, immunophenotypic analyses could identify subtypes of CLL with high or low expression of the CD38 cell surface antigen (6,8,9), and a correlation between CD38 expression and disease course has been noted. To gain insights into the various CLL subtypes, GEP analyses were undertaken to identify the genes that distinguish IgV-mutated from IgV-unmutated CLLs (21,22), CD38$^+$ from CD38$^-$ CLLs (24), or CLL subgroups defined by patient survival or disease staging (23,29). The outcome of these studies was somewhat surprising, as they demonstrated in each case that all CLLs display a common GEP (see previous section), indicating that CLL is a phenotypically homogeneous disease.

Nevertheless, applying a more stringent supervised analysis and using purified tumor cells, it was possible to identify a small set of genes that were differentially expressed between somatically mutated and unmutated CLLs (21,22). This pattern of genes could be used to classify an independent panel of CLL cases into the two genetically defined CLL subgroups at a high-confidence level, indicating that the IgV-mutated and IgV-unmutated CLL subgroups display a subtle, but consistent, phenotypic difference. It was essential to use purified CLL cells to generate the classifiers (21,22), probably because of cellular contamination of non-tumor cells in unpurified samples. These signatures, however, were then able to successfully classify CLL samples of an unpurified panel (21,22). What did we learn from the identity of the differentially expressed genes between the IgV-mutated and IgV-unmutated subgroups? Compared with IgV-mutated CLLs, the IgV-unmutated subgroup seems to express higher mRNA levels of genes that are normally activated upon in vitro B-cell receptor (BCR)-mediated stimulation (22), suggesting that IgV-unmutated CLLs are subjected to continuous BCR signaling in vivo. Moreover, this study identified ZAP-70, a member of the Syk-ZAP-70 protein tyrosine kinase family involved in T-cell activation, as being specifically associated with an expression in the IgV-unmutated CLL subtype (22). While the potential role of this kinase in the physiology of the unmutated subtype remains to be determined, the discovery of ZAP-70 as a marker protein associated with the IgV-unmutated CLL subtype had an immediate impact on diagnosis. Flow cytometry–based assays that measure ZAP-70 protein levels have been established by several groups (30–32) and are now routinely used in many hospitals as a surrogate for the determination of the IgV mutational status. A study suggests that ZAP-70 expression might be a better prognostic marker for prediction of the clinical course of CLL than the IgV gene mutational status (31), perhaps reflecting a direct role of ZAP-70 in the pathophysiology of a subset of CLL. However, since ZAP-70 expression is variable among CLL cases, it is not always clear whether the intensity of ZAP-70 as measured in the flow cytometry–based assay can be considered present or absent. Presently, it seems that the combination of both ZAP-70 protein levels and IgV mutational status of a CLL case represents the best predictor of the clinical course. Obviously, a lot of effort is put into the development of an easy and reliable assay that can discriminate IgV-mutated from IgV-unmutated cases. Possible candidates include the genes LPL and ADAM29, whose expression is upregulated in unmutated and somatically mutated CLLs, respectively (33). Several other candidates that were identified in global GEP analyses are currently being evaluated for their potential value in discriminating the two subtypes. The ultimate goal would be to identify a small set of gene products whose differential expression can be analyzed in a simple flow cytometrical assay.

While the gene expression pattern discriminating IgV somatically mutated and unmutated CLLs allows classification of the vast majority of cases into either subgroup, it is not absolute. CLL cases that carry a rearrangement of the VH3-21 gene segment show a low overall poor survival regardless of the level of IgV hypermutation (34); VH3-21-expressing cases can be somatically mutated or unmutated. Molecular analysis of the rearranged antibody genes revealed that these CLL cases also show a restricted VDJ-junctional repertoire, and the corresponding heavy chains furthermore show a tendency to be associated with a specific λ light chain gene. Indeed, a GEP analysis supports the claim that most VH3-21-bearing CLLs show a gene expression profile that is largely distinct from that of VH3-21-negative cases (35). Taken together, these observations suggest a predominant role for a common antigen in the pathogenesis of VH3-21-expressing CLL cases. A critical involvement of antigen in CLL development had previously been suggested on the basis of the results of large-scale IgV gene repertoire analyses, which showed that certain IgV gene segments are almost exclusively expressed either by unmutated (such as VH1-69) or by mutated (such as VH3-07) CLLs (36). The case of the VH3-21 gene segment suggests that it appears to be the particular antigen receptor rather than the level of IgV somatic hypermutation as such that correlates with good or bad clinical prognosis.

In several published GEP-based studies on CLL, biostatistical analyses suggested the existence of clinically defined subgroups. Thus, a subgroup of CLL was identified that predominantly comprised patients with a more favorable clinical course with longer progression-free survival (24). Other studies described a set of genes that correlated with clinical staging (29), or the identification of genes that distinguished Rai stage 0 from stage 4 patients in the respective panels (23). In accordance with the commonly observed homogeneous gene expression pattern of CLL, in each of these studies, the expression differences between the corresponding subgroups were very small. The relevance of the respective patterns for diagnosis/prognosis remains to be evaluated by testing them in a classification analysis on an independent panel of CLL cases.

Finally, two independent analyses that have measured the expression of microRNAs in genetically characterized CLL cases commonly found the microRNAs miR-223, miR-29b, and miR29c to be specifically upregulated in patients with IgV-mutated CLLs (27,28). It will be interesting to see whether the expression of these, and perhaps additional, not yet identified, microRNAs may provide novel insights into the biology of CLL subtypes and/or represent suitable markers of subtype identification or may have prognostic relevance.

CELLULAR ORIGIN OF CLL

Global GEP, which simultaneously measures the expression of thousands of marker genes of a cell population, turned out to be a useful tool in dissecting the cellular origin of CLL. Although it had early on been recognized that CLL is a tumor derived from mature B cells, the normal cellular counterpart of this entity remained elusive. In the human, the B-cell compartment comprises functionally distinct subpopulations that can be identified by their immunophenotype and by the level of somatic hypermutation in their rearranged IgV genes (37,38). Naïve B cells express unmutated IgV genes and, upon antigen activation in the course of a T cell–dependent immune response, differentiate into GC B cells that undergo somatic hypermutation. Following several rounds of mutation and selection, B cells with improved antigen binding develop into either plasma cells or memory B cells. The latter respond quickly to repeated antigen encounter by differentiating into plasma cells secreting highly specific antibodies. A subset of B cells in the human with unmutated IgV genes are characterized by the expression of the CD5 antigen (39,40). While in the mouse, these cells are functionally distinct from the B cells participating in T cell–dependent immune responses, their role and significance in the human is less clear.

The expression of the CD5 cell surface antigen on the CLL tumor cells initially pointed toward a phenotypic relation of the tumor precursor to the $CD5^+$ B cell. Functional characteristics of mouse $CD5^+$ B cells, most notably, their long life span (41) and the fact that they tend to outgrow as a monoclonal population in old mice (42) contributed to the notion that CLL tumor cells and $CD5^+$ B cells are related. However, the immunophenotype of the tumor cells ($CD5^+CD23^+CD27^+$, low surface Ig expression) is distinct from that of $CD5^+$ B cells and also from that of any other known normal B cell (1,2). The picture became more complex with the realization that CLL cases can have somatically mutated or unmutated IgV genes (3–5). Since the level of somatic hypermutation in a rearranged antibody gene is an indication of the developmental stage of the B cell, it was assumed that the normal counterpart of an unmutated CLL case may represent a naïve B cell, whereas IgV-mutated CLLs may originate from the malignant transformation of a B cell that had previously acquired somatic hypermutations during the GC reaction.

More specific comparison of gene expression data from CLL with those of the various normal B-cell subsets suggests that all CLLs are mostly related in their gene expression profile to that derived from $CD27^+$ B cells (21), which comprises a heterogeneous subset of antigen-experienced B cells and includes classical memory B cells and also marginal zone B cells. The CLL profile did not show similarity to those derived from $CD5^+$ cord blood, $CD27^-$ (naïve), or GC B cells (21,22) (Fig. 2).

The vast majority of $CD27^+$ B cells express somatically mutated IgV genes, while $CD27^-$ B cells are almost exclusively unmutated (43,44). Only a subset of $CD27^+$ cells carry unmutated IgV genes, which are thought to represent either GC-derived memory B cells that have not acquired hypermutations or B cells that have responded to T cell–independent antigens. $CD27^+$ B cells can express all Ig isotypes (43,45); subsets of $CD27^+$ B cells are found in PB of healthy humans that are IgG, IgM-only, or IgM^+IgD^+.

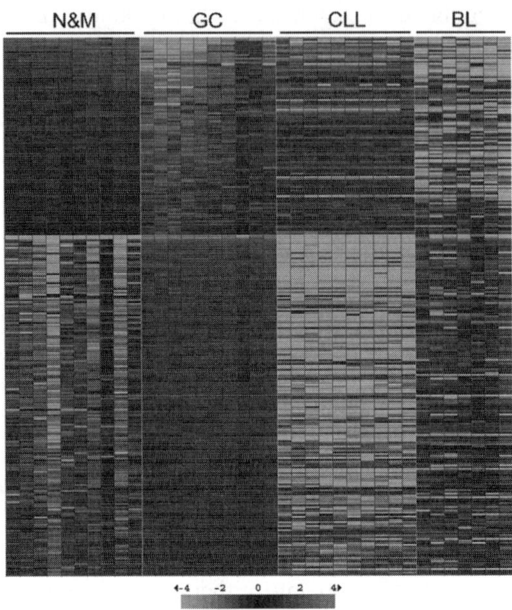

Figure 2 Visualization of the histological derivation of CLL and Burkitt lymphoma by GEP. Genes differentially expressed between naïve and memory B cells (N&M) on the one hand and GC B cells (GC B) on the other were identified by supervised pattern discovery analysis. The expression level of the respective genes in CLL and Burkitt lymphoma (BL) is shown along with the differentially expressed genes. The relatedness of the tumor cases to either the GC B cells or the non-GC B cells is visible from the expression values coded in shades of gray and can be quantitatively expressed by statistical analysis (not shown). Upregulated and downregulated genes are identified by darker and lighter gray tones, respectively. *Abbreviations*: CLL, chronic lymphocytic leukemia; GC, germinal center (*See Color Insert*).

Moreover, immunophenotypic analyses demonstrated the differential expression of certain cell surface markers on these cells, such as CD80 (46,47). Together with the observation that in vitro, phenotypically distinct CD27$^+$ subsets respond differently to activation stimuli (48–51), this indicates that the CD27$^+$ population comprises functionally diverse B-cell subsets. IgM-expressing, somatically mutated CD27$^+$ cells respond to T-independent antigens (50,51), suggesting that these cells might represent marginal zone B cells, which comprise a subset of cells that are rapidly activated to secret Ig against invading microorganisms (52). The developmental origin of those IgM-expressing, somatically mutated B cells is presently unclear. On the one hand, they may represent memory B cells that have undergone the GC reaction without switching their isotype (43,44), on the other hand, it has been suggested that this subset is generated in an antigen-independent fashion by an extrafollicular developmental pathway (53,54). Thus, the CD27$^+$ population may comprise "classical" memory B cells generated in the GC reaction, antigen-experienced cells selected to respond to T-independent antigens, and, possibly a somatically mutated B-cell subset that is generated in a developmental pathway not involving antigen or T cells. Since in the peripheral lymphoid organs, CD27$^+$ B cells are located in the marginal zone, one may characterize these cells collectively as marginal zone B cells. In vitro, CD27$^+$ cells, in contrast to CD27$^-$ cells, and irrespective of their isotype, respond very fast by differentiating into antibody-secreting cells (48,49,51).

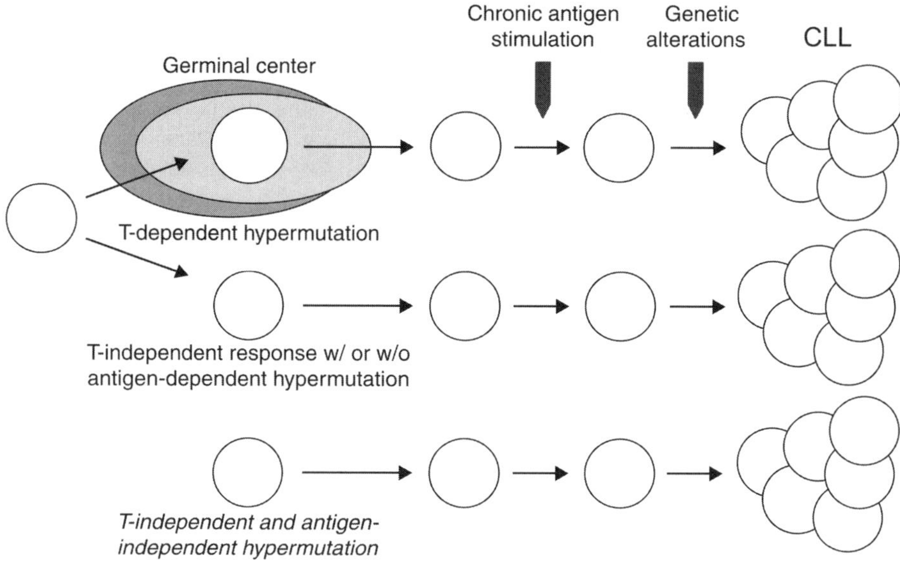

Figure 3 A model of the hypothetical pathways leading to CLL development. Antigen-inexperienced naïve B cells are driven into the GC B-cell response or into a T cell–independent response (*branches on top*). A separate pathway (*branch on bottom*) has been proposed in which somatically mutated B cells are generated in a T cell–independent and antigen-independent fashion (see text). After the B cell has undergone the GC- or the T-independent responses, the cells differentiate into memory/marginal zone B cells. These cells may then be subjected to chronic antigen stimulation, during which they may acquire genetic alterations that cause oncogenic transformation, eventually leading to CLL development. *Abbreviations*: CLL, chronic lymphocytic leukemia; GC, germinal center.

Thus, despite their uncertain developmental origin, all marginal zone B cells may have a common function in protecting the body against invading pathogens by quickly differentiating into plasma cells.

Taken together, it emerges that memory/marginal zone B cells display features that are consistent with a putative CLL precursor cell. All CLLs express CD27 on the cell surface (55), and the pattern of Ig isotype distribution among CLL cases (class switch, IgM-only, IgM$^+$IgD$^+$) resembles that of CD27$^+$ cells (56). Moreover, the IgV genes of both mutated and unmutated CLLs show evidence of antigenic selection, suggesting an important role for antigen in CLL pathogenesis (56). Taken together, the available evidence is compatible with the notion that CLL may develop through the oncogenic transformation of a memory/marginal zone B cell (Fig. 3).

RELATION OF CLL TO OTHER MATURE B-CELL MALIGNANCIES

The observation that CLL tumor cells show phenotypic relatedness to memory/marginal zone B cells suggests that the multistep process of tumorigenesis begins in these cells (21) (Fig. 3). This notion is further supported by the specific pattern of cytogenetic abnormalities in CLL that is markedly different from that found in most types of mature B-cell malignancies (10). Burkitt lymphoma, follicular lymphoma, and DLBCL are characterized by recurrent balanced chromosomal translocations, typically involving the Ig loci and a specific proto-oncogene. These translocations are a consequence of errors during the processes of VDJ recombination, Ig class switch recombination, or somatic hypermutation (57,58). CLL, on the other hand, does not exhibit chromosomal translocations occurring during the Ig loci remodeling processes, but instead shows chromosomal deletions and amplifications (10) similar to those found in solid tumors [although the occurrence of nonrecurrent, imbalanced chromosomal translocations in a subgroup of CLL has been reported (59)]. The absence in CLL of chromosomal translocations involving the Ig loci indicates that the causative mechanisms, class switch recombination, and somatic hypermutation are presumably not active in the tumor precursor cell. This in turn suggests that the chromosomal alterations associated with CLL pathogenesis occur in the antigen-experienced B cell after completion of these DNA-modifying processes, and that they may originate from errors during the continuous proliferation of the precursor cell, possibly caused by chronic antigen stimulation (Fig. 3).

The normal cellular counterpart of most types of mature B-cell malignancies is thought to be a GC B cell (e.g., follicular lymphoma, Burkitt lymphoma, some DLBCLs) or a post-GC B cell that has acquired a crucial oncogenic hit during the GC reaction (some DLBCLs) (57,58). The notion that CLL originates from a different cell type and through distinct oncogenic mechanisms is further supported by the results of an unsupervised hierarchical cluster analysis of various types of non-Hodgkin lymphomas, where CLL clusters separately from the lymphomas of putative GC origin (18,21,22). This analysis further showed that CLL clusters along with hairy cell leukemia (25). The morphology and phenotype of hairy cell leukemia is clearly distinct from that of any other B-cell malignancy (60). However, as for CLL, the GEP of hairy cell leukemia was found to resemble most closely that of $CD27^+$ B cells (25). An additional similarity between the two entities is their lack of chromosomal translocations (61,62). Together, these observations suggest that CLL and HCL both originate from the oncogenic transformation of $CD27^+$ B cells. Different transformation mechanisms might give rise to the distinct phenotypes and pathophysiologies of the two malignancies, or the targets of malignant transformation in CLL or hairy cell leukemia may represent different cell types of the heterogeneous $CD27^+$ population. Taken together, the results from the comparative GEP analysis led to the concept that CLL and HCL may belong to a subgroup of B-cell malignancies that originate from the oncogenic transformation of antigen-experienced B cells.

INSIGHTS INTO THE PHYSIOLOGY OF CLL
BY GEP-BASED APPROACHES

The salient features of GEP make this technology an extremely attractive tool for the identification of genes whose expression levels move specifically as the result of a stimulation of a particular signaling pathway, or of drugs interfering with specific cellular pathways. Thereby, one straightforward experimental approach is to devise a defined in vitro system in which, e.g., a transcription factor is upregulated in an inducible fashion. Indeed, GEP has been used early on to identify the specific gene expression signatures resulting from the activity of certain proto-oncogenes or transcription factors, such as c-Myc or BCL6, yielding new insights into their targets and their effects on cell physiology (63,64). Other works have exploited the power of GEP to measure the response of cells derived from specific lymphoma subtypes to an NFκB-inhibitory drug (65) or the effects of the activation of a cell surface receptor such as the TNF receptor family member CD40 in normal B cells (66,67). Since CD40 is also expressed on the CLL tumor cells, an understanding of the molecular consequences of CD40 stimulation on

CLL versus normal B cells may yield insights into the pathophysiology of the cells. Indeed, a comparison of the GEP data derived from CD40-stimulated CLL versus normal resting B cells found that CLL tumor cells show increased expression of pro-survival and antiproliferative genes relative to the normal B cells (67). These observations suggested that CD40 stimulation may have an adverse effect in the response of CLL cells to cytotoxic drugs, which is important information since activation of CLL cells through CD40 enhances their susceptibility to recognition by immune cells.

Fludarabine is commonly used as a cytotoxic drug in the treatment of CLL. GEP of CLL tumor cells derived from patients who have received fludarabine show an upregulation of known p53 target genes (68). The same gene expression changes were observed when treating CLL cells with this drug in vitro. Importantly, the comparative analysis of p53-proficient and p53-deficient cell lines demonstrated that a large number of the fludarabine signature genes were indeed p53 target genes (68). The findings of this study demonstrate that fludarabine treatment activates the p53 pathway in vivo and provides a molecular explanation for the circumstance that fludarabine treatment can result in the selection of p53-null CLL cells that are more resistant to cytotoxic drugs.

GEP has been used to study changes in the transcriptomes of CLL tumor cells in the response to pharmacological inhibitors. Thus, a study investigated the in vitro cytotoxicity of a newly developed cyclin-dependent kinase inhibitor in CLL cases with and without mutations in the *ATM* or *TP53* genes (65), with the aim to potentially identify a drug that could be effective in the treatment of CLL cases that are resistant to current cytotoxic treatment regimen. The results of the GEP analysis showed a downregulation of genes involved in survival and DNA repair, and is expected to guide further studies aimed at using this inhibitor to induce apoptosis in CLL. Another study found that pharmacological inhibitors of the NF-κB pathway have a potential in apoptosis induction of CLL cells, but not normal B cells (69). Toward this aim, GEP were generated that identified potential new NF-κB target genes in CLL.

Finally, a GEP-based approach was employed to investigate the possible effects of the CLL tumor cells on other (nonmalignant) immune cells. Thus, T cells derived from untreated CLL patients displayed a distinct GEP compared with that of normal controls, and was cell-cell contact dependent, indicating that the tumor cells actively cause changes in the physiology of T cells in CLL patients that impair their normal function (70). Results from the gene expression data give insights into the cellular pathways that are affected in these cells and may help to identify treatment strategies that would selectively enhance T-cell immunity in CLL patients.

Clearly, the combination of well-controlled in vitro experiments that are aimed at investigating an agent's effect on the CLL tumor cells and the unbiased measurement of the corresponding global gene expression changes represents a powerful methodological approach to yield new clues into CLL pathophysiology.

SUMMARY AND CONCLUDING REMARKS

The results obtained from global GEP analyses provided new insights into several aspects of CLL physiology. All CLLs, regardless of their level of IgV somatic hypermutation, display a common GEP, indicating a derivation of CLL from a developmentally related precursor cell. Comparison of the GEPs obtained from CLL with B-cell subpopulation–specific signatures suggests a phenotypic relatedness of CLL to CD27$^+$ B cells, which comprise a heterogeneous cell population of antigen-experienced B cells. This, together with the observation that among B cell–derived tumors, CLL exhibits a unique cytogenetic profile, suggests that the oncogenic transformation is initiated in these cells. Subgroups of CLL, foremost the IgV gene somatically mutated and unmutated cases, express a small but robust set of differentially expressed genes that allow their classification into the corresponding subtypes in most instances. While the determination of the level of IgV somatic hypermutation provides important information for clinical evaluation of the respective CLL case, evidence suggests that CLL subgroups differing in their clinical prognosis may be primarily defined by their recognition of particular antigens rather than by the level of IgV hypermutation. GEP-based approaches are ideal tools for the identification of CLL- or subgroup-specific genes as well as cellular pathways that are affected upon exposition to cytotoxic drugs, and are expected to improve our understanding of CLL pathophysiology.

Clearly, several aspects of CLL pathophysiology still await clarification. How is the CLL precursor cell driven toward CLL development? What are the putative antigen(s) involved in this step? Is the severity of the clinical course dependent on the specific nature of the antigen? Since no common genetic alterations have as yet been identified for this disease, is there a common pathogenetic mechanism involved in the initial steps of CLL development? In the not so distant future, results stemming from genome-wide approaches including GEP, high-throughput genomic analysis to identify novel genetic aberrations, and a more comprehensive characterization of the "miRnome" are likely to be integrated and are hoped to improve our understanding of CLL pathogenesis.

ACKNOWLEDGMENTS

I thank Riccardo Dalla-Favera, Andrea Califano, Gustavo Stolovitzky, Yuhai Tu, and Katia Basso for their essential involvement in some of the gene expression profiling experiments described here.

REFERENCES

1. Kipps TJ. Chronic lymphocytic leukemia. Curr Opin Hematol 1998; 5(4):244–253.
2. Caligaris-Cappio F, Hamblin TJ. B-cell chronic lymphocytic leukemia: a bird of a different feather. J Clin Oncol 1999; 17(1):399–408.
3. Schroeder HW Jr., Dighiero G. The pathogenesis of chronic lymphocytic leukemia: analysis of the antibody repertoire. Immunol Today 1994; 15(6):288–294.
4. Oscier DG, Thompsett A, Zhu D, et al. Differential rates of somatic hypermutation in V(H) genes among subsets of chronic lymphocytic leukemia defined by chromosomal abnormalities. Blood 1997; 89(11):4153–4160.
5. Fais F, Ghiotto F, Hashimoto S, et al. Chronic lymphocytic leukemia B cells express restricted sets of mutated and unmutated antigen receptors. J Clin Invest 1998; 102(8):1515–1525.
6. Damle RN, Wasil T, Fais F, et al. Ig V gene mutation status and CD38 expression as novel prognostic indicators in chronic lymphocytic leukemia. Blood 1999; 94(6):1840–1847.
7. Hamblin TJ, Davis Z, Gardiner A, et al. Unmutated Ig V(H) genes are associated with a more aggressive form of chronic lymphocytic leukemia. Blood 1999; 94(6):1848–1854.
8. Hamblin TJ, Orchard JA, Gardiner A, et al. Immunoglobulin V genes and CD38 expression in CLL. Blood 2000; 95(7):2455–2457.
9. Hamblin TJ, Orchard JA, Ibbotson RE, et al. CD38 expression and immunoglobulin variable region mutations are independent prognostic variables in chronic lymphocytic leukemia, but CD38 expression may vary during the course of the disease. Blood 2002; 99(3):1023–1029.
10. Döhner H, Stilgenbauer S, Dohner K, et al. Chromosome aberrations in B-cell chronic lymphocytic leukemia: reassessment based on molecular cytogenetic analysis. J Mol Med 1999; 77(2):266–281.

11. Brown PO, Botstein D. Exploring the new world of the genome with DNA microarrays. Nat Genet 1999; 21(1 suppl):33–37.
12. Lockhart DJ, Dong H, Byrne MC, et al. Expression monitoring by hybridization to high-density oligonucleotide arrays. Nat Biotechnol 1996; 14(13):1675–1680.
13. Eisen MB, Spellman PT, Brown PO, et al. Cluster analysis and display of genome-wide expression patterns. Proc Natl Acad Sci U S A 1998; 95(25):14863–14868.
14. Golub TR, Slonim DK, Tamayo P, et al. Molecular classification of cancer: class discovery and class prediction by gene expression monitoring. Science 1999; 286(5439):531–537.
15. Califano A, Stolovitzky G, Tu Y. Analysis of gene expression microarrays for phenotype classification. Proc Int Conf Intell Syst Mol Biol 2000; 8:75–85.
16. Shaffer AL, Rosenwald A, Staudt LM. Lymphoid malignancies: the dark side of B-cell differentiation. Nat Rev Immunol 2002; 2(12):920–932.
17. Ebert BL, Golub TR. Genomic approaches to hematologic malignancies. Blood 2004; 104(4): 923–932.
18. Alizadeh AA, Eisen MB, Davis RE, et al. Distinct types of diffuse large B-cell lymphoma identified by gene expression profiling. Nature 2000; 403(6769):503–511.
19. Rosenwald A, Wright G, Chan WC, et al. The use of molecular profiling to predict survival after chemotherapy for diffuse large-B-cell lymphoma. N Engl J Med 2002; 346(25):1937–1947.
20. Shipp MA, Ross KN, Tamayo P, et al. Diffuse large B-cell lymphoma outcome prediction by gene-expression profiling and supervised machine learning. Nat Med 2002; 8(1):68–74.
21. Klein U, Tu Y, Stolovitzky GA, et al. Gene expression profiling of B cell chronic lymphocytic leukemia reveals a homogeneous phenotype related to memory B cells. J Exp Med 2001; 194(11):1625–1638.
22. Rosenwald A, Alizadeh AA, Widhopf G, et al. Relation of gene expression phenotype to immunoglobulin mutation genotype in B cell chronic lymphocytic leukemia. J Exp Med 2001; 194(11):1639–1647.
23. Jelinek DF, Tschumper RC, Stolovitzky GA, et al. Identification of a global gene expression signature of B-chronic lymphocytic leukemia. Mol Cancer Res 2003; 1(5):346–361.
24. Dürig J, Nuckel H, Huttmann A, et al. Expression of ribosomal and translation-associated genes is correlated with a favorable clinical course in chronic lymphocytic leukemia. Blood 2003; 101(7):2748–2755.
25. Basso K, Liso A, Tiacci E, et al. Gene expression profiling of hairy cell leukemia reveals a phenotype related to memory B cells with altered expression of chemokine and adhesion receptors. J Exp Med 2004; 199(1):59–68.
26. Wang J, Coombes KR, Highsmith WE, et al. Differences in gene expression between B-cell chronic lymphocytic leukemia and normal B cells: a meta-analysis of three microarray studies. Bioinformatics 2004; 20(17):3166–3178.
27. Calin GA, Liu CG, Sevignani C, et al. MicroRNA profiling reveals distinct signatures in B cell chronic lymphocytic leukemias. Proc Natl Acad Sci U S A 2004; 101(32):11755–11760.
28. Fulci V, Chiaretti S, Goldoni M, et al. Quantitative technologies establish a novel microRNA profile of chronic lymphocytic leukemia. Blood 2007; 109(11):4944–4951.
29. Stratowa C, Loffler G, Lichter P, et al. CDNA microarray gene expression analysis of B-cell chronic lymphocytic leukemia proposes potential new prognostic markers involved in lymphocyte trafficking. Int J Cancer 2001; 91(4):474–480.
30. Crespo M, Bosch F, Villamor N, et al. ZAP-70 expression as a surrogate for immunoglobulin-variable-region mutations in chronic lymphocytic leukemia. N Engl J Med 2003; 348(18): 1764–1775.
31. Rassenti LZ, Huynh L, Toy TL, et al. ZAP-70 compared with immunoglobulin heavy-chain gene mutation status as a predictor of disease progression in chronic lymphocytic leukemia. N Engl J Med 2004; 351(9):893–901.
32. Orchard JA, Ibbotson RE, Davis Z, et al. ZAP-70 expression and prognosis in chronic lymphocytic leukaemia. Lancet 2004; 363(9403):105–111.
33. Oppezzo P, Vasconcelos Y, Settegrana C, et al. The LPL/ADAM29 expression ratio is a novel prognosis indicator in chronic lymphocytic leukemia. Blood 2005; 106(2):650–657.

34. Tobin G, Thunberg U, Johnson A, et al. Chronic lymphocytic leukemias utilizing the VH3-21 gene display highly restricted Vlambda2-14 gene use and homologous CDR3s: implicating recognition of a common antigen epitope. Blood 2003; 101(12):4952–4957.

35. Falt S, Merup M, Tobin G, et al. Distinctive gene expression pattern in VH3-21 utilizing B-cell chronic lymphocytic leukemia. Blood 2005; 106(2):681–689.

36. Chiorazzi N, Rai KR, Ferrarini M. Chronic lymphocytic leukemia. N Engl J Med 2005; 352(8): 804–815.

37. MacLennan IC. Germinal centers. Annu Rev Immunol 1994; 12:117–139.

38. Rajewsky K. Clonal selection and learning in the antibody system. Nature 1996; 381 (6585):751–758.

39. Brezinschek HP, Foster SJ, Brezinschek RI, et al. Analysis of the human VH gene repertoire. Differential effects of selection and somatic hypermutation on human peripheral CD5(+)/IgM+ and CD5(−)/IgM+ B cells. J Clin Invest 1997; 99(10):2488–2501.

40. Fischer M, Klein U, Küppers R. Molecular single-cell analysis reveals that CD5-positive peripheral blood B cells in healthy humans are characterized by rearranged Vkappa genes lacking somatic mutation. J Clin Invest 1997; 100(7):1667–1676.

41. Kantor AB, Stall AM, Adams S, et al. De novo development and self-replenishment of B cells. Int Immunol 1995; 7(1):55–68.

42. Forster I, Gu H, Rajewsky K. Germline antibody V regions as determinants of clonal persistence and malignant growth in the B cell compartment. EMBO J 1988; 7(12):3693–3703.

43. Klein U, Rajewsky K, Küppers R. Human immunoglobulin (Ig)M+IgD+ peripheral blood B cells expressing the CD27 cell surface antigen carry somatically mutated variable region genes: CD27 as a general marker for somatically mutated (memory) B cells. J Exp Med 1998; 188(9): 1679–1689.

44. Tangye SG, Liu YJ, Aversa G, et al. Identification of functional human splenic memory B cells by expression of CD148 and CD27. J Exp Med 1998; 188(9):1691–1703.

45. Agematsu K, Hokibara S, Nagumo H, et al. CD27: a memory B-cell marker. Immunol Today 2000; 21(5):204–206.

46. Dono M, Zupo S, Leanza N, et al. Heterogeneity of tonsillar subepithelial B lymphocytes, the splenic marginal zone equivalents. J Immunol 2000; 164(11):5596–5604.

47. Bar-Or A, Oliveira EM, Anderson DE, et al. Immunological memory: contribution of memory B cells expressing costimulatory molecules in the resting state. J Immunol 2001; 167(10): 5669–5677.

48. Agematsu K, Nagumo H, Yang FC, et al. B cell subpopulations separated by CD27 and crucial collaboration of CD27+ B cells and helper T cells in immunoglobulin production. Eur J Immunol 1997; 27(8):2073–2079.

49. Kindler V, Zubler RH. Memory, but not naive, peripheral blood B lymphocytes differentiate into Ig-secreting cells after CD40 ligation and costimulation with IL-4 and the differentiation factors IL-2, IL-10, and IL-3. J Immunol 1997; 159(5):2085–2090.

50. Dono M, Zupo S, Massara R, et al. In vitro stimulation of human tonsillar subepithelial B cells: requirement for interaction with activated T cells. Eur J Immunol 2001; 31(3):752–756.

51. Werner-Favre C, Bovia F, Schneider P, et al. IgG subclass switch capacity is low in switched and in IgM-only, but high in IgD+IgM+, post-germinal center (CD27+) human B cells. Eur J Immunol 2001; 31(1):243–249.

52. Martin F, Kearney JF. Marginal-zone B cells. Nat Rev Immunol 2002; 2(5):323–335.

53. Weller S, Braun MC, Tan BK, et al. Human blood IgM "memory" B cells are circulating splenic marginal zone B cells harboring a prediversified immunoglobulin repertoire. Blood 2004; 104(12):3647–3654.

54. Kruetzmann S, Rosado MM, Weber H, et al. Human immunoglobulin M memory B cells controlling Streptococcus pneumoniae infections are generated in the spleen. J Exp Med 2003; 197(7):939–945.

55. van Oers MH, Pals ST, Evers LM, et al. Expression and release of CD27 in human B-cell malignancies. Blood 1993; 82(11):3430–3436.

56. Chiorazzi N, Ferrarini M. B cell chronic lymphocytic leukemia: lessons learned from studies of the B cell antigen receptor. Annu Rev Immunol 2003; 21:841–894.
57. Küppers R, Klein U, Hansmann ML, et al. Cellular origin of human B-cell lymphomas. N Engl J Med 1999; 341(20):1520–1529.
58. Küppers R, Dalla-Favera R. Mechanisms of chromosomal translocations in B cell lymphomas. Oncogene 2001; 20(40):5580–5594.
59. Mayr C, Speicher MR, Kofler DM, et al. Chromosomal translocations are associated with poor prognosis in chronic lymphocytic leukemia. Blood 2006; 107(2):742–751.
60. Harris NL, Jaffe ES, Stein H, et al. A revised European-American classification of lymphoid neoplasms: a proposal from the International Lymphoma Study Group. Blood 1994; 84(5): 1361–1392.
61. Haglund U, Juliusson G, Stellan B, et al. Hairy cell leukemia is characterized by clonal chromosome abnormalities clustered to specific regions. Blood 1994; 83(9):2637–2645.
62. Sambani C, Trafalis DT, Mitsoulis-Mentzikoff C, et al. Clonal chromosome rearrangements in hairy cell leukemia: personal experience and review of literature. Cancer Genet Cytogenet 2001; 129(2):138–144.
63. Tamayo P, Slonim D, Mesirov J, et al. Interpreting patterns of gene expression with self-organizing maps: methods and application to hematopoietic differentiation. Proc Natl Acad Sci U S A 1999; 96(6):2907–2912.
64. Shaffer AL, Yu X, He Y, et al. BCL-6 represses genes that function in lymphocyte differentiation, inflammation, and cell cycle control. Immunity 2000; 13(2):199–212.
65. Alvi AJ, Austen B, Weston VJ, et al. A novel CDK inhibitor, CYC202 (R-roscovitine), overcomes the defect in p53-dependent apoptosis in B-CLL by down-regulation of genes involved in transcription regulation and survival. Blood 2005; 105(11):4484–4491.
66. Basso K, Klein U, Niu H, et al. Tracking CD40 signaling during germinal center development. Blood 2004; 104(13):4088–4096.
67. Gricks CS, Zahrieh D, Zauls AJ, et al. Differential regulation of gene expression following CD40 activation of leukemic compared to healthy B cells. Blood 2004; 104(13):4002–4009.
68. Rosenwald A, Chuang EY, Davis RE, et al. Fludarabine treatment of patients with chronic lymphocytic leukemia induces a p53-dependent gene expression response. Blood 2004; 104(5): 1428–1434.
69. Pickering BM, de Mel S, Lee M, et al. Pharmacological inhibitors of NF-kappaB accelerate apoptosis in chronic lymphocytic leukaemia cells. Oncogene 2007; 26(8):1166–1177.
70. Gorgun G, Holderried TA, Zahrieh D, et al. Chronic lymphocytic leukemia cells induce changes in gene expression of CD4 and CD8 T cells. J Clin Invest 2005; 115(7):1797–1805.

3

Molecular Pathogenesis

Arianna Bottoni and Carlo M. Croce
Human Cancer Genetics, Department of Molecular Virology, Immunology, and Medical Genetics, Ohio State University, Columbus, Ohio, U.S.A.

George A. Calin
Departments of Experimental Therapeutics and Cancer Genetics, University of Texas M.D. Anderson Cancer Center, Houston, Texas, U.S.A.

INTRODUCTION

Chronic lymphocytic leukemia (CLL) is a common hematologic malignancy with high prevalence in the West (1). In the 1990 decade, the incidence of CLL in the United States equals to 5.17 per 100,000 person-years, only surpassed by incidence of diffuse large B-cell lymphoma and multiple myeloma (2). The vast majority of CLL is B-CLL. CLL B cells are mature CD5+/CD19+/CD23+ B lymphocytes that express low levels of surface immunoglobulins (Ig) such as IgM or IgD (3). Some patients die from the disease within a few months of the diagnosis, whereas others live for 20 years or more (4). The clinical staging systems devised by Rai et al. (5) and Binet et al. (6) are useful methods to identify patients with short survival. However, these staging systems cannot be used to predict the individual risk of disease progression and survival in the early stages of CLL (Binet stage A or Rai stage 0 to 2 disease) in most patients. Conventional cytogenetics is of limited clinical value because of the low mitotic activity of the leukemic cells, which are nondividing G0 cells (7). Recent advances in the molecular dissection of CLL proved that the molecular pathogenesis of this disease is very complicated and further proved the basis of a new dogma in molecular biology (for extensive reviews on these topics see Refs. 8–10) (Fig. 1, Table 1). Further strengthening the importance of the genetic component in CLL, a high level of familial aggregation was described in this disease (11).

CHROMOSOMAL ABERRATIONS IN CLL:
THE MARKERS OF HIDDEN GENES

Genomic aberrations are common in CLL and often contribute to deregulation of cell cycle (12). Chromosomal aberrations are identified in approximately 80% of CLL patients by fluorescence in situ hybridization (FISH) and by interphase cytogenetics (13). The

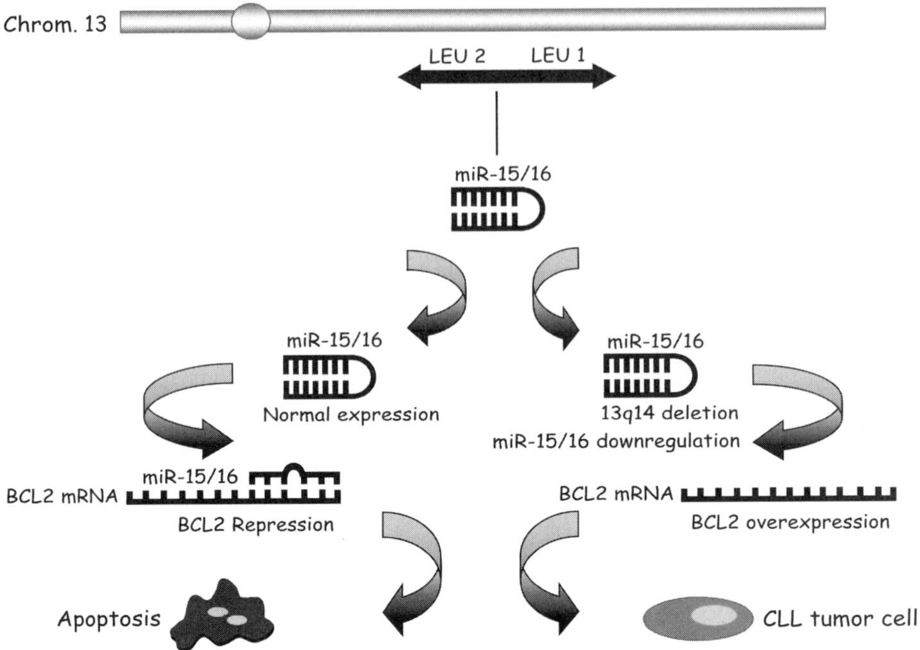

Figure 1 CLL is the best-known model of interplay between noncoding RNAs and protein-coding genes. During the initiation and progression of B cell, CLL alteration in at least three different types of genes, PCGs, miRNAs, and UCGs, were identified. Complex regulatory interactions between miRNAs and PCGs and between miRNAs and UCGs occur and are specific to good or bad prognosis CLL, respectively. For example, deletions of *miR-15* and *miR-16* on chromosome 13 and the deregulation of BCL2 interaction are more frequent in patients with good prognosis, while the downregulation of *miR-29/miR-181* families of genes and the deregulation of the TCL1 interaction are more frequent in patients with bad prognosis. *Abbreviations*: CLL, chronic lymphocytic leukemia; PCGs, protein-coding genes; miRNAs, microRNAs; UCGs, ultraconserved genes.

most frequent abnormalities are deletions involving chromosome band 13q14 (53%), followed by deletions of the genomic region 11q22.3-q23.1 (19%), trisomy 12 (15%), deletions of 6q21-q23 (9%), and deletions/mutations of the *TP53* tumor suppressor gene at 17p13 (8%) (14).

Chromosome 12 harbors many genes involved in cell cycle control, while 17p deletion (17p-) and 11q deletion (11q-) are prognostic factors identifying subgroups of patients with rapid disease progression and short survival times in multivariate analysis, whereas 13q deletion (13q-) as the sole aberration is associated with favorable outcome (15). In CLL, trisomy is associated with overexpression of p27, cyclin dependent kinase 4 (CDK4), BCL2-associated X protein (BAX) and E2F transcription factor 1 (E2F1) (16).

Although in CLL and related disorders, loss of the short arm of chromosome 17, to which the p53 tumor suppressor gene is localized, is not a frequent chromosome aberration, further studies showed the evidence for a role of p53 in this disease. A study screening for p53 mutations in CLL found mutations in 15% patients with CLL (17), and in further studies, p53 gene mutations were found at a frequency of 10% to 15% (18,19). Point mutations coupled with deletion of the second allele is one of the characteristics of a recessively acting tumor suppressor gene such as p53 (20). The majority of 11q- cases show a decreased synthesis of ataxia teleangiectasia mutated (ATM), which results in p53 dysfunction (21). 13q

Table 1 miRNAs Involved in CLL: Targets and Molecular Pathways

miRNA	Chromosome location	Target genes	Molecular function
miR-15a, miR-16-1	13q14	Oncogene BCL2	Apoptosis
miR-21	17q23.1	Tumor suppressor PDCD4	Transformation, invasion, metastasis
		Tumor suppressor phosphatese and tensin homolog (PTEN)	Angiogenesis and tumor growth
		Tropomypsin-1 (TPM1)	Tumor growth
miR-29 family	Various	Methyltransferase 3A and 3B	DNA methylation
		Oncogene TCL1	Cell survival, proliferation, and death
		Oncogene MCL-1	Apoptosis
miR-150	19q13.33	Transcription factor C-Myb	Lymphocyte development and response
miR-155	21q21.3	Tumor protein 53–induced nuclear protein (TP53INP1)	Apoptosis
miR-181 family	Various	Oncogene TCL1	Cell survival, proliferation, and death

Abbreviations: miRNA, microRNA; CLL, chronic lymphocytic leukemia.

deletion is usually accompanied by an increase in the expression of AKT (protein kinase B), which promotes cell survival through different mechanisms (22). Further studies supported the hypothesis that CLL is a genetic disease where the main alterations occur at the level of transcriptional/posttranscriptional regulation in malignant cells' genome because of deregulations of a new class of genes named microRNAs (miRNAs) (23).

miRNAs IN THE PATHOGENESIS OF CLL

miRNAs are a family of small RNAs, which encode tiny transcripts of about 19 to 25 nucleotides (nt). With over 200 members per species in higher eukaryotes, miRNAs are one of the largest gene families, accounting for $\sim 1\%$ of the genome (24). Transcription of miRNA genes is mediated by RNA polymerase II (pol II), which yields primary transcripts, named pri-miRNAs. These transcripts are usually several kilobases long and contain a local hairpin structure. This stem-loop structure is cleaved by the nuclear RNase III Drosha to release the precursor of miRNA, pre-miRNA. Following nuclear processing by Drosha, pre-miRNAs are exported to the cytoplasm. Once there, they are subjected to the second processing step by Dicer (another RNase III enzyme) to generate the final ~ 22-nt product (25). In animals, single-stranded miRNA binds specific mRNA through sequences that are imperfectly complementary to the target mRNA, mainly to the $3'$-untraslated region (UTR). The bound mRNA remains untranslated, resulting in reduced levels of the corresponding protein, or can be degraded, resulting in reduced levels of the corresponding mRNA (26).

miRNAs as Tumor Supressors in CLL

The first report linking miRNAs and cancer was in CLL (27). In CLL, nonrandom chromosomal abnormalities are consistent and frequently isolated, suggesting an important role for the genes located in those specific regions. Hemizygous and/or

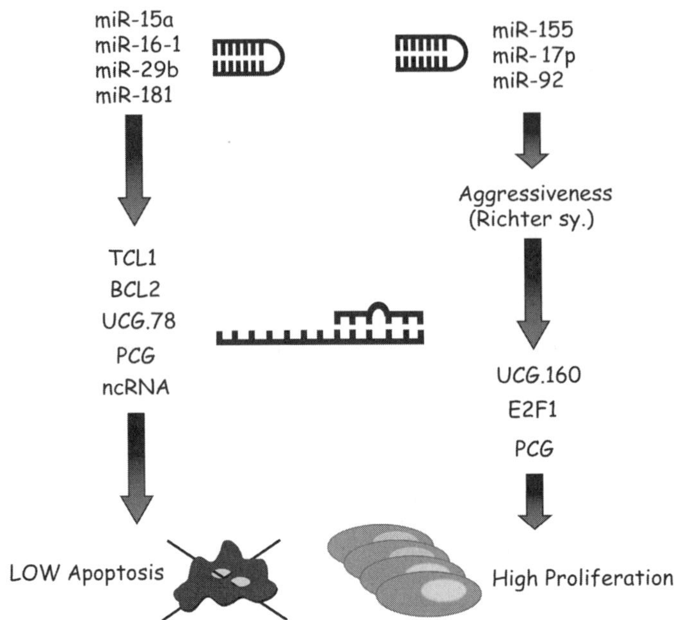

Figure 2 Chromosomal alterations and miRNA loci in CLL. The most frequently identified regions of loss of heterozygosity at chromosome 13 is shown. The genomic regions are not drawn at scale. The functional consequences are presented on the left side. In the former case, the downregulation of *miR-15a* and *miR-16-1* induces overexpression of the antiapoptotic BCL2 protein in leukemia cells. The arrows and the bars represent stimulatory and inhibitory signals, respectively. *Abbreviations*: miRNA, microRNA; CLL, chronic lymphocytic leukemia.

homozygous loss at 13q14.3 occur in more than half of the cases and constitute the most frequent chromosomal abnormality in CLL, suggesting that one or more tumor suppressor genes at 13q14.3 are involved in the pathogenesis of these human tumors. Two clustered miRNAs located exactly in the smallest region of deletion at 13q14.3, named *miR-15a* and *miR-16-1*, were found expressed at high levels in normal CD5+ B lymphocytes, while Northern blot analysis showed that both miRNAs were downregulated in the majority of cases of CLL (about 70%) (Fig. 2). Further strengthening the possible tumor suppressor roles of these two miRNAs, a germline mutation (a C/T substitution located in the 3′ flanking sequence of *miR-16-1*) was identified in the *miR-16-1/miR-15a* primary transcript. This mutation was associated with deletion of the normal allele and caused low levels of expression of the transcript of *miR-15* and *miR-16* associated with reduced miR gene expression (28).

    miR-15a and *miR-16* expression was found downregulated in pituitary adenomas too. These miRNAs' expression correlates with a greater tumor diameter, suggesting that these genes may influence tumor growth (29), confirming their potential role as tumor suppressor genes.

    The genome-wide expression profiling of miRNAs in human CLL was analyzed by using a microarray containing hundreds of human precursor and mature miRNA oligonucleotide probes. By this approach, significant differences in miRNome expression were found between CLL samples and normal CD5 B cells. At least two distinct clusters of CLL samples were associated with the presence or absence of expression of the tyrosine kinase zeta chain–associated protein kinase 70 (Zap-70), a predictor of early disease progression (30). These findings suggest that miRNA expression patterns have relevance to the biologic and clinical behavior of this leukemia.

It is known that CLL is characterized by the clonal expansion of CD5+ B cells. Most of the leukemic cells (>90%) are nondividing and at the G0/G1 phase of the cell cycle. CLL cells are also quite resistant to apoptosis. The malignant, mostly nondividing B cells of CLL overexpress BCL2 (31). BCL2 is a central player in the genetic program of eukaryotic cells, favoring survival by inhibiting cell death (32). By analyzing homology between *miR-15* and *miR-16* and the BCL2 mRNA sequence, it was found that the first nine nucleotides from the 5′ ends of both miRNAs are complementary to specific sequences of the BCL2 cDNA. The analyses of CLL samples and normal CD5+ B lymphocytes showed an inverse correlation between the expression of *miR-15a*, *miR-16-1*, and Bcl2. In normal CD5+ B cells, the levels of both miRNAs were high, and the Bcl2 protein was expressed at low levels. However, most leukemic B cells had low levels of *miR-15a* and *miR-16-1* associated with high-level expression of Bcl2. Thus, in CLL cases, a concordant downregulation of *miR-15a* and *miR-16-1* and overexpression of the Bcl2 protein were observed (Fig. 2) (33).

This interaction has an important functional consequence: the activation of the intrinsic apoptosis pathway. BCL2 downregulation by *miR-15a* and *miR-16-1* triggers apoptosis, and the levels of these two miRNAs are important for cell survival. Therefore, as *miR-15a* and *miR-16-1* are antisense BCL2 interactors, these two miRNAs could be tested as therapeutic agents in CLL and in BCL2-overexpressing tumors.

Many animal models were used to study the molecular mechanism of B-CLL. The New Zealand Black (NZB) strain is a naturally occurring model of late-onset CLL characterized by B-cell hyperproliferation and autoimmunity early in life, followed by progression to CLL, and it has been studied extensively as a model for CLL. The region of synteny with mouse is the human 13q14 region, associated with human CLL, containing miRNAs, *miR-15a*, and *miR-16-1*. DNA sequencing of multiple NZB tissues identified a point mutation in the 3′ flanking sequence of the identical miRNA, *miR-16-1*. Levels of *miR-16* were decreased in NZB lymphoid tissue. Exogenous *miR-16* delivered to an NZB malignant B-1 cell line resulted in cell cycle alterations and increased apoptosis. Linkage of the *miR-15a* and *miR-16-1* complex and the development of B-lymphoproliferative disorders (B-LPD) in this spontaneous mouse model suggest that the altered expression of the *miR-15a* and *miR-16-1* is the main molecular lesion in CLL (34).

Lately, in deleted regions in zebra fish cDNA, 38 orthologues of human genes were identified, and syntenic regions for the human deletions were described in the zebra fish genome. Within chromosome 9 in the zebra fish genome, five genes and two miRNAs were identified with shared synteny to the deleted regions in B-CLL (two genes to human chromosome 11, three to human chromosome 13, and two chromosome 13 miRNAs). This region on zebra fish chromosome 9 maps to the deleted regions for both human chromosomes, suggesting a common ancestry for B-CLL tumor suppressor genes. Zebra fish miRNAs, *dre-miR-15a-2* and *dre-miR-16c*, orthologous to the 13q14.3 miRNAs *miR-15a* and *miR-16-1*, respectively, lie within this region. Two of the zebra fish orthologues (fk54b05, fw91a08) for the human genes ARGHAP20 and FDX from the 11q22-23 deleted region also lie on the same region of zebra fish chromosome 9. Similarly, zebra fish orthologues for the genes P2RY5 and CYSLTR2, adjacent to retinoblastoma 1 (RB1) on human chromosome 13, lie on chromosome 21 within the region syntenic with the human 11q22-23 region of deletion. Mutagenesis screens for zebra fish mutants of genes within the syntenic regions will aid in the characterization of those genes at 13q14 and 11q22-23 involved in neoplastic limphoproliferation (35).

Further strengthening the importance of these findings, at 11q23, the second most common deleted region in CLL that strongly correlated with a bad prognosis (36), two miRNAs were localized, *miR-34b* and *miR-34c*. Very recently, it was found that both of them are targets of p53 and cooperate in control of cell proliferation and adhesion-independent growth (37).

miRNAs as TCL1 Interactors

The functional role of miRNAs in aggressive CLL was not clearly defined until very recently when it was reported that expression of T-cell leukemia 1 (TCL1) oncogene in B-CLL is regulated by *miR-29* and *miR-181* (38). TCL1 encodes a critical molecule in the pathogenesis of leukemias. The TCL1 oncogene was discovered as a target of translocations and inversions in mature T-cell prolymphocytic leukemia (PLL). It encodes a molecule, which plays an important role in the pathogenesis of CLL.

In CLL, TCL1 overexpression is correlated not only with the aggressive phenotype but also with 11q deletion. Therefore, three groups of CLL samples were analyzed to evaluate TCL1 and miRNA expression: indolent CLL, aggressive CLL, and aggressive CLL showing 11q deletion. miRNA microarray revealed three characteristic miRNA expression patterns differentiating these groups. The expression levels of two miRNA families, *miR-29* and *miR-181*, generally inversely correlated with TCL1 expression in the examined CLL samples. Thus, TCL1 expression is regulated by *miR-29* and *miR-181* members. Interestingly, neither *miR-29* nor *miR-181* are located at 11q, indicating that an important transcriptional activator of these two miRNAs might be located at 11q. Because *miR-29* and *miR-181* are natural TCL1 inhibitors, these miRNAs may be candidates for therapeutic agents in B-CLL overexpressing TCL1. Although the involvement of TCL1 in B-CLL is clear, the molecular mechanism linking TCL1 and B-CLL remains poorly understood. The role of *miR-181* and *miR-29* as antisense regulators of TCL1 provided a novel mechanism involved in overexpression of this gene in B-CLL.

Although deregulation of a specific gene in certain types of cancer suggests a potential oncogenic role, the final proof of this requires the generation of animal models showing that the same malignant phenotype results from the deregulation of a specific oncogene. A transgenic mouse expressing TCL1 under the control of a VH promoter–Emiu enhancer allowed forced overexpression of the transgene in immature and mature B cells (39,40). These mice developed non-clonal expansions of B220+/CD5+ B cells. The phenotype of these leukemic cells was very similar to that seen in human CLL. These results conclusively demonstrated that deregulation of TCL1 is a causal event in the pathogenesis of CLL.

Since TCL1 overexpression is observed in aggressive human CLL, it was important to determine whether CLL-like disease in Em-TCL1 mice is similar to the aggressive form of human CLL. A recent report studied how the extent of VHDJH and VLJL rearrangements in a series of TCL1-driven B-CLL derived from Em-TCL1 mice resemble those found in patients with CLL (41). The main conclusion of this study was that the TCL1 transgenic mice show the IgV region rearrangements characteristic of the more aggressive subtype of human CLL. Studies performed on these animal models clearly demonstrated that there are three molecular mechanisms in B-CLL: a pathway downstream TCL1, a BCL2 apoptotic pathway, and a nuclear factor-kappa B (NF-kB) pathway. All of these pathways are critical in the origination of this common leukemia (42).

Multiple miRNAs are Involved in CLL

Recently, by using new techniques such as microarray and real-time PCR, the study of miRNAs was strongly improved.

By cloning many miRNAs genes and then by real-time PCR, the expression of miRNAs in CLL and their healthy counterpart was provided. Both approaches showed that *miR-21* and *miR-155* are dramatically overexpressed in patients with CLL. *MiR-150* and *miR-92* are also significantly deregulated in these patients (43). Also, by cloning small RNAs from CLL cells, an independent group identified a consistent under-expression of *miR-181a*, *let-7a*, and *miR-30d* and confirmed the differential expression of miR-16-1 in the two prognostic groups of CLL (44).

Also, by real-time polymerase chain reaction (PCR), the miRNA expression profile on CLL and acute lymphocytic leukemia (ALL) samples was performed and compared with pooled CD19+ samples from healthy individuals. The most highly expressed miRNAs in ALL were *miR-128b*, *miR-204*, *miR-218*. *miR-331*, and *miR-181b-1*, and *miR-331*, *miR-29a*, *miR-195*, *miR-34a*, *and miR-29c* in were the most expressed in CLL. The *miR-17-92* cluster was also found to be up-regulated in ALL, as previously reported for some types of lymphomas. The target analysis for *miR-331* showed that suppressor of cytokine signaling-1 (SOCS1) is one of its putative targets. SOCS1 is involved in signal transducers and activators of transcription (STAT) activation, which promotes cell proliferation and survival. Therefore, *miR-331* could be involved in these processes and suggests the possible role of these miRNAs in hematopoiesis and leukemogenesis (45).

miR-143 and *miR-145* were also found decreased in B-cell malignancies including CLL, B-cell lymphomas, Epstein-Barr virus (EBV)-transformed B-cell lines, and Burkitt lymphoma cell lines. These miRNAs may contribute to carcinogenesis in B-cell malignancies by a newly defined mechanism and could be useful as biomarkers since they differentiate B-cell malignant cells from normal cells (46).

ULTRACONSERVED GENES AND CLL

Ultraconserved regions (UCRs) are a subset of conserved sequences that are located in both intra- and intergenic regions. They are completely conserved between orthologous regions of the human, rat, and mouse genomes (47). Further proofs of the importance of UCRs are based on analysis performed on mice with targeted mutations. The lack of ultraconserved elements or highly conserved sequences in these mice, resulted in viable animals that developed apparently normal phenotypes (48,49).

Recently, the status of UCRs in a large panel of human leukemias and carcinomas was investigated, and the existence of a relationship between the genomic location of these sequences and the known regions involved in cancers was proved. A large fraction of genomic transcribed UCRs (T-UCRs) or ultraconserved genes (UCGs) encode a particular set of noncoding RNAs (ncRNAs) whose expression is altered in CLL patients. miRNAs play a functional role in the transcriptional regulation of cancer-associated UCRs in leukemias. Furthermore, differentially expressed T-UCRs can alter the functional characteristics of malignant cells as the inhibition of an overexpressed UCR induces apoptosis in colon cancer cells. Many T-UCRs were found abnormally expressed in human CLL at statistically significant levels. The finding that another class of ncRNAs, the T-UCRs, are consistently altered at the genomic level in a high percentage of analyzed leukemias and carcinomas supports a model in which both coding and noncoding genes are involved and cooperate in human tumorigenesis (Fig. 1) (50). Furthermore, correlations between the expression of UCRs and miRNAs in CLL patients raise the intriguing possibility of complex functional regulatory pathways in which two or more types of ncRNAs interact and influence the phenotype. This offers the prospect of defining tumor-specific signatures of ncRNAs that are associated with diagnosis, prognosis, and response to treatment.

ACKNOWLEDGMENTS

Dr. Calin is supported by the CLL Global Research Foundation, by an MD Anderson Trust grant, and by a Regent scholarship, and Dr. Croce is supported by Program Project Grants from the National Cancer Institute.

REFERENCES

1. Chiorazzi N, Rai KR, Ferrarini M. Chronic lymphocytic leukemia. N Engl J Med 2005; 352(8): 804–815.
2. Morton LM, Wang SS, Devesa SS, et al. Lymphoma incidence patterns by WHO subtype in the United States, 1992–2001. Blood 2006; 107(1):265–276.
3. Matutes E, Polliack A. Morphological and immunophenotypic features of chronic lymphocytic leukemia. Rev Clin Exp Hematol 2000; 4(1):22–47.
4. Rozman C, Montserrat E. Chronic lymphocytic leukemia. N Engl J Med 1995; 333(16): 1052–1057. Erratum in: N Engl J Med 1995; 333(22):1515.
5. Rai KR, Sawitsky A, Cronkite EP, et al. Clinical staging of chronic lymphocytic leukemia. Blood 1975; 46(2):219–234.
6. Binet JL, Lepoprier M, Dighiero G, et al. A clinical staging system for chronic lymphocytic leukemia: prognostic significance. Cancer 1977; 40(2):855–864.
7. Gahrton G, Robert KH, Friberg K, et al. Nonrandom chromosomal aberrations in chronic lymphocytic leukemia revealed by polyclonal B-cell-mitogen stimulation. Blood 1980; 56(4):640–647.
8. Calin GA, Croce CM. MicroRNA-cancer connection: the beginning of a new tale. Cancer Res 2006; 66(15):7390–7394.
9. Calin GA, Croce CM. MicroRNAs and chromosomal abnormalities in cancer cells. Oncogene 2006; 25(46):6202–6210.
10. Calin GA, Croce CM. MicroRNA signatures in human cancers. Nat Rev Cancer 2006; 6(11):857–866.
11. Caporaso N, Marti GE, Goldin L. Perspectives on familial chronic lymphocytic leukemia: genes and the environment. Semin Hematol 2004; 41(3):201–206.
12. Danilov AV, Danilova OV, Klein AK, et al. Molecular pathogenesis of chronic lymphocytic leukemia. Curr Mol Med 2006; 6(6):665–675.
13. Zenz T, Döhner H, Stilgenbauer S. Genetics and risk-stratified approach to therapy in chronic lymphocytic leukemia. Best Pract Res Clin Haematol 2007; 20(3):439–453.
14. Dohner H, Stilgenbauer S, Döhner K, et al. Chromosome aberrations in B-cell chronic lymphocytic leukemia: reassessment based on molecular cytogenetic analysis. J Mol Med 1999; 77(2):266–281.
15. Dohner H, Stilgenbauer S, Benner A, et al. Genomic aberrations and survival in chronic lymphocytic leukemia. N Engl J Med 2000; 343(26):1910–1916.
16. Nourse J, Firpo E, Flanagan WM, et al. Interleukin-2-mediated elimination of the p27Kip1 cyclin-dependent kinase inhibitor prevented by rapamycin. Nature 1994; 372(6506):570–5733.
17. Gaidano G, Ballerini P, Gong JZ, et al. p53 mutations in human lymphoid malignancies: association with Burkitt lymphoma and chronic lymphocytic leukemia. Proc Natl Acad Sci U S A 1991; 88(12):5413–5417.
18. Fenaux P, Preudhomme C, Lai JL, et al. Mutations of the p53 gene in B-cell chronic lymphocytic leukemia: a report on 39 cases with cytogenetic analysis. Leukemia 1992; 6(4):246–250.

19. El Rouby S, Thomas A, Costin D, et al. p53 gene mutation in B-cell chronic lymphocytic leukemia is associated with drug resistance and is independent of MDR1/MDR3 gene expression. Blood 1993; 82(11):3452–3459.
20. Carter A, Lin K, Sherrington PD, et al. Imperfect correlation between p53 dysfunction and deletion of TP53 and ATM in chronic lymphocytic leukaemia. Leukemia 2006; 20(4):737–740.
21. Manning BD, Cantley LC. AKT/PKB signaling: navigating downstream. Cell 2007; 129(7): 1261–1274.
22. Dohner H, Fischer K, Bentz M, et al. p53 gene deletion predicts for poor survival and non-response to therapy with purine analogs in chronic B-cell leukemias. Blood 1995; 85(6): 1580–1589.
23. Calin GA, Croce CM. Genomics of chronic lymphocytic leukemia microRNAs as new players with clinical significance. Semin Oncol 2006; 33(2):167–173.
24. Ambros V. microRNAs: tiny regulators with great potential. Cell 2001; 107(7):823–826.
25. Kim VN. MicroRNA biogenesis: coordinated cropping and dicing. Nat Rev Mol Cell Biol 2005; 6(5):376–385.
26. Bartel DP. MicroRNAs: genomics, biogenesis, mechanism, and function. Cell 2004; 116(2): 281–297.
27. Calin GA, Dumitru CD, Shimizu M, et al. Frequent deletions and down-regulation of micro-RNA genes miR-15 and miR-16 at 3q14 in chronic lymphocytic leukemia. Proc Natl Acad Sci U S A 2002; 99(24):15524–15529.
28. Calin GA, Ferracin M, Cimmino A, et al. A MicroRNA signature associated with prognosis and progression in chronic lymphocytic leukemia. N Engl J Med 2005; 353(17):1793–801. Erratum in: N Engl J Med 2006; 355(5):533.
29. Bottoni A, Piccin D, Tagliati F, et al. miR-15a and miR-16-1 down-regulation in pituitary adenomas. J Cell Physiol 2005; 204(1):280–285.
30. Calin GA, Liu CG, Sevignani C, et al. MicroRNA profiling reveals distinct signatures in B cell chronic lymphocytic leukemias. Proc Natl Acad Sci U S A 2004; 101(32):11755–11760.
31. Kitada S, Andersen J, Akar S, et al. Expression of apoptosis-regulating proteins in chronic lymphocytic leukemia: correlations with In vitro and In vivo chemoresponses. Blood 1998; 91(9):3379–3389.
32. Cory S, Adams JM. The Bcl2 family: regulators of the cellular life-or-death switch. Nat Rev Cancer 2002; 2(9):647–656.
33. Cimmino A, Calin GA, Fabbri M, et al. miR-15 and miR-16 induce apoptosis by targeting BCL2. Proc Natl Acad Sci U S A 2005; 102(39):13944–13949 [Epub 2005]. Erratum in: Proc Natl Acad Sci U S A 2006; 103(7):2464.
34. Raveche ES, Salerno E, Scaglione BJ, et al. Abnormal microRNA-16 locus with synteny to human 13q14 linked to CLL in NZB mice. Blood 2007; 109(12):5079–5086.
35. Auer RL, Riaz S, Cotter FE. The 13q and 11q B-cell chronic lymphocytic leukaemia-associated regions derive from a common ancestral region in the zebrafish. Br J Haematol 2007; 137(5): 443–453.
36. Döhner H, Stilgenbauer S, Benner A, et al. Genomic aberrations and survival in chronic lymphocytic leukemia. N Engl J Med 2000; 343(26):1910–1916.
37. Corney DC, Flesken-Nikitin A, Godwin AK, et al. MicroRNA-34b and MicroRNA-34c are targets of p53 and cooperate in control of cell proliferation and adhesion-independent growth. Cancer Res 2007; 67(18):8433–8438.
38. Pekarsky Y, Santanam U, Cimmino A, et al. Tcl1 expression in chronic lymphocytic leukemia is regulated by miR-29 and miR-181. Cancer Res 2006; 66(24):11590–115933.
39. Bichi R, Shinton SA, Martin ES, et al. Human chronic lymphocytic leukemia modeled in mouse by targeted TCL1 expression. Proc Natl Acad Sci U S A 2002; 99(10):6955–6960.
40. Hoyer KK, French SW, Turner DE, et al. Dysregulated TCL1 promotes multiple classes of mature B cell lymphoma. Proc Natl Acad Sci U S A 2002; 99(22):14392–14397.
41. Pekarsky Y, Zanesi N, Aqeilan R, et al. Tcl1 as a model for lymphomagenesis. Hematol Oncol Clin North Am 2004; 18(4):863–879.
42. Pekarsky Y, Calin GA, Aqeilan R. Chronic lymphocytic leukemia: molecular genetics and animal models. Curr Top Microbiol Immunol 2005; 294:51–70.

43. Fulci V, Chiaretti S, Goldoni M, et al. Quantitative technologies establish a novel microRNA profile of chronic lymphocytic leukemia. Blood 2007; 109(11):4944–4951.
44. Marton S, Garcia MR, Robello C, et al. Small RNAs analysis in CLL reveals a deregulation of miRNA expression and novel miRNA candidates of putative relevance in CLL pathogenesis. Leukemia 2008; 22(2):330–338 [Epub November 8, 2007].
45. Zanette DL, Rivadavia F, Molfetta GA, et al. miRNA expression profiles in chronic lymphocytic and acute lymphocytic leukemia. Braz J Med Biol Res 2007; 40(11):1435–1440.
46. Akao Y, Nakagawa Y, Kitade Y, et al. Downregulation of microRNAs-143 and -145 in B-cell malignancies. Cancer Sci 2007; 98(12):1914–1920 [Epub September 24, 2007].
47. Bejerano G, Pheasant M, Makunin I, et al. Ultraconserved elements in the human genome. Science 2004; 304(5675):1321–13255.
48. Nobrega MA, Ovcharenko I, Afzal V, et al. Scanning human gene deserts for long-range enhancers. Science 2003; 302(5644):413.
49. Rigoutsos T, Huynh K, Miranda A, et al. Short blocks from the noncoding parts of the human genome have instances within nearly all known genes and relate to biological processes. Proc Natl Acad Sci U S A 2006; 103:6605–6610.
50. Calin GA, Liu CG, Ferracin M, et al. Ultraconserved regions encoding ncRNAs are altered in human leukemias and carcinomas. Cancer Cell 2007; 12(3):215–229.

4

Chronic Lymphocytic Leukemia and the B-Cell Receptor

Marta Muzio
Unit and Laboratory of Lymphoid Malignancies, Department of Oncology, San Raffaele Scientific Institute, Milano, Italy

Federico Caligaris-Cappio
Unit and Laboratory of Lymphoid Malignancies, Department of Oncology, Università Vita-Salute San Raffaele and San Raffaele Scientific Institute, Milano, Italy

INTRODUCTION

Accumulating evidence support the view that the monoclonal B-cell receptor (BCR) of leukemic lymphocytes plays a crucial role in the selection and survival of chronic lymphocytic leukemia (CLL) cells (1,2). At the molecular level, malignant cells preferentially use specific immunoglobulin heavy chain variable (IGHV) genes; in more than half of the cases, they carry somatic mutations in the IGHV genes (3,4); over 20% of the cases express highly homologous ("stereotyped") complementarity-determining region 3 (CDR3) sequences (5–12). At the functional level, CLL cells show a heterogeneous pattern of responsiveness to BCR cross-linking, and some of them resemble anergic lymphocytes (1,2). To better define the molecular framework of antigenic stimulation in CLL cells, we will herein dissect step by step the mechanisms of regulation of BCR activity: first, we will analyze the nature of the membrane-associated BCR chains; second, we will discuss the BCR signal transduction pathways in normal and malignant B lymphocytes; third, we will describe distinct BCR coreceptors and costimulatory molecules, and; finally, we will propose a model where all the described BCR regulatory molecules concur to modulate antigen responsiveness or anergy in clinically different CLL subsets.

THE BCR COMPLEX ON CLL CELLS

The BCR belongs to the family of multichain immune recognition receptors (MIRR), which includes the T-cell receptor (TCR) and distinct receptors for the Fc portions of IgG (FcγRI, FcγRIIA, FcγRIIC, FcγRIIIA). This family of receptors shares an oligomeric structure, which uses different membrane-spanning subunits for antigen recognition and signal transduction. The BCR is a multiproteic structure composed of a variable antigen-binding subunit (the membrane immunoglobulin or mIg, also referred to as surface Ig or sIg) and a signaling subunit containing a disulfide-linked heterodimer of Igα (CD79α) and Igβ (CD79β) (13,14). Immunoglobulins of any isotype can function as the sIg component of the BCR; while immature B lymphocytes express only sIgM, mature B lymphocytes coexpress sIgM and sIgD, and memory B cells may express different isotypes, including IgG and IgA.

In 1971, the presence of Ig on the surface of CLL cells was identified (15); from those studies, it was also clear that CLL lymphocytes are monoclonal and that the majority of cases are IgM^+ (15,16). The presence of IgD on the surface of IgM-positive CLL cells was subsequently reported in most cases (17,18) and demonstrated to have the same idiotypic specificity as the coexpressed IgM (19). The analysis of a large cohort of patients revealed that there was no survival difference between those with IgM^+IgD^+ and IgM^+IgD^- (20).

sIgG-positive cases were also reported, although at a very low frequency (20–25); on the basis of the fact that few IgM^+ cells are present in IgG^+ patients, it was suggested that these cells might represent progenitors of CLL that undergo intraclonal differentiation and diversification (26). IgG+ individuals carry somatically mutated IGHV genes, and accordingly tend to have an indolent disease (27,28). Rare surface IgA-positive cases exist, as demonstrated also by DNA sequence analysis (20,23).

CD79α and CD79β are members of the Ig superfamily and contain an extracellular Ig-like domain, a single transmembrane region, and a cytoplasmatic tail containing an immunoreceptor tyrosine-based activation motif (ITAM) sequence that accounts for signal transduction after BCR ligation (29–31). The cytoplasmic tails of both Igα and Igβ play a fundamental role in BCR signaling, as no signaling has been detected in a cell line transduced with a mutated Igβ cytoplasmic tail (32). CD79α and CD79β also mediate apoptosis induced by the BCR stimulation (33,34), influence Ag internalization and presentation (34), and are essential for newly synthesized Ig molecules to translocate to the cell membrane (13,14,35,36). As expected, Igβ knockout mice show a complete block in B-cell development at pro-B-cell stage, likely because the BCR cannot reach the cell membrane in the absence of a complete Igα/Igβ heterodimer (37). In contrast, transgenic mice with a truncated Igα cytoplasmic tail have apparent normal B-cell development. However, the B-cell number in these mice is drastically reduced, and B lymphocytes are not able to respond to antigens that are presented in a T-independent manner (38), indicating a defective B-cell function.

By using a monoclonal antibody, which identifies an epitope on the extracellular domain of CD79β (39), it was shown that most malignant B cells in CLL patients express different levels of this molecule on the cell membrane (40,41). After transfection of CD79β, B-cell lines show an increase of IgM expression on their cell surface (42). Given that, the diminished levels of BCR on the membrane of CLL cells have been associated with the reduced amounts of CD79β mRNA or with the occurrence of somatic mutations predicted to affect CD79β expression (43). Some of these mutations were described to alter signaling when transfected in Jurkat cells (44). However, other studies did not confirm causal mutations of the CD79β gene in CLL cells (45–47). Rather, they indicate a role for an alternative splicing isoform of CD79β called δCD79β, which was identified in human B cells and cell lines (48,49); this variant lacks exon 3, which encodes the extracellular Ig-like domain. This mRNA isoform is expressed in CLL cells and may be responsible for the reduced BCR expression on the cell surface (45,50).

CD79β expression in CLL is higher in cells that carry trisomy 12 (51) and correlates with IGHV mutational status, but does not serve as an independent predictor of clinical severity (52). That notwithstanding, it has been proposed as an additional marker for the assessment of minimal residual disease (MRD) (53).

Different from the β isoform, normal CD79α levels were initially reported in CLL cells (43); however, additional studies determined that lower levels of surface BCR in CLL may be associated with glycosylation and folding defects of CD79α (54,55).

BCR SIGNALING IN NORMAL B CELLS

Mature B lymphocytes express a unique BCR on the cell surface that, after recognition of a specific antigen, triggers a cascade of signaling events, which lead to cell activation, survival, and differentiation; the BCR also mediates antigen processing and presentation. However, in immature B lymphocytes, BCR signaling can also trigger an apoptotic program that eliminates potentially autoreactive B lymphocytes (13,29,56); the fate of the cells depends on the activity of coreceptors and on the affinity and amount of antigens (56–58). All this is achieved by activating specific genetic programs that result from the transcription of several genes. In particular, BCR engagement propagates the signal inside the cells by activating a cascade of protein kinases (PKs) that eventually direct distinct transcription factors to enter the nucleus and to regulate gene expression (56,59–61).

We will herein briefly describe some of the key molecules involved in BCR signaling that have also been studied in CLL cells. Specifically, we will first describe the protein tyrosine kinases (PTKs) lyn, Syk, and ZAP70, and the proximal adaptor molecule HS1. Second, we will focus on PI3K, phospholipase Cγ2 (PLCγ2), and mitogen-activated protein kinase (MAPK) parallel pathways. Third, we will discuss the activation of distinct transcription factors, including nuclear factor k-B (NF-kB) and NF-AT. A schematic representation of BCR signal transduction pathway is shown in Figure 1.

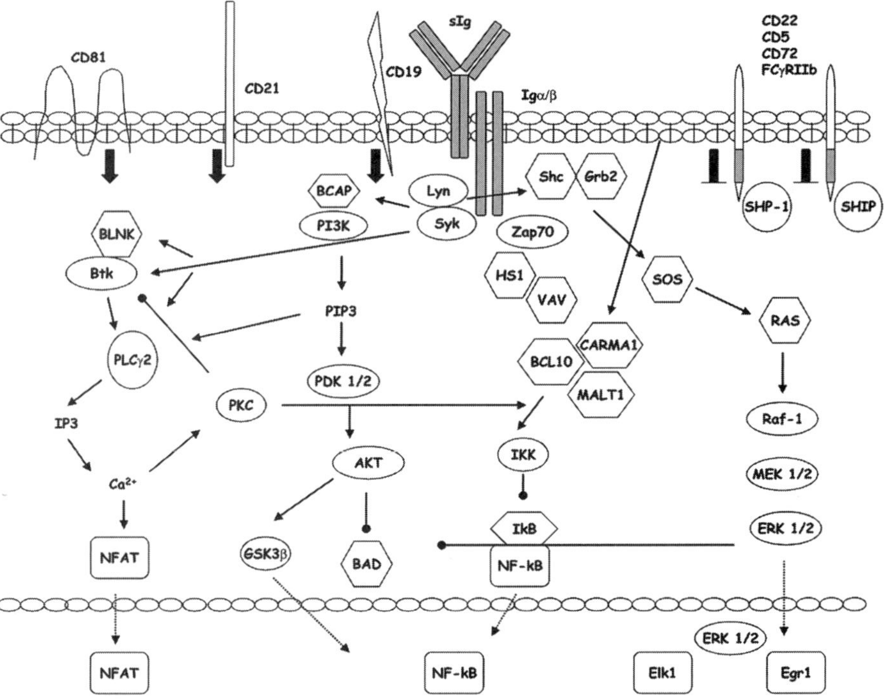

Figure 1 BCR-signaling pathway. A schematic representation of BCR-induced signaling pathway is reported. Kinases are drawn as ovals; phosphatases as circles; transcription factors as rectangles; and adapters as hexagons. *Abbreviation*: BCR, B-cell receptor.

Proximal BCR-Signaling Mediators

The Src family includes nine closely related tyrosine-specific PKs involved in the regulation of very different cellular events such as cell division, cell differentiation, and cell aggregation. They are expressed by different cell types, but B lymphocytes express mainly lyn and Blk (60,62).

Lyn tyrosine kinase is expressed in all blood cells except T cells. After antigen binding to the BCR, it translocates into lipid rafts, where it is dephosphorylated on inhibitory Tyr-507 by CD45 (this site is constitutively phosphorylated by the tyrosine kinase CSK); at the same time, it autophosphorylates on activatory Tyr-396 (this site is subsequently dephosphorylated by the phosphatase SHP-1). Lyn is now able to activate the signaling subunits of the BCR through phosphorylation of Igα and CD19. That notwithstanding, lyn-deficient mice (lyn$^{-/-}$) have normal B-cell development in bone marrow; this might indicate that, in the absence of lyn, its function can be replaced by other Src family kinases. In addition to its positive function, lyn also has a negative regulatory function on the signaling process (57,63). Accordingly, lyn$^{-/-}$ mice show enhanced activation of the downstream signaling pathway (MAPK pathway) and increased proliferation response to anti-IgM antibody stimulation, indicating that in this case the role of lyn is not redundant and cannot be compensated by other Src family members (64). Taken together, these results demonstrate that lyn is required in maintaining the balance between negative and positive signals driven by antigen stimulation.

Syk is a 72-kDa kinase containing two Src homology 2 (SH2) domains, which allow binding to phosphorylated CD79α and CD79β, followed by a kinase domain. Syk knockout mice die shortly after birth because of hemorrhage, indicating that Syk has nonredundant functions in utero. Also, the vast majority of B cells in these animals are not able to differentiate in mature peripheral B lymphocytes, even though CD79α and CD79β are phosphorylated after BCR stimulation (65). When Syk binds to CD79α and CD79β through the tyrosine residues previously phosphorylated by lyn, it can phosphorylate two additional ITAM tyrosine residues on Igα and Igβ. The tandem SH2 domains of Syk then bind to the doubly phosphorylated ITAM (ppITAM), fixing the kinase in an open and active conformation (66). Further phosphorylation of near ITAM sequences occurs, and this event causes positive amplification of Syk-BCR signal. This process is counterbalanced by the activity of phosphatases like SHP-1, which exerts its activity not only by dephosphorylation of Syk substrates but also by preventing Syk activation (67). Syk is also negatively regulated by lyn activity, which phosphorylates Syk in an inhibitory site (68).

Downstream substrates of Syk include Btk kinase (belonging to the Tec family), the PLCγ2, and the adaptor molecules B-cell linker (BLNK) and BCAP (phosphoinositide-3-kinase adaptor protein 1) (69).

ZAP70 (ζ chain-associated protein) was originally identified as a T-cell-specific kinase, which plays a key role in transducing signals from the TCR. ZAP-70 is also expressed by normal and malignant human B-cell subsets of different maturational stage (70). It is structurally homologous to Syk with several consensus sites for phosphorylation and activation. Accordingly, ZAP70 likely plays a role similar to Syk in B lymphocytes where both kinases are expressed; preliminary studies in cell lines suggested that ZAP70 may have a role in BCR signaling irrespective of its kinase activity (71); however, more functional studies are required to assess its molecular role in normal and malignant B cells.

HS1 is an intracellular protein expressed in cells of lymphohemopoietic origin (72). It was originally identified in B lymphocytes as a major substrate of BCR-induced phosphorylation after Ag stimulation (73). Genetically modified mice confirmed that in both B and T lymphocytes HS1 is involved in the processes of Ag-receptor-induced clonal expansion and deletion (74). In T lymphocytes, HS1 binds Vav and is recruited to the immunological synapse where it plays a crucial role in cytoskeleton organization (75).

Phosphatidylinositol 3-kinase Pathway

Phosphatidylinositide kinases (PIKs) modify plasma membrane lipids to create second messenger compounds crucial to intracellular signal transduction. In particular, phosphatidylinositol 3-kinase (PI3K) is responsible for the phosphorylation of PI, PIP, and PIP2, resulting in the generation of phosphatidyl inositol 3,4,5 tryphosphate (PIP3). The most-studied PI3K is PI3Kα, a heterodimer made up of a catalytic subunit (p110α) and a regulatory subunit (p85α). A key serine/threonine kinase that is a substrate of PI3K cascade and that mediates its action is protein kinase B (PKB), also known as Akt. The phosphorylation of Akt is often used as a surrogate marker of PI3K activity because direct measurement of 3-phosphoinositide levels is technically difficult. The phosphorylation and subsequent activation of Akt in two residues (Ser-308 and Thr-473) is mediated by PDK1 and PDK2, respectively (PIP3-dependent kinase 1 and 2) (76,77). Akt substrates include IkB kinase (IKK), GSK3β, and the proapoptotic protein BAD (78–80) (see next paragraph on transcription factors).

Phospholypase Cγ2 and Calcium Signaling

There are at least four families of PLCs, but the most expressed isoform in B lymphocytes is PLCγ2, a 150-kDa protein consisting of a plexstrin-homology (PH) domain at the N-terminus, followed by a catalytic domain, two tandem SH2 domains, an SH3 domain, and a second catalytic domain (81). PLCs hydrolyze plasma membrane PIP2 molecules into diacylglycerol (DAG) and IP3. IP3 binds its specific receptor located in the endoplasmic reticulum membrane, inducing calcium release from intracellular organelles into the cytosol. The increase in cytoplasmic Ca^{2+} concentration and DAG leads to the activation of PKC and distinct transcription factors, which are dependent on ions oscillation (see below) (82).

MAPK Cascade

The MAPK pathway is one of the most conserved signaling pathways among eukaryotes and controls basic cellular events like proliferation, differentiation, survival, and apoptosis. In this pathway, different PKs trigger a cascade of signals by sequential phosphorylation events in a hierarchical way. In general, a G-protein (guanine nucleotide-binding molecule) works upstream of an MAPK kinase kinase (MAPKKK), which phosphorylates and activates an MAPK kinase (MAPKK) that eventually leads to the activation of the downstream kinase MAPK. One of the best-characterized MAPK pathways involves as terminal effector the kinases ERK1 and ERK2 (extracellular signal-regulated kinase 1 and 2); others include JNK and p38 MAPK, which will not be further discussed here (83–85).

Ras activation after BCR stimulation is driven by SHC recruitment by phosphorylated ITAM in CD79α and CD79β. SHC is then phosphorylated and forms a complex with growth factor receptor-binding protein 2 (Grb2), which binds to the Ras-specific GEF, Sos. Ras belongs to a superfamily of monomeric GTPases that switches between two isoforms: one, inactive GDP-bound form, and one, active GTP-bound form (83–86).

The activated GTP form of Ras protein interacts with the Raf kinase via its Ras-binding domain (RBD), thus mediating its membrane localization and activation.

Activation of Raf-1 involves complex changes in phosphorylation and protein-protein and protein-lipid interactions (87,88). Activated Raf-1 directly phosphorylates and activates MEK1/2. Following activation, MEK1/2 phosphorylates ERK1/2. ERK is the most downstream protein of the MAPK pathway that acts directly on apoptosis regulators (i.e., BAD) and transcription factors, including Elk1 and Egr1 (85,89,90).

Transcription Factors

The NF-AT family of transcription factors plays a central role in inducible gene transcription during immune responses and includes five different proteins: NF-AT1 (also called NFATc2 or NFATp), NF-AT2 (also called NFATc1 or NFATc), NFAT3, NFAT4, and NFAT5. They are all DNA-binding molecules containing an Rel-homology region (RHR) and an NFAT-homology region (NHR); accordingly, they act as transcription factors (91,92). In nonstimulated lymphocytes, NF-AT is present in the cytoplasm in an inactive form; after BCR triggering, it is activated in three sequential steps: dephosphorylation by the Ca^{2+}/calmodulin-activated phosphatase calcineurin, nuclear translocation, and increased affinity for target DNA sequences. The nuclear localization signal (NLS) and a DNA recognition region are exposed by dephosphorylation. All these steps are blocked by treating the cells with CsA (cyclosporine A) or FK506, both specific calcineurin inhibitors (93–95). In the nucleus, activated NF-AT cooperates with AP-1 transcription factor for DNA binding and gene transcription of cytokines and cytokine receptors (96,97).

The NF-kB/Rel family of transcription factors includes five members: Rel A (p65), Rel B, c-Rel, NF-kB1 (p50 and its precursor p105), and NF-kB2 (p52 and its precursor p100) (98,99). NF-kB activity is regulated by IkB inhibitory proteins that retain NF-kB/Rel dimer in the cytoplasm, thus keeping it inactive. Signals triggered by BCR induce IKK activation via PLCγ and PKC; activated IKK phosphorylates IkB and targets it for ubiquitination and proteasome-mediated degradation, with consequent exposition of NLS present on NF-kB and translocation of this transcription factor to the nucleus, where it activates the transcription of several target genes, including cytokines, antiapoptotic molecules, and costimulatory proteins, thus regulating differentiation, survival, and proliferation (80,100).

IgM- and IgD-Signaling Pathways

Experiments with transgenic mice indicated that the δ heavy chain fully substitutes a μ heavy chain, and vice versa, in B-cell development and function (101–105). In contrast, transfection of IgD into IgM-only murine cell lines results into different signaling capacity of the two sIg isotypes (106,107). However, IgM-only cells have an immature profile as compared with IgM^+IgD^+ cells, and this might have an impact on the signaling outcome. Although sIgM and sIgD have identical ability to activate B cells, stimulation of resting B lymphocytes with anti-IgM or IgD induces qualitatively similar but quantitatively different signaling pathways and kinases activation (108,109). This may be explained by the evidence that an IgD molecule can be expressed on the surface in two different ways. In the canonical way, mIgD is associated with Igα and Igβ. In the alternative way, IgD is GPI-linked to membrane lipids and activates cAMP-dependent signaling pathways that are not induced by classic BCR triggering (110,111). Thus, high antigen concentrations or affinity would allow saturating receptor occupancy, stimulation of both subsets of sIgD, and the achievement of an optimal response.

BCR SIGNALING IN CLL CELLS

We will now focus on the signaling pathways that are activated by BCR cross-linking in CLL cells and discuss their possible involvement in the pathogenesis of the disease with particular emphasis on the correlations that have been reported between signaling molecules and clinical parameters. First, we will describe the functional consequences of antigen or antigen-like stimulation of leukemic cells. Second, we will analyze the expression pattern and activation status of distinct BCR-signaling mediators.

BCR Signaling

If CLL cells are treated in vitro with anti-IgM antibodies, a variety of heterogeneous responses can be obtained in terms of signaling or cell fate decision (112,113). Overall, a subset of patients (here referred to as "responders") show several cellular modification after BCR ligation; in contrast, the cells of "nonresponders" show no major differences after anti-IgM treatment. Most studies demonstrated that sIgM ligation induces apoptosis in responder patients (114–116), while others proposed that it induces proliferation (112,117). Subsequently, it was proposed that the apoptosis versus proliferation decision was dependent on the use of respectively soluble or cross-linked anti-IgM antibodies (118); this was further supported by the fact that immobilized antibodies induced a sustained signaling as compared with soluble antibodies (118).

As for signal transduction, several biochemical parameters were analyzed to assess stimulation of CLL cells after sIgM ligation; by using as readouts Ca^{2+} flux (113,114,119–122), the Syk and lyn activation, or levels of total phosphotyrosine proteins (120–124), several groups demonstrated two subsets of patients who either respond or do not respond to sIgM ligation.

In an effort to reconcile BCR responsiveness to biological prognostic factors, several groups proposed that ZAP70, which tends to be highly expressed by CLL cells from patients with aggressive disease, directly enhances IgM signaling in CLL cells (71,125,126). In contrast, another group proposed that IgM-induced survival is restricted to progressive CLL irrespective of ZAP70 expression (127). CD38 expression can also distinguish two groups of patients with CLL whose cells show differences in response to anti-IgM and propensity to apotosis (115,128). Differential signaling via surface IgM, in terms of Ca^{2+} mobilization and Syk phosphorylation, is associated with the VH gene mutational status; however, it is a reversible phenomenon, suggesting that the state of unresponsiveness of the cells reflects a state of reversible anergy because of previous engagement of putative antigen in vivo (128,129). Finally, HS1 is prevalently phosphorylated in a subset of CLL patients with a poor prognosis (130). Given the emerging role of HS1 in regulating cytoskeleton organization, it may represent a functional link between BCR stimulation and migration of the cells in normal and malignant B lymphocytes (131). All this evidence further supports the hypothesis that an ongoing antigen stimulation is occurring in a subset of patients with CLL and an aggressive course of disease.

Differences in the outcome of IgM and IgD signaling were observed in CLL cells treated with anti-IgM or anti-IgD antibodies. Anti-IgM induced apoptosis, while anti-IgD induced plasma cell differentiation; the signaling pathways were similar but with different kinetics (116,132,133).

Rare IgG-positive cases of CLL were also analyzed for their BCR-signaling ability in terms of Ca^{2+} release and Syk phosphorylation; 9 of 14 patients were responders irrespective of the expression of CD38 and ZAP70. However, signaling capacity correlated with the levels of sIgG expression (28). It should be underlined that sIgG, in contrast to sIgM and sIgD isotypes, has a longer cytoplasmic tail, which is capable of differential signaling and which is not influenced by negative regulation from CD22 (see below) (134).

The temporal genetic program following BCR ligation was analyzed in normal and malignant CLL cells; at late time points after BCR stimulation, a specific genetic program could be found in CLL cells as compared with normal B lymphocytes; this genetic program may indeed explain the altered balance between proliferation and death in healthy or malignant cells (135).

BCR-Signaling Molecules

Several groups analyzed different signaling pathways that originate from the BCR in CLL cells and found that some of them are constitutively activated in CLL patients regardless of the heterogeneity of their disease progression. Specifically, NF-AT and NF-kB transcription factors were found to be active in B cells from patients with CLL (136,137). Constitutive NF-kB activation can also be mediated by GSK3β activity (138) and was suggested as the molecular mechanism that protects CLL from spontaneous apoptosis (139,140). Lyn may also play a role in regulating CLL cell survival; of interest, it was reported to be aberrantly expressed and activated in patients (141). Constitutive activation of p38 MAPK was reported (142,143). Controversy surrounds the activation of Akt kinase and the PI3K pathway: constitutive activation of PKC and PI3K but not of Akt in CLL cells was demonstrated by one group (142) and Akt constitutive activation was shown by another group (144). However, all these data do not explain the differential ability of cells from different patients to be activated by an antigen-like stimulation. We recently determined the phosphorylation levels of ERK as a prototype BCR-induced signaling molecule. We found that a subset of CLL cases show constitutive activation of the MAPK-signaling pathway regardless of the actual engagement of the BCR. These biochemical features resemble the pattern found in murine anergic B lymphocytes and might be responsible for the different functional behavior of the leukemic cell in patients with different clinical profiles (145) (see below).

It has recently been proposed that PKCβ2 is responsible for differential responsiveness of the cells after sIgM ligation: in some patients, high levels of expression of PKCβ2 would inhibit BCR signaling in terms of calcium release and survival (146). From another perspective, two different groups analyzed gene expression profiles of CLL patients and found that many genes belonging to the BCR-signaling pathway are differentially expressed, further supporting a role of BCR in the pathogenesis of the disease (147–149).

BCR CORECEPTORS IN NORMAL AND LEUKEMIC CELLS

A broader definition of the BCR-signaling complex also includes coreceptors and immune inhibitory receptors that modulate its activity in a positive or negative manner. The pairing of activation and inhibition is necessary to modulate the immune response and may also play a role in regulating CLL cell fate. Membrane-associated CD19, CD21, and CD81 take part in the BCR proximal-signaling cascade and lower the threshold of antigen required for BCR to signal. The main inhibitory receptors in normal and leukemic cells are CD5, CD72, CD22, and FcγRIIb. We will also describe the CD38 molecule, which has no homology to the previously described proteins, but has been demonstrated to act as a bona fide BCR coreceptor.

Activating Coreceptors

CD19 and CD21 are mainly expressed by B lymphocytes, while CD81 is widely expressed. CD19 intracellular domain synergistically signals with Igα and Igβ. The simultaneous interaction of the complement receptor CD21 (also called CR2) with C3d-tagged antigens enhances signaling through BCR by transducing a signal to CD19 and CD81 (150). Lyn is then able to activate the signaling subunit of the BCR via phosphorylation of Igα and CD19; this creates a signal amplification loop, since CD19 associates with different signaling proteins, including Vav and PI3K (151). CD81 is a member of the TM4 superfamily and is predicted to have four transmembrane regions, short N and C terminal regions, and two extracellular regions (152). It binds to several different molecules, including CD19 and CD21 on B cells, thus acting as a BCR coreceptor (153).

The levels of expression of CD21 in CLL cells have no prognostic importance (20), nor do the levels of expression of CD19 and CD81. Accordingly, flow cytometry analysis of CD81 and CD19 are included in different protocols for the assessment of MRD (154,155).

Inhibitory Coreceptors

Distinct transmembrane receptors inhibit the signaling pathways originating from the BCR through their intracellular immunoreceptor tyrosine-based inhibitory motif (ITIM) domain (156). The ITIM that is present in the cytoplasmic domain of inhibitory receptors is capable of inhibiting signaling by two different mechanisms: after tyrosine phosphorylation (which occurs upon ligand-induced clustering), ITIM can bind to either SHP-1 or SHIP phosphatases. The tyrosine phosphatases SHP-1 dephosphorylates critical residues in BCR-signaling molecules, including Ig-ITAM, Syk, and PLCγ, while the inositol phosphatase SHIP blocks recruitment of key molecules to the cell membrane (i.e., PH domain-containing proteins Btk and PLCγ).

CD5

This transmembrane protein is expressed by B1 lymphocytes localized in the mouse peritoneal cavity. While B1 cells undergo apoptosis after BCR cross-linking, B1 cells from CD5-deficient mice respond to the same stimulation with increased proliferation (157). This result, together with the observation that CD5 is constitutively associated with SHP-1 in B1 murine lymphocytes, indicates that CD5 may play a negative role in BCR signaling (158). In addition, lyn$^{-/-}$ B1 lymphocytes show no phosphorylation of tyrosine residues in the CD5 cytoplasmic domain, nor association between CD5 and SHP-1, demonstrating that lyn is necessary for CD5 inhibitory activity (159).

Normal human tonsil B cells undergo apoptosis after CD5 ligation. However, CD5 induces differential apoptosis in two groups of CLL patients (responders and nonresponders): responders have high levels of expression of CD38, IgM, CD5, and CD79β (160,161); CD5 signal flows through CD79α and CD79β and subsequent translocation of CD79α/β and CD5 itself into lipid rafts (161). Accordingly, high expression of the truncated splicing version of CD79β results in resistance to CD5-triggered apoptosis (161). As expected, CD5$^+$ lymphocytes are more sensitive than CD5–human B lymphocytes to IgM-induced apoptosis (162). In contrast, another group found that responders have low levels of CD5 and CD72 expression (163). Finally, it was proposed that prolonged incubation with anti-CD5 antibodies increases survival of B cells from a subset of patients with CLL, while in the remaining patients, the cells undergo apoptosis (164). Microarray analysis of a CD5-transfected B-cell line revealed several gene families that are commonly activated in CLL cells, suggesting that CD5 is constitutively active (165); indeed CD5 was found to be constitutively phosphorylated in leukemic cells (165). Proposed ligands for CD5 include the Ig framework region sequences (166), GP40–80 (167–169) and CD72 (170).

CD72

Expression of CD72 is restricted to B-cell lineage and is turned off in antibody-secreting plasma cells (171). B Cells from CD72-deficient mice are hyperresponsive to BCR aggregation, demonstrating that CD72 has an inhibitory role (172).

That notwithstanding, anti-CD72 antibodies were initially shown to deliver costimulatory signals to CLL cells (173). Recently, CD72 was identified as a lymphocyte receptor for the class IV semaphorin CD100, thus representing a novel potential element of regulation of B-cell signaling (174). Given the fact that two of the putative ligands for CD72, CD5 and CD100, are expressed by CLL cells, it is tempting to speculate that they may create a feedback regulation loop on the clone itself (175,176).

CD22

CD22 (SIGLEC2) is a B-cell-restricted cell surface protein expressed at high levels-only in mature B lymphocytes. After BCR ligation, lyn phosphorylates the tyrosine residues present in the three ITIM sequences of CD22, allowing the creation of docking sites for the protein phosphatase SHP-1, which is a negative regulator of BCR signaling (177). The levels of expression of CD22 in CLL cells have no prognostic importance (20).

FcγRIIb

The low-affinity receptor for IgG is known as a blocker of antigen-induced BCR signaling. This effect is mediated by ITIM phosphorylation by lyn. Only when phosphorylated is the cytoplasmic domain of FcγRIIb able to recruit SHIP, which mediates the block of BCR-signaling pathway. FcγRIIb was found to be differentially expressed during B-cell maturation and in B-cell lymphomas (178).

CLL cells express levels of FcγRIIb similar to those of normal B lymphocytes (178). FcγRIIb signals in CLL cells by inhibiting ERK activation induced by BCR (179), but it does not induce apoptosis as reported in murine B cells (179,180). Since a number of CLL cells express polyreactive BCR, it is possible that malignant cells may interact with several IgG immune complexes that may activate the FcγRIIb inhibitory pathway.

CD38

CD38 is a multifunctional ectoenzyme widely expressed in cells and tissues especially in leukocytes. It is expressed at different stages of B-cell development, absent in memory cells, and highly expressed in plasma cells and the germinal centers (181,182). CD38 also functions as a signaling receptor in cell adhesion by inducing calcium increase and tyrosine phosphorylation after binding to CD31 expressed by stromal cells (182–184). CD38-deficient mice completely lose tissue-associated NAD+ glycohydrolase activity and show an altered humoral immune response with a marked deficiency in antibody responses to T-cell-dependent protein antigens and augmented antibody responses to T-cell-independent type 2 polysaccharide antigen (185). Along this line of research, it has been shown that CD38 acts as a coreceptor for BCR; transfection of CD38 in a murine CD38-negative cell line augments BCR signaling (186); in fact, CD38 signaling is dependent on BCR and not on its cytoplasmic tail (186).

CD38 acts as an autonomous signaling molecule by inducing Ca^{2+} flux, lipid raft formation, and proliferation (187); cocapping of CD38 with CD79α/β, IgM, and IgD further supports its role as a BCR coreceptor (187). CD38 expression identifies a subset of CLL cells that are enriched in proliferating cells (188). Moreover, CD38 ligation triggers ZAP70 phosphorylation (189), and the coexpression of the two molecules labels a subset of CLL cells with a high migratory potential and proliferation capacity (188,189); this may explain why CD38 expression appears to be higher on CLL cells present in lymph nodes as compared with those accumulating in peripheral blood (PB) or bone marrow (BM) (190). Interestingly, phosphorylation of the cytoskeleton adaptor protein HS1 also correlates with CD38 expression in CLL (130).

In patients with CLL, the expression of CD38 has prognostic significance (see chap. 7) (191). CD38 is an independent prognostic marker that correlates with a shorter median survival (192–195). Its expression also identifies a group of patients with CLL that are responsive to anti-IgM in terms of Ca^{2+} release, PTK activation, and apoptosis (115,128).

BCR COSTIMULATION IN NORMAL AND LEUKEMIC CELLS

The notion that relevant events of CLL stimulation occur in tissues has led to a tissue-oriented model of CLL natural history (196), which is based on two compartments and their interactions with different elements of the tissue environments. The accumulation compartment that is mainly represented in the PB is likely nourished by a "proliferation" compartment, which is represented by focal aggregates of proliferating cells that form the proliferation centers (PCs) in lymph nodes and BM (197,198). Within and around the PC, malignant CLL cells are interspersed with numerous T lymphocytes; many express CD4 and CD40L and are in close contact with the proliferating malignant B cells (199).

Three concurring signals are required for human B-cell maturation: BCR ligation, T-cell help, and toll-like receptor costimulation (200–202). The in vitro stimulation of CLL cells from PB through CD40 mimics some events that likely occur in the PC; cells are rescued from apoptosis and increase their proliferation and differentiation (199,203–207). In fact, CLL cells can progress in vitro to the final stages of B-cell maturation in the presence of T-cell help and cytokines (208–210). Several data highlight the role of T cells in supporting the clonal growth and suggest that within PC T cells provide a short-term support to malignant B cells, which influences their proliferative activity (196,211,212). The absolute number of T cells is increased in patients with CLL (213), and T-cell subsets are redistributed: $CD4^+$ T cells predominate in BM and lymph nodes (214) where they tend to concentrate into PC (198). However, it was also reported that in the PB of CLL patients there were less T-helper cells (215), which also showed functional defects (216), suggesting that a defective costimulation may lead to somewhat anergic peripheral cells.

Toll-like receptors recognize a set of different microbial components with a certain degree of specificity (217,218). In particular, TLR 1, 2, 4, 5, and 6 act on the surface of the cell to detect pathogens and to signal activation. TLR2 can form heterodimers with TLR1 or TLR6 to recognize specific bacterial lipoproteins. TLR3, TLR7, and TLR9 are located inside intracellular endosomal compartments and can detect nucleic acids previously internalized (219). Despite the hypothesis that CLL cells may recognize and be regulated by microbial-derived costimulatory signals, little information is available on which TLR are expressed by leukemic cells and which microbial components they can detect in the microenvironment. TLR9 and TLR7 expression and function have been recently addressed on CLL cells with the aim of augmenting their immunogenic profile for immunotherapy or their sensitivity to apoptosis for chemotherapy (220). Further studies are needed to address the full TLR repertoire on CLL cells and their functional role in costimulation and activation of the leukemic clone.

B-CELL ANERGY

Several pieces of evidence described so far indicate that stimulation through the BCR is a central event in the natural history of CLL (1). However, CLL cells are heterogeneous in their ability to respond to stimulation via the antigen receptor. At least half of the cases can be stimulated in vitro through their sIg, and the responsive cases have an unfavorable clinical prognosis. In contrast, the remaining CLL cases (mainly with an indolent clinical course) are unresponsive to BCR cross-linking, as determined by the absence of global tyrosine phosphorylation (120,128,129), thereby recalling B cells anergized in vivo after chronic stimulation by an antigen (221).

Anergy has been mainly studied in murine models, taking advantage of double transgenic mice expressing a single-idiotype immunoglobulin and its cognate antigen. These studies identified some functional features restricted to anergic B cells such as attenuated BCR signal transduction, reduced sIgM expression, and limited lifespan. At the molecular level, tolerant B lymphocytes have a constitutive level of phospho-tyrosines in cell lysates, showing activated ERK that cannot be further induced. NF-AT transcription factor is translocated to the nucleus and is constitutively active in anergic B cells (222,223). Interestingly, all B lymphocytes responding to antigenic stimulation activate the same molecules during a normal immune response.

The term "B-cell anergy" in the human immune system has been primarily used to describe the overall failure to respond to stimulation through the immunoglobulin receptor; there is no molecular definition. We have recently observed that a distinct number of CLL cases tend to reproduce the same biochemical signature of mouse anergic B cells (145).

It has been reported that continuous binding of antigen and subsequent receptor signaling are essential for the maintenance of anergy in B lymphocytes, excluding the possibility that anergy may be induced after transient exposure to antigen and then "remembered" with time (224). This is in accordance with a recent report showing that anergized IgM responses can be restored following in vitro incubation, suggesting the possibility for direct engagement of putative antigen in vivo (129). This would necessitate the presence of a functional-signaling cascade, as confirmed by results from our own and other groups that show the constitutive activation of distinct kinase pathways in different subsets of patients with CLL (128,145).

CONCLUSIONS

Chronic antigenic stimulation by both microbial and self-antigens is implicated in the onset and progression of several chronic B-cell malignancies. All experimental data indicate that CLL B cells have had some sort of antigenic exposure. However, irrespective of its phenotypic homogeneity, CLL is clinically heterogeneous. Some patients have an

Scenario A: Chronic BCR ligation (Anergy)

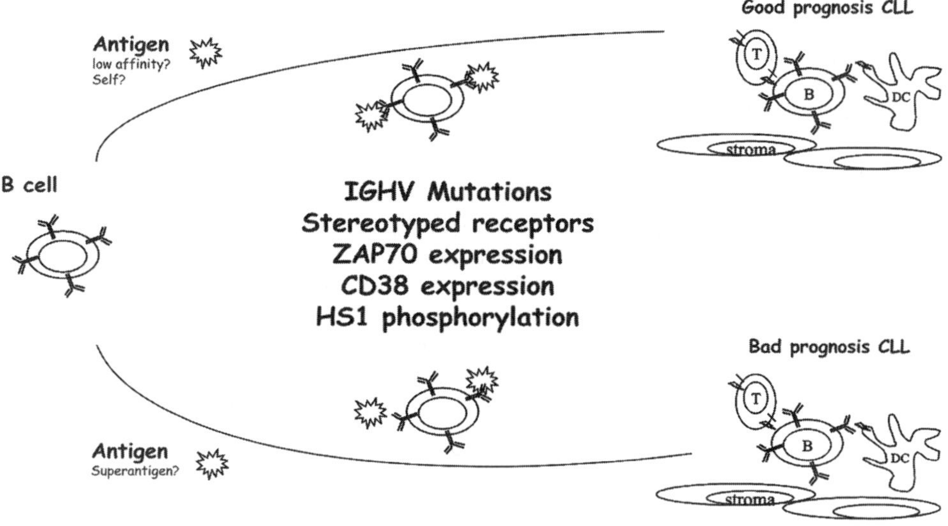

Scenario B: Ongoing BCR stimulation (Activation)

Figure 2 CLL and BCR: a tentative model. *Abbreviations*: CLL, chronic lymphocytic leukemia; BCR, B-cell receptor.

aggressive disease, others an indolent course. A number of biologically defined prognostic factors are used as markers to dissect the clinical heterogeneity (Fig. 2). As also discussed in this chapter, the biological function of these markers (IGHV mutational status, stereotyped sequences, ZAP70, and CD38 expression, HS1 phosphorylation) is again directing our attention toward the BCR and its stimulation.

CLL cells differ significantly in their in vitro capacity to signal through the BCR, with some cases (most unmutated) carrying more competent BCRs and others (usually mutated) appearing to be unresponsive. This may depend on the nature of the antigen and on the affinity of the receptor. It is not unreasonable to postulate that in some cases a persistent antigenic stimulation might promote CLL survival and growth via sIg-mediated signals, while in other cases antigen interaction might lead to receptor desensitization and to an anergic state (Fig. 2). The former would lead to an aggressive disease; the latter would translate into a more indolent clinical behavior.

If it is reasonable to consider that the functional response of CLL cells to BCR stimulation proceeds with the same modalities and along the same pathways used by normal B cells; it follows that the important players are the quality and the nature of the stimuli received through the BCR. Important abnormalities may involve the connections that link BCR stimulation, cell activation, and the cytoskeleton modification that the cell has to acquire to both proliferate and circulate (131). In this context, it is possible that the signal transduction may lead to a stimulated, hyperactivated leukemic cell that is unable to complete a cell division unless located in the specific environment of tissue PC. Over time, the development of further genomic aberrations may stop the need for Ag triggering or may mimic the consequences of Ag stimulation.

REFERENCES

1. Stevenson FK, Caligaris-Cappio F. Chronic lymphocytic leukemia: revelations from the B-cell receptor. Blood 2004; 103(12):4389–4395.
2. Chiorazzi N, Ferrarini M. B cell chronic lymphocytic leukemia: lessons learned from studies of the B cell antigen receptor. Annu Rev Immunol 2003; 21:841–894.
3. Damle RN, Wasil T, Fais F, et al. Ig V gene mutation status and CD38 expression as novel prognostic indicators in chronic lymphocytic leukemia. Blood 1999; 94(6):1840–1847.
4. Hamblin TJ, Davis Z, Gardiner A, et al. Unmutated Ig V(H) genes are associated with a more aggressive form of chronic lymphocytic leukemia. Blood 1999; 94(6):1848–1854.
5. Ghia P, Stamatopoulos K, Belessi C, et al. Geographic patterns and pathogenetic implications of IGHV gene usage in chronic lymphocytic leukemia: the lesson of the IGHV3-21 gene. Blood 2005; 105(4):1678–1685.
6. Ghiotto F, Fais F, Valetto A, et al. Remarkably similar antigen receptors among a subset of patients with chronic lymphocytic leukemia. J Clin Invest 2004; 113(7):1008–1016.
7. Messmer BT, Albesiano E, Efremov DG, et al. Multiple distinct sets of stereotyped antigen receptors indicate a role for antigen in promoting chronic lymphocytic leukemia. J Exp Med 2004; 200(4):519–525.
8. Stamatopoulos K, Belessi C, Moreno C, et al. Over 20% of patients with chronic lymphocytic leukemia carry stereotyped receptors: Pathogenetic implications and clinical correlations. Blood 2007; 109(1):259–270.
9. Tobin G, Thunberg U, Karlsson K, et al. Subsets with restricted immunoglobulin gene rearrangement features indicate a role for antigen selection in the development of chronic lymphocytic leukemia. Blood 2004; 104(9):2879–2885.
10. Widhopf GF 2nd, Rassenti LZ, Toy TL, et al. Chronic lymphocytic leukemia B cells of more than 1% of patients express virtually identical immunoglobulins. Blood 2004; 104(8):2499–2504.
11. Tobin G, Thunberg U, Johnson A, et al. Somatically mutated Ig V(H)3-21 genes characterize a new subset of chronic lymphocytic leukemia. Blood 2002; 99(6):2262–2264.
12. Murray F, Darzentas N, Hadzidimitriou A, et al. Stereotyped patterns of somatic hypermutation (SHM) in subsets of patients with chronic lymphocytic leukemia (CLL): implications for the role of antigen selection in leukemogenesis. Blood 110(11):229a, 2007.
13. Reth M. Antigen receptors on B lymphocytes. Annu Rev Immunol 1992; 10:97–121.
14. van Noesel CJ, Lankester AC, van Lier RA. Dual antigen recognition by B cells. Immunol Today 1993; 14(1):8–11.
15. Grey HM, Rabellino E, Pirofsky B. Immunoglobulins on the surface of lymphocytes. IV. Distribution in hypogammaglobulinemia, cellular immune deficiency, and chronic lymphatic leukemia. J Clin Invest 1971; 50(11):2368–2375.
16. Aisenberg AC, Bloch KJ. Immunoglobulins on the surface of neoplastic lymphocytes. N Engl J Med 1972; 287(6):272–276.
17. Kubo RT, Grey HM, Pirofsky B. IgD: a major immunoglobulin on the surface of lymphocytes from patients with chronic lymphatic leukemia. J Immunol 1974; 112(5):1952–1954.
18. Fu SM, Winchester RJ, Kunkel HG. Occurrence of surface IgM, IgD, and free light chains of human lymphocytes. J Exp Med 1974; 139(2):451–456.
19. Fu SM, Winchester RJ, Feizi T, et al. Idiotypic specificity of surface immunoglobulin and the maturation of leukemic bone-marrow-derived lymphocytes. Proc Natl Acad Sci U S A 1974; 71(11):4487–4490.
20. Geisler CH, Larsen JK, Hansen NE, et al. Prognostic importance of flow cytometric immunophenotyping of 540 consecutive patients with B-cell chronic lymphocytic leukemia. Blood 1991; 78(7):1795–1802.
21. Stevenson FK, Hamblin TJ, Stevenson GT, et al. Extracellular idiotypic immunoglobulin arising from human leukemic B lymphocytes. J Exp Med 1980; 152(6):1484–1496.
22. Rubartelli A, Sitia R, Zicca A, et al. Differentiation of chronic lymphocytic leukemia cells: correlation between the synthesis and secretion of immunoglobulins and the ultrastructure of the malignant cells. Blood 1983; 62(2):495–504.

23. Friedman DF, Moore JS, Erikson J, et al. Variable region gene analysis of an isotype-switched (IgA) variant of chronic lymphocytic leukemia. Blood 1992; 80(9):2287–2297.
24. Dhaliwal HS, Ling NR, Bishop S, et al. Expression of immunoglobin G on blood lymphocytes in chronic lymphocytic leukaemia. Clin Exp Immunol 1978; 31(2):226–236.
25. Kimby E, Mellstedt H, Bjorkholm M, et al. Surface immunoglobulin pattern of the leukaemic cell population in chronic lymphocytic leukaemia (CLL) in relation to disease activity. Hematol Oncol 1985; 3(4):261–269.
26. Dono M, Hashimoto S, Fais F, et al. Evidence for progenitors of chronic lymphocytic leukemia B cells that undergo intraclonal differentiation and diversification. Blood 1996; 87(4):1586–1594.
27. Ligler FS, Kettman JR, Smith RG, et al. Immunoglobulin phenotype on B cells correlates with clinical stage of chronic lymphocytic leukemia. Blood 1983; 62(2):256–263.
28. Potter KN, Mockridge CI, Neville L, et al. Structural and functional features of the B-cell receptor in IgG-positive chronic lymphocytic leukemia. Clin Cancer Res 2006; 12(6):1672–1679.
29. Clark MR, Campbell KS, Kazlauskas A, et al. The B cell antigen receptor complex: association of Ig-alpha and Ig-beta with distinct cytoplasmic effectors. Science 1992; 258(5079): 123–126.
30. Lin J, Justement LB. The MB-1/B29 heterodimer couples the B cell antigen receptor to multiple src family protein tyrosine kinases. J Immunol 1992; 149(5):1548–1555.
31. Sanchez M, Misulovin Z, Burkhardt AL, et al. Signal transduction by immunoglobulin is mediated through Ig alpha and Ig beta. J Exp Med 1993; 178(3):1049–1055.
32. Teh YM, Neuberger MS. The immunoglobulin (Ig)alpha and Igbeta cytoplasmic domains are independently sufficient to signal B cell maturation and activation in transgenic mice. J Exp Med 1997; 185(10):1753–1758.
33. Tseng J, Eisfelder BJ, Clark MR. B-cell antigen receptor-induced apoptosis requires both Ig alpha and Ig beta. Blood 1997; 89(5):1513–1520.
34. Bonnerot C, Lankar D, Hanau D, et al. Role of B cell receptor Ig alpha and Ig beta subunits in MHC class II-restricted antigen presentation. Immunity 1995; 3(3):335–347.
35. Pleiman CM, D'Ambrosio D, Cambier JC. The B-cell antigen receptor complex: structure and signal transduction. Immunol Today 1994; 15(9):393–399.
36. Venkitaraman AR, Williams GT, Dariavach P, et al. The B-cell antigen receptor of the five immunoglobulin classes. Nature 1991; 352(6338):777–781.
37. Gong S, Nussenzweig MC. Regulation of an early developmental checkpoint in the B cell pathway by Ig beta. Science 1996; 272(5260):411–414.
38. Torres RM, Flaswinkel H, Reth M, et al. Aberrant B cell development and immune response in mice with a compromised BCR complex. Science 1996; 272(5269):1804–1808.
39. Okazaki M, Luo Y, Han T, et al. Three new monoclonal antibodies that define a unique antigen associated with prolymphocytic leukemia/non-Hodgkin's lymphoma and are effectively internalized after binding to the cell surface antigen. Blood 1993; 81(1):84–94.
40. Zomas AP, Matutes E, Morilla R, et al. Expression of the immunoglobulin-associated protein B29 in B cell disorders with the monoclonal antibody SN8 (CD79b). Leukemia 1996; 10(12): 1966–1970.
41. Moreau EJ, Matutes E, A'Hern RP, et al. Improvement of the chronic lymphocytic leukemia scoring system with the monoclonal antibody SN8 (CD79b). Am J Clin Pathol 1997; 108(4): 378–382.
42. Minuzzo S, Indraccolo S, Tosello V, et al. Heterogeneous intracellular expression of B-cell receptor components in B-cell chronic lymphocytic leukaemia (B-CLL) cells and effects of CD79b gene transfer on surface immunoglobulin levels in a B-CLL-derived cell line. Br J Haematol 2005; 130(6):878–889.
43. Thompson AA, Talley JA, Do HN, et al. Aberrations of the B-cell receptor B29 (CD79b) gene in chronic lymphocytic leukemia. Blood 1997; 90(4):1387–1394.
44. Gordon MS, Kato RM, Lansigan F, et al. Aberrant B cell receptor signaling from B29 (Igbeta, CD79b) gene mutations of chronic lymphocytic leukemia B cells. Proc Natl Acad Sci U S A 2000; 97(10):5504–5509.

45. Alfarano A, Indraccolo S, Circosta P, et al. An alternatively spliced form of CD79b gene may account for altered B-cell receptor expression in B-chronic lymphocytic leukemia. Blood 1999; 93(7):2327–2335.

46. Payelle-Brogard B, Magnac C, Mauro FR, et al. Analysis of the B-cell receptor B29 (CD79b) gene in familial chronic lymphocytic leukemia. Blood 1999; 94(10):3516–3522.

47. Payelle-Brogard B, Magnac C, Alcover A, et al. Defective assembly of the B-cell receptor chains accounts for its low expression in B-chronic lymphocytic leukaemia. Br J Haematol 2002; 118(4):976–985.

48. Hashimoto S, Chiorazzi N, Gregersen PK. Alternative splicing of CD79a (Ig-alpha/mb-1) and CD79b (Ig-beta/B29) RNA transcripts in human B cells. Mol Immunol 1995; 32(9):651–659.

49. Koyama M, Nakamura T, Higashihara M, et al. The novel variants of mb-1 and B29 transcripts generated by alternative mRNA splicing. Immunol Lett 1995; 47(3):151–156.

50. Cragg MS, Chan HT, Fox MD, et al. The alternative transcript of CD79b is overexpressed in B-CLL and inhibits signaling for apoptosis. Blood 2002; 100(9):3068–3076.

51. Schlette E, Medeiros LJ, Keating M, et al. CD79b expression in chronic lymphocytic leukemia. Association with trisomy 12 and atypical immunophenotype. Arch Pathol Lab Med 2003; 127(5):561–566.

52. Cajiao I, Sargent R, Elstrom R, et al. Igbeta(CD79b) mRNA expression in chronic lymphocytic leukaemia cells correlates with immunoglobulin heavy chain gene mutational status but does not serve as an independent predictor of clinical severity. Am J Hematol 2007; 82(8):712–720.

53. Garcia Vela J, Delgado I, Benito L, et al. CD79b expression in B cell chronic lymphocytic leukemia: its implication for minimal residual disease detection. Leukemia 1999; 13(10): 1501–1505.

54. Bell PB, Rooney N, Bosanquet AG. CD79a detected by ZL7.4 separates chronic lymphocytic leukemia from mantle cell lymphoma in the leukemic phase. Cytometry 1999; 38(3):102–105.

55. Vuillier F, Dumas G, Magnac C, et al. Lower levels of surface B-cell-receptor expression in chronic lymphocytic leukemia are associated with glycosylation and folding defects of the mu and CD79a chains. Blood 2005; 105(7):2933–2940.

56. Niiro H, Clark EA. Regulation of B-cell fate by antigen-receptor signals. Nat Rev Immunol 2002; 2(12):945–956.

57. Healy JI, Goodnow CC. Positive versus negative signaling by lymphocyte antigen receptors. Annu Rev Immunol 1998; 16:645–670.

58. DeFranco AL. The complexity of signaling pathways activated by the BCR. Curr Opin Immunol 1997; 9(3):296–308.

59. Gauld SB, Dal Porto JM, Cambier J. B Cell Antigen Receptor Sci STKE (Connections Map Pathway) 2002; http://stke.sciencemag.org/cgi/cm/stkecm; CMP_6909.

60. Kurosaki T. Genetic analysis of B cell antigen receptor signaling. Annu Rev Immunol 1999; 17:555–592.

61. Skaggs BJ, Clark MR. Proximal B cell receptor signaling pathways. Signal Transduct 2004; 5–6:173–194.

62. Gauld SB, Cambier JC. Src-family kinases in B-cell development and signaling. Oncogene 2004; 23(48):8001–8006.

63. Xu Y, Harder KW, Huntington ND, et al. Lyn tyrosine kinase: accentuating the positive and the negative. Immunity 2005; 22(1):9–18.

64. Chan VW, Meng F, Soriano P, et al. Characterization of the B lymphocyte populations in Lyn-deficient mice and the role of Lyn in signal initiation and down-regulation. Immunity 1997; 7(1):69–81.

65. Cornall RJ, Cheng AM, Pawson T, et al. Role of Syk in B-cell development and antigen-receptor signaling. Proc Natl Acad Sci U S A 2000; 97(4):1713–1718.

66. Rowley RB, Burkhardt AL, Chao HG, et al. Syk protein-tyrosine kinase is regulated by tyrosine-phosphorylated Ig alpha/Ig beta immunoreceptor tyrosine activation motif binding and autophosphorylation. J Biol Chem 1995; 270(19):11590–1594.

67. Rolli V, Gallwitz M, Wossning T, et al. Amplification of B cell antigen receptor signaling by a Syk/ITAM positive feedback loop. Mol Cell 2002; 10(5):1057–1069.

68. Hong JJ, Yankee TM, Harrison ML, et al. Regulation of signaling in B cells through the phosphorylation of Syk on linker region tyrosines. A mechanism for negative signaling by the Lyn tyrosine kinase. J Biol Chem 2002; 277(35):31703–1714.
69. Ishiai M, Kurosaki M, Pappu R, et al. BLNK required for coupling Syk to PLC gamma 2 and Rac1-JNK in B cells. Immunity 1999; 10(1):117–125.
70. Scielzo C, Camporeale A, Geuna M, et al. ZAP-70 is expressed by normal and malignant human B-cell subsets of different maturational stage. Leukemia 2006; 20(4):689–695.
71. Gobessi S, Laurenti L, Longo PG, et al. ZAP-70 enhances B-cell-receptor signaling despite absent or inefficient tyrosine kinase activation in chronic lymphocytic leukemia and lymphoma B cells. Blood 2007; 109(5):2032–2039.
72. Kitamura D, Kaneko H, Miyagoe Y, et al. Isolation and characterization of a novel human gene expressed specifically in the cells of hematopoietic lineage. Nucleic Acids Res 1989; 17(22):9367–9379.
73. Yamanashi Y, Okada M, Semba T, et al. Identification of HS1 protein as a major substrate of protein-tyrosine kinase(s) upon B-cell antigen receptor-mediated signaling. Proc Natl Acad Sci U S A 1993; 90(8):3631–3635.
74. Taniuchi I, Kitamura D, Maekawa Y, et al. Antigen-receptor induced clonal expansion and deletion of lymphocytes are impaired in mice lacking HS1 protein, a substrate of the antigen-receptor-coupled tyrosine kinases. Embo J 1995; 14(15):3664–3678.
75. Gomez TS, McCarney SD, Carrizosa E, et al. HS1 functions as an essential actin-regulatory adaptor protein at the immune synapse. Immunity 2006; 24(6):741–752.
76. Coffer PJ, Jin J, Woodgett JR. Protein kinase B (c-Akt): a multifunctional mediator of phosphatidylinositol 3-kinase activation. Biochem J 1998; 335(Pt 1):1–13.
77. Alessi DR, Andjelkovic M, Caudwell B, et al. Mechanism of activation of protein kinase B by insulin and IGF-1. Embo J 1996; 15(23):6541–6551.
78. Mitsiades CS, Mitsiades N, Koutsilieris M. The Akt pathway: molecular targets for anti-cancer drug development. Curr Cancer Drug Targets 2004; 4(3):235–256.
79. Datta SR, Dudek H, Tao X, et al. Akt phosphorylation of BAD couples survival signals to the cell-intrinsic death machinery. Cell 1997; 91(2):231–241.
80. Ozes ON, Mayo LD, Gustin JA, et al. NF-kappaB activation by tumour necrosis factor requires the Akt serine-threonine kinase. Nature 1999; 401(6748):82–85.
81. Kurosaki T, Maeda A, Ishiai M, et al. Regulation of the phospholipase C-gamma2 pathway in B cells. Immunol Rev 2000; 176:19–29.
82. Dolmetsch RE, Xu K, Lewis RS. Calcium oscillations increase the efficiency and specificity of gene expression. Nature 1998; 392(6679):933–936.
83. Zebisch A, Czernilofsky AP, Keri G, et al. Signaling through RAS-RAF-MEK-ERK: from basics to bedside. Curr Med Chem 2007; 14(5):601–623.
84. McKay MM, Morrison DK. Integrating signals from RTKs to ERK/MAPK. Oncogene 2007; 26(22):3113–3121.
85. Kuida K, Boucher DM. Functions of MAP kinases: insights from gene-targeting studies. J Biochem (Tokyo) 2004; 135(6):653–656.
86. D'mbrosio D, Hippen KL, Cambier JC. Distinct mechanisms mediate SHC association with the activated and resting B cell antigen receptor. Eur J Immunol 1996; 26(8):1960–1965.
87. Mason CS, Springer CJ, Cooper RG, et al. Serine and tyrosine phosphorylations cooperate in Raf-1, but not B-Raf activation. Embo J 1999; 18(8):2137–2148.
88. Sun H, King AJ, Diaz HB, et al. Regulation of the protein kinase Raf-1 by oncogenic Ras through phosphatidylinositol 3-kinase, Cdc42/Rac and Pak. Curr Biol 2000; 10(5):281–284.
89. Holmstrom TH, Schmitz I, Soderstrom TS, et al. MAPK/ERK signaling in activated T cells inhibits CD95/Fas-mediated apoptosis downstream of DISC assembly. Embo J 2000; 19(20):5418–5428.
90. Hayakawa J, Ohmichi M, Kurachi H, et al. Inhibition of BAD phosphorylation either at serine 112 via extracellular signal-regulated protein kinase cascade or at serine 136 via Akt cascade sensitizes human ovarian cancer cells to cisplatin. Cancer Res 2000; 60(21):5988–5994.

91. Macian F. NFAT proteins: key regulators of T-cell development and function. Nat Rev Immunol 2005; 5(6):472–484.

92. Rao A, Luo C, Hogan PG. Transcription factors of the NFAT family: regulation and function. Annu Rev Immunol 1997; 15:707–747.

93. Martinez-Martinez S, Redondo JM. Inhibitors of the calcineurin/NFAT pathway. Curr Med Chem 2004; 11(8):997–1007.

94. Hogan PG, Chen L, Nardone J, et al. Transcriptional regulation by calcium, calcineurin, and NFAT. Genes Dev 2003; 17(18):2205–2232.

95. Dumont FJ. FK506, an immunosuppressant targeting calcineurin function. Curr Med Chem 2000; 7(7):731–748.

96. Macian F, Lopez-Rodriguez C, Rao A. Partners in transcription: NFAT and AP-1. Oncogene 2001; 20(19):2476–2489.

97. Luo C, Burgeon E, Rao A. Mechanisms of transactivation by nuclear factor of activated T cells-1. J Exp Med 1996; 184(1):141–147.

98. Karin M. Nuclear factor-kappaB in cancer development and progression. Nature 2006; 441(7092): 431–436.

99. Hacker H, Karin M. Regulation and function of IKK and IKK-related kinases. Sci STKE 2006; 2006(357):re13.

100. Sen R. Control of B lymphocyte apoptosis by the transcription factor NF-kappaB. Immunity 2006; 25(6):871–883.

101. Iglesias A, Lamers M, Kohler G. Expression of immunoglobulin delta chain causes allelic exclusion in transgenic mice. Nature 1987; 330(6147):482–484.

102. Lutz C, Ledermann B, Kosco-Vilbois MH, et al. IgD can largely substitute for loss of IgM function in B cells. Nature 1998; 393(6687):797–801.

103. Nitschke L, Kosco MH, Kohler G, et al. Immunoglobulin D-deficient mice can mount normal immune responses to thymus-independent and -dependent antigens. Proc Natl Acad Sci U S A 1993; 90(5):1887–1891.

104. Roes J, Rajewsky K. Immunoglobulin D (IgD)-deficient mice reveal an auxiliary receptor function for IgD in antigen-mediated recruitment of B cells. J Exp Med 1993; 177(1):45–55.

105. Brink R, Goodnow CC, Crosbie J, et al. Immunoglobulin M and D antigen receptors are both capable of mediating B lymphocyte activation, deletion, or anergy after interaction with specific antigen. J Exp Med 1992; 176(4):991–1005.

106. Ales-Martinez JE, Warner GL, Scott DW. Immunoglobulins D and M mediate signals that are qualitatively different in B cells with an immature phenotype. Proc Natl Acad Sci U S A 1988; 85(18):6919–6923.

107. Tisch R, Roifman CM, Hozumi N. Functional differences between immunoglobulins M and D expressed on the surface of an immature B-cell line. Proc Natl Acad Sci U S A 1988; 85(18): 6914–6918.

108. Cambier JC, Monroe JG. B cell activation. V. Differentiation signaling of B cell membrane depolarization, increased I-A expression, G0 to G1 transition, and thymidine uptake by anti-IgM and anti-IgD antibodies. J Immunol 1984; 133(2):576–581.

109. Burkhardt AL, Brunswick M, Bolen JB, et al. Anti-immunoglobulin stimulation of B lymphocytes activates src-related protein-tyrosine kinases. Proc Natl Acad Sci U S A 1991; 88(16):7410–7414.

110. Wienands J, Reth M. Glycosyl-phosphatidylinositol linkage as a mechanism for cell-surface expression of immunoglobulin D. Nature 1992; 356(6366):246–248.

111. Chaturvedi A, Siddiqui Z, Bayiroglu F, et al. A GPI-linked isoform of the IgD receptor regulates resting B cell activation. Nat Immunol 2002; 3(10):951–957.

112. Hivroz C, Geny B, Brouet JC, et al. Altered signal transduction secondary to surface IgM cross-linking on B-chronic lymphocytic leukemia cells. Differential activation of the phosphatidylinositol-specific phospholipase C. J Immunol 1990; 144(6):2351–2358.

113. Hivroz C, Grillot-Courvalin C, Labaume S, et al. Cross-linking of membrane IgM on B CLL cells: dissociation between intracellular free Ca2+ mobilization and cell proliferation. Eur J Immunol 1988; 18(11):1811–1817.

114. McConkey DJ, Aguilar-Santelises M, Hartzell P, et al. Induction of DNA fragmentation in chronic B-lymphocytic leukemia cells. J Immunol 1991; 146(3):1072–1076.
115. Zupo S, Isnardi L, Megna M, et al. CD38 expression distinguishes two groups of B-cell chronic lymphocytic leukemias with different responses to anti-IgM antibodies and propensity to apoptosis. Blood 1996; 88(4):1365–1374.
116. Zupo S, Massara R, Dono M, et al. Apoptosis or plasma cell differentiation of CD38-positive B-chronic lymphocytic leukemia cells induced by cross-linking of surface IgM or IgD. Blood 2000; 95(4):1199–1206.
117. Bernal A, Pastore RD, Asgary Z, et al. Survival of leukemic B cells promoted by engagement of the antigen receptor. Blood 2001; 98(10):3050–3057.
118. Petlickovski A, Laurenti L, Li X, et al. Sustained signaling through the B-cell receptor induces Mcl-1 and promotes survival of chronic lymphocytic leukemia B cells. Blood 2005; 105(12): 4820–4827.
119. Michel F, Merle-Beral H, Legac E, et al. Defective calcium response in B-chronic lymphocytic leukemia cells. Alteration of early protein tyrosine phosphorylation and of the mechanism responsible for cell calcium influx. J Immunol 1993; 150(8 Pt 1):3624–3633.
120. Lankester AC, van Schijndel GM, van der Schoot CE, van Oers MH, van Noesel CJ, van Lier RA. Antigen receptor nonresponsiveness in chronic lymphocytic leukemia B cells. Blood 1995; 86(3):1090–1097.
121. Semichon M, Merle-Beral H, Lang V, Bismuth G. Normal Syk protein level but abnormal tyrosine phosphorylation in B-CLL cells. Leukemia 1997; 11(11):1921–1928.
122. Allsup DJ, Kamiguti AS, Lin K, et al. B-cell receptor translocation to lipid rafts and associated signaling differ between prognostically important subgroups of chronic lymphocytic leukemia. Cancer Res 2005; 65(16):7328–7337.
123. Lankester AC, Schijndel GM, Pakker NG, et al. Antigen receptor function in chronic lymphocytic leukemia B cells. Leuk Lymphoma 1996; 24(1–2):27–33.
124. Kawauchi K, Ogasawara T, Yasuyama M. Activation of extracellular signal-regulated kinase through B-cell antigen receptor in B-cell chronic lymphocytic leukemia. Int J Hematol 2002; 75(5):508–513.
125. Chen L, Apgar J, Huynh L, et al. ZAP-70 directly enhances IgM signaling in chronic lymphocytic leukemia. Blood 2005; 105(5):2036–2041.
126. Chen L, Widhopf G, Huynh L, et al. Expression of ZAP-70 is associated with increased B-cell receptor signaling in chronic lymphocytic leukemia. Blood 2002; 100(13):4609–4614.
127. Deglesne PA, Chevallier N, Letestu R, et al. Survival response to B-cell receptor ligation is restricted to progressive chronic lymphocytic leukemia cells irrespective of Zap70 expression. Cancer Res 2006; 66(14):7158–7166.
128. Lanham S, Hamblin T, Oscier D, et al. Differential signaling via surface IgM is associated with VH gene mutational status and CD38 expression in chronic lymphocytic leukemia. Blood 2003; 101(3):1087–1093.
129. Mockridge CI, Potter KN, Wheatley I, et al. Reversible anergy of sIgM-mediated signaling in the two subsets of CLL defined by VH-gene mutational status. Blood 2007; 109(10):4424–4431.
130. Scielzo C, Ghia P, Conti A, et al. HS1 protein is differentially expressed in chronic lymphocytic leukemia patient subsets with good or poor prognoses. J Clin Invest 2005; 115(6):1644–1650.
131. Muzio M, Scielzo C, Frenquelli M, et al. HS1 complexes with cytoskeleton adapters in normal and malignant chronic lymphocytic leukemia B cells. Leukemia 2007; 21(9):2067–2070.
132. Mongini PK, Blessinger C, Posnett DN, et al. Membrane IgD and membrane IgM differ in capacity to transduce inhibitory signals within the same human B cell clonal populations. J Immunol 1989; 143(5):1565–1574.
133. Zupo S, Cutrona G, Mangiola M, et al. Role of surface IgM and IgD on survival of the cells from B-cell chronic lymphocytic leukemia. Blood 2002; 99(6):2277–2278.
134. Silver K, Cornall RJ. Isotype control of B cell signaling. Sci STKE 2003; 2003(184):pe21.
135. Vallat LD, Park Y, Li C, et al. Temporal genetic program following B-cell receptor cross-linking: altered balance between proliferation and death in healthy and malignant B cells. Blood 2007; 109(9):3989–3997.

136. Schuh K, Avots A, Tony HP, et al. Nuclear NF-ATp is a hallmark of unstimulated B cells from B-CLL patients. Leuk Lymphoma 1996; 23(5–6):583–592.
137. Furman RR, Asgary Z, Mascarenhas JO, et al. Modulation of NF-kappa B activity and apoptosis in chronic lymphocytic leukemia B cells. J Immunol 2000; 164(4):2200–2206.
138. Ougolkov AV, Bone ND, Fernandez-Zapico ME, Kay NE, Billadeau DD. Inhibition of glycogen synthase kinase-3 activity leads to epigenetic silencing of nuclear factor kappaB target genes and induction of apoptosis in chronic lymphocytic leukemia B-cells. Blood 2007; 110(2):735–742.
139. Cuni S, Perez-Aciego P, Perez-Chacon G, et al. A sustained activation of PI3K/NF-kappaB pathway is critical for the survival of chronic lymphocytic leukemia B cells. Leukemia 2004; 18(8):1391–1400.
140. Endo T, Nishio M, Enzler T, et al. BAFF and APRIL support chronic lymphocytic leukemia B-cell survival through activation of the canonical NF-kappaB pathway. Blood 2007; 109(2): 703–710.
141. Contri A, Brunati AM, Trentin L, et al. Chronic lymphocytic leukemia B cells contain anomalous Lyn tyrosine kinase, a putative contribution to defective apoptosis. J Clin Invest 2005; 115(2):369–378.
142. Ringshausen I, Schneller F, Bogner C, et al. Constitutively activated phosphatidylinositol-3 kinase (PI-3K) is involved in the defect of apoptosis in B-CLL: association with protein kinase Cdelta. Blood 2002; 100(10):3741–3748.
143. Sainz-Perez A, Gary-Gouy H, Portier A, et al. High Mda-7 expression promotes malignant cell survival and p38 MAP kinase activation in chronic lymphocytic leukemia. Leukemia 2006; 20(3):498–504.
144. Plate JM. PI3-kinase regulates survival of chronic lymphocytic leukemia B-cells by preventing caspase 8 activation. Leuk Lymphoma 2004; 45(8):1519–1529.
145. Muzio M, Apollonio B, Scielzo C, et al. Constitutive activation of distinct BCR-signaling pathways in a subset of CLL patients: a molecular signature of anergy. Blood 2008 Feb 21; [Epub ahead of print].
146. Abrams ST, Lakum T, Lin K, et al. B-cell receptor signaling in chronic lymphocytic leukemia cells is regulated by overexpressed active protein kinase CbetaII. Blood 2007; 109(3): 1193–1201.
147. Kienle DL, Korz C, Hosch B, et al. Evidence for distinct pathomechanisms in genetic subgroups of chronic lymphocytic leukemia revealed by quantitative expression analysis of cell cycle, activation, and apoptosis-associated genes. J Clin Oncol 2005; 23(16):3780–3792.
148. Kienle D, Benner A, Krober A, et al. Distinct gene expression patterns in chronic lymphocytic leukemia defined by usage of specific VH genes. Blood 2006; 107(5):2090–2093.
149. Rodriguez A, Villuendas R, Yanez L, et al. Molecular heterogeneity in chronic lymphocytic leukemia is dependent on BCR signaling: clinical correlation. Leukemia 2007; 21(9): 1984–1991.
150. Rickert RC. Regulation of B lymphocyte activation by complement C3 and the B cell coreceptor complex. Curr Opin Immunol 2005; 17(3):237–243.
151. Fujimoto M, Fujimoto Y, Poe JC, et al. CD19 regulates Src family protein tyrosine kinase activation in B lymphocytes through processive amplification. Immunity 2000; 13(1):47–57.
152. Wright MD, Tomlinson MG. The ins and outs of the transmembrane 4 superfamily. Immunol Today 1994; 15(12):588–594.
153. Fearon DT, Carter RH. The CD19/CR2/TAPA-1 complex of B lymphocytes: linking natural to acquired immunity. Annu Rev Immunol 1995; 13:127–149.
154. Rawstron AC, de Tute R, Jack AS, Hillmen P. Flow cytometric protein expression profiling as a systematic approach for developing disease-specific assays: identification of a chronic lymphocytic leukaemia-specific assay for use in rituximab-containing regimens. Leukemia 2006; 20(12):2102–2110.
155. Rawstron AC, Villamor N, Ritgen M, et al. International standardized approach for flow cytometric residual disease monitoring in chronic lymphocytic leukaemia. Leukemia 2007; 21(5):956–964.

156. Ravetch JV, Lanier LL. Immune inhibitory receptors. Science 2000; 290(5489):84–89.

157. Bikah G, Carey J, Ciallella JR, et al. CD5-mediated negative regulation of antigen receptor-induced growth signals in B-1 B cells. Science 1996; 274(5294):1906–1909.

158. Sen G, Bikah G, Venkataraman C, et al. Negative regulation of antigen receptor-mediated signaling by constitutive association of CD5 with the SHP-1 protein tyrosine phosphatase in B-1 B cells. Eur J Immunol 1999; 29(10):3319–3328.

159. Ochi H, Watanabe T. Negative regulation of B cell receptor-mediated signaling in B-1 cells through CD5 and Ly49 co-receptors via Lyn kinase activity. Int Immunol 2000; 12(10): 1417–1423.

160. Pers JO, Berthou C, Porakishvili N, et al. CD5-induced apoptosis of B cells in some patients with chronic lymphocytic leukemia. Leukemia 2002; 16(1):44–52.

161. Renaudineau Y, Nedellec S, Berthou C, et al. Role of B-cell antigen receptor-associated molecules and lipid rafts in CD5-induced apoptosis of B CLL cells. Leukemia 2005; 19(2): 223–229.

162. Pers JO, Jamin C, Le Corre R, Lydyard PM, Youinou P. Ligation of CD5 on resting B cells, but not on resting T cells, results in apoptosis. Eur J Immunol 1998; 28(12):4170–4176.

163. Cioca DP, Kitano K. Apoptosis induction by hypercross-linking of the surface antigen CD5 with anti-CD5 monoclonal antibodies in B cell chronic lymphocytic leukemia. Leukemia 2002; 16(3):335–343.

164. Perez-Chacon G, Vargas JA, Jorda J, et al. CD5 provides viability signals to B cells from a subset of B-CLL patients by a mechanism that involves PKC. Leuk Res 2007; 31(2):183–193.

165. Gary-Gouy H, Sainz-Perez A, Marteau JB, et al. Natural phosphorylation of CD5 in chronic lymphocytic leukemia B cells and analysis of CD5-regulated genes in a B cell line suggest a role for CD5 in malignant phenotype. J Immunol 2007; 179(7):4335–4344.

166. Pospisil R, Fitts MG, Mage RG. CD5 is a potential selecting ligand for B cell surface immunoglobulin framework region sequences. J Exp Med 1996; 184(4):1279–1284.

167. Biancone L, Bowen MA, Lim A, et al. Identification of a novel inducible cell-surface ligand of CD5 on activated lymphocytes. J Exp Med 1996; 184(3):811–819.

168. Bikah G, Lynd FM, Aruffo AA, et al. A role for CD5 in cognate interactions between T cells and B cells, and identification of a novel ligand for CD5. Int Immunol 1998; 10(8):1185–1196.

169. Calvo J, Places L, Padilla O, et al. Interaction of recombinant and natural soluble CD5 forms with an alternative cell surface ligand. Eur J Immunol 1999; 29(7):2119–2129.

170. Van de Velde H, von Hoegen I, Luo W, et al. The B-cell surface protein CD72/Lyb-2 is the ligand for CD5. Nature 1991; 351(6328):662–665.

171. Gordon J. B-cell signalling via the C-type lectins CD23 and CD72. Immunol Today 1994; 15(9):411–417.

172. Pan C, Baumgarth N, Parnes JR. CD72-deficient mice reveal nonredundant roles of CD72 in B cell development and activation. Immunity 1999; 11(4):495–506.

173. Cerutti A, Trentin L, Zambello R, et al. The CD5/CD72 receptor system is coexpressed with several functionally relevant counterstructures on human B cells and delivers a critical signaling activity. J Immunol 1996; 157(5):1854–1862.

174. Kumanogoh A, Watanabe C, Lee I, et al. Identification of CD72 as a lymphocyte receptor for the class IV semaphorin CD100: a novel mechanism for regulating B cell signaling. Immunity 2000; 13(5):621–631.

175. Granziero L, Circosta P, Scielzo C, et al. CD100/Plexin-B1 interactions sustain proliferation and survival of normal and leukemic CD5+ B lymphocytes. Blood 2003; 101(5): 1962–1969.

176. Gagro A, Dasic G, Sabioncello A, et al. Phenotypic analysis of receptor-ligand pairs on B-cells in B-chronic lymphocytic leukemia. Leuk Lymphoma 1997; 25(3–4):301–311.

177. Tamir I, Dal Porto JM, Cambier JC. Cytoplasmic protein tyrosine phosphatases SHP-1 and SHP-2: regulators of B cell signal transduction. Curr Opin Immunol 2000; 12(3):307–315.

178. Camilleri-Broet S, Cassard L, Broet P, et al. FcgammaRIIB is differentially expressed during B cell maturation and in B-cell lymphomas. Br J Haematol 2004; 124(1):55–62.

179. Gamberale R, Fernandez-Calotti P, Sanjurjo J, et al. Signaling capacity of FcgammaRII isoforms in B-CLL cells. Leuk Res 2005; 29(11):1277–1284.

180. Pearse RN, Kawabe T, Bolland S, et al. SHIP recruitment attenuates Fc gamma RIIB-induced B cell apoptosis. Immunity 1999; 10(6):753–760.

181. Jackson DG, Bell JI. Isolation of a cDNA encoding the human CD38 (T10) molecule, a cell surface glycoprotein with an unusual discontinuous pattern of expression during lymphocyte differentiation. J Immunol 1990; 144(7):2811–2815.

182. Deaglio S, Vaisitti T, Aydin S, et al. In-tandem insight from basic science combined with clinical research: CD38 as both marker and key component of the pathogenetic network underlying chronic lymphocytic leukemia. Blood 2006; 108(4):1135–1144.

183. Deaglio S, Morra M, Mallone R, et al. Human CD38 (ADP-ribosyl cyclase) is a counter-receptor of CD31, an Ig superfamily member. J Immunol 1998; 160(1):395–402.

184. Deaglio S, Mallone R, Baj G, et al. CD38/CD31, a receptor/ligand system ruling adhesion and signaling in human leukocytes. Chem Immunol 2000; 75:99–120.

185. Cockayne DA, Muchamuel T, Grimaldi JC, et al. Mice deficient for the ecto-nicotinamide adenine dinucleotide glycohydrolase CD38 exhibit altered humoral immune responses. Blood 1998; 92(4):1324–1333.

186. Lund FE, Yu N, Kim KM, et al. Signaling through CD38 augments B cell antigen receptor (BCR) responses and is dependent on BCR expression. J Immunol 1996; 157(4):1455–1467.

187. Deaglio S, Capobianco A, Bergui L, et al. CD38 is a signaling molecule in B-cell chronic lymphocytic leukemia cells. Blood 2003; 102(6):2146–2155.

188. Damle RN, Temburni S, Calissano C, et al. CD38 expression labels an activated subset within chronic lymphocytic leukemia clones enriched in proliferating B cells. Blood 2007; 110(9): 3352–3359.

189. Deaglio S, Vaisitti T, Aydin S, et al. CD38 and ZAP-70 are functionally linked and mark CLL cells with high migratory potential. Blood 2007; 110(12):4012–4021.

190. Jaksic O, Paro MM, Kardum Skelin I, et al. CD38 on B-cell chronic lymphocytic leukemia cells has higher expression in lymph nodes than in peripheral blood or bone marrow. Blood 2004; 103(5):1968–1969.

191. Matrai Z. CD38 as a prognostic marker in CLL. Hematology (Amsterdam, Netherlands) 2005; 10(1):39–46.

192. Del Poeta G, Maurillo L, Venditti A, et al. Clinical significance of CD38 expression in chronic lymphocytic leukemia. Blood 2001; 98(9):2633–2639.

193. Ibrahim S, Keating M, Do KA, et al. CD38 expression as an important prognostic factor in B-cell chronic lymphocytic leukemia. Blood 2001; 98(1):181–186.

194. Hamblin TJ, Orchard JA, Ibbotson RE, et al. CD38 expression and immunoglobulin variable region mutations are independent prognostic variables in chronic lymphocytic leukemia, but CD38 expression may vary during the course of the disease. Blood 2002; 99(3):1023–1029.

195. Durig J, Naschar M, Schmucker U, et al. CD38 expression is an important prognostic marker in chronic lymphocytic leukaemia. Leukemia 2002; 16(1):30–35.

196. Ghia P, Caligaris-Cappio F. The origin of B-cell chronic lymphocytic leukemia. Semin Oncol 2006; 33(2):150–156.

197. Caligaris-Cappio F. Role of the microenvironment in chronic lymphocytic leukaemia. Br J Haematol 2003; 123(3):380–388.

198. Ghia P, Granziero L, Chilosi M, et al. Chronic B cell malignancies and bone marrow microenvironment. Semin Cancer Biol 2002; 12(2):149–155.

199. Granziero L, Ghia P, Circosta P, et al. Survivin is expressed on CD40 stimulation and interfaces proliferation and apoptosis in B-cell chronic lymphocytic leukemia. Blood 2001; 97(9):2777–2783.

200. Ruprecht CR, Lanzavecchia A. Toll-like receptor stimulation as a third signal required for activation of human naive B cells. Eur J Immunol 2006; 36(4):810–816.

201. Pasare C, Medzhitov R. Toll-like receptors: linking innate and adaptive immunity. Microbes Infect 2004; 6(15):1382–1387.

202. Lanzavecchia A, Sallusto F. Toll-like receptors and innate immunity in B-cell activation and antibody responses. Curr Opin Immunol 2007; 19(3):268–274.
203. Malisan F, Fluckiger AC, Ho S, et al. B-chronic lymphocytic leukemias can undergo isotype switching in vivo and can be induced to differentiate and switch in vitro. Blood 1996; 87(2): 717–724.
204. Fluckiger AC, Rossi JF, Bussel A, et al. Responsiveness of chronic lymphocytic leukemia B cells activated via surface Igs or CD40 to B-cell tropic factors. Blood 1992; 80(12): 3173–3181.
205. Buske C, Gogowski G, Schreiber K, et al. Stimulation of B-chronic lymphocytic leukemia cells by murine fibroblasts, IL-4, anti-CD40 antibodies, and the soluble CD40 ligand. Exp Hematol 1997; 25(4):329–337.
206. Kitada S, Zapata JM, Andreeff M, et al. Bryostatin and CD40-ligand enhance apoptosis resistance and induce expression of cell survival genes in B-cell chronic lymphocytic leukaemia. Br J Haematol 1999; 106(4):995–1004.
207. Romano MF, Lamberti A, Tassone P, et al. Triggering of CD40 antigen inhibits fludarabine-induced apoptosis in B chronic lymphocytic leukemia cells. Blood 1998; 92(3):990–995.
208. Fu SM, Chiorazzi N, Kunkel HG, et al. Induction of in vitro differentiation and immunoglobulin synthesis of human leukemic B lymphocytes. J Exp Med 1978; 148(6): 1570–1578.
209. Totterman TH, Nilsson K, Sundstrom C. Phorbol ester-induced differentiation of chronic lymphocytic leukaemia cells. Nature 1980; 288(5787):176–178.
210. Gordon J, Mellstedt H, Aman P, et al. Phenotypic modulation of chronic lymphocytic leukemia cells by phorbol ester: induction of IgM secretion and changes in the expression of B cell-associated surface antigens. J Immunol 1984; 132(1):541–547.
211. Caligaris-Cappio F, Hamblin TJ. B-cell chronic lymphocytic leukemia: a bird of a different feather. J Clin Oncol 1999; 17(1):399–408.
212. Chiorazzi N, Rai KR, Ferrarini M. Chronic lymphocytic leukemia. N Engl J Med 2005; 352(8):804–815.
213. Serrano D, Monteiro J, Allen SL, et al. Clonal expansion within the CD4+CD57+ and CD8+CD57+ T cell subsets in chronic lymphocytic leukemia. J Immunol 1997; 158(3): 1482–1489.
214. Pizzolo G, Chilosi M, Ambrosetti A, et al. Immunohistologic study of bone marrow involvement in B-chronic lymphocytic leukemia. Blood 1983; 62(6):1289–1296.
215. Davey FR, Kurec AS, Tomar RH, et al. Serum immunoglobulins and lymphocyte subsets in chronic lymphocytic leukemia. Am J Clin Pathol 1987; 87(1):60–65.
216. Chiorazzi N, Fu SM, Montazeri G, et al. T cell helper defect in patients with chronic lymphocytic leukemia. J Immunol 1979; 122(3):1087–1090.
217. Muzio M, Mantovani A. Toll-like receptors. Microbes Infect 2000; 2(3):251–255.
218. Akira S. TLR signaling. Curr Top Microbiol Immunol 2006; 311:1–16.
219. Akira S. Toll-like receptors: lessons from knockout mice. Biochem Soc Trans 2000; 28(5): 551–556.
220. Spaner DE, Masellis A. Toll-like receptor agonists in the treatment of chronic lymphocytic leukemia. Leukemia 2007; 21(1):53–60.
221. Gauld SB, Merrell KT, Cambier JC. Silencing of autoreactive B cells by anergy: a fresh perspective. Curr Opin Immunol 2006; 18(3):292–297.
222. Healy JI, Dolmetsch RE, Timmerman LA, et al. Different nuclear signals are activated by the B cell receptor during positive versus negative signaling. Immunity 1997; 6(4):419–428.
223. Merrell KT, Benschop RJ, Gauld SB, et al. Identification of anergic B cells within a wild-type repertoire. Immunity 2006; 25(6):953–962.
224. Gauld SB, Benschop RJ, Merrell KT, et al. Maintenance of B cell anergy requires constant antigen receptor occupancy and signaling. Nat Immunol 2005; 6(11):1160–1167.

5

Etiology of CLL: The Role of MBL

Paolo Ghia
*Unit and Laboratory of Lymphoid Malignancies, Department of Oncology,
Università Vita-Salute San Raffaele and Istituto Scientifico San Raffaele,
Milano, Italy*

Andrew C. Rawstron
*Department of Haematology, St. James's Institute of Oncology, HMDS,
Leeds Teaching Hospitals, Leeds, U.K.*

CLL: EPIDEMIOLOGY AND ETIOLOGY

Chronic lymphocytic leukemia (CLL) is the most common form of leukemia among older adults in western countries, accounting for around 30% of all leukemias (1), though in a proportion of cases it can present with lymphoadenomegaly with a limited, if any, peripheral blood involvement (defined as "Small Lymphocytic Lymphoma" - SLL). Data from the United States Surveillance, Epidemiology, and End Results (SEER) Registry estimate the U.S. incidence between 1996 and 2000 to be 3.7 per 100,000 individuals per year, being rather stable over the past decades (2,3). The median age at diagnosis is 72 years (4), though, in recent years, one-third of new cases are diagnosed before the age of 55 years (5), indicating an increase in the incidence among younger individuals. Given the long median survival of the disease (around 10 years), prevalence of CLL is 0.03% to 0.05%, i.e., 30 to 50 individuals affected among 100,000 citizens. Overall, CLL diagnosis may be underestimated because of underreporting and incomplete case ascertainment (6), which did not change over the last 40 years (3). Age-adjusted incidence rates for CLL/SLL were 70% to 90% higher among males than females, with a sex ratio of about 1.5–2:1 (1). Although male gender is an important risk factor for most hematological malignancies (7,8), the causal factors underlying this association are unknown. Occupational exposures are always of potential concern in male-predominant cancers.

ETIOLOGY

The etiology of CLL is mostly unknown, though advanced age, Caucasian race, and family history of CLL or other lymphoproliferative malignancies have consistently been recognized as risk factors for CLL (2,5,8–12), indicating a genetic and familial predisposition in the pathogenesis of the disease. In particular, age-adjusted incidence rates for CLL/

SLL are 25% to 28% and 69% to 80% lower among African-Americans and Asian/Pacific islanders, respectively, as compared with Caucasians (13). These race-specific differences in incidence rates in the United States are similar to those present in the native populations in the countries of origin (8) Interestingly, the low incidence rates persist among emigrants to the United States from Asian countries and their descendants, excluding an environmental or lifestyle influence (9,11,14–16).

In addition, over the past 60 years, it has been repeatedly observed that a family history of CLL or other lymphoproliferative disease (LPD) is one of the strongest risk factors for development of CLL (13,17,18), with around 5% to 10% of CLL cases being familial, i.e., two or more individuals within the same family are affected (19,20). First relatives of CLL patients have an overall risk to develop the same disease between two and seven times higher than the general population (21). This familial predisposition is accompanied by the so-called anticipation phenomenon (20,22–24), i.e., an earlier onset and a more severe course of the disease in the descendants. In terms of clinical, molecular, and biological features, familial CLL shares a high similarity with the sporadic cases.

Beside genetic and familial factors predisposing to CLL, very little is known in terms of causal factors determining the onset of the disease (6). Several studies of populations exposed to any known environmental factor have evaluated diverse environmental and occupational exposures such as chemical compounds, pesticides, viruses, ionizing radiation, and nonionizing power-frequency magnetic fields, but have not found consistent associations (25,26). These studies do not allow any final conclusions to be drawn because of several limitations particularly applying when CLL is studied. As previously mentioned, CLL is rare in particular populations (e.g., Japanese atomic bomb survivors) (27,28), has a very long natural history with a prolonged subclinical phase, and is frequently misclassified in death certificate, leading to the grouping of CLL with other leukemias or lymphomas (29–31). More recently, a case-control study of leukemia incidence among uranium miners found a positive association of CLL with cumulative radon exposure (32), and an ecological study of radon exposure in Iowa, a SEER catchment area, demonstrated a weak association with CLL (33). In addition, an excess of risks of CLL and related LPD may be present in farmers and in other agricultural occupations (34), as suggested by several observations (35–39), though no particular linkage with specific agricultural chemical exposures has been studied (36,38,40). Excesses of lymphocytic leukemia (41) and non-Hodgkin lymphoma (NHL) (42) have been also reported in a few studies of rubber workers and petroleum workers (43), suggesting a possible role for solvents and other chemicals, e.g., benzene and butadiene.

Taken together, these preliminary observations strongly indicate the need for new epidemiological studies primarily focused on CLL with lifetime follow-up of exposed cohorts to allow for long latency to finally assess the role of agriculture and occupational chemical and radiation exposure in the pathogenesis of the disease.

CLL is not more frequent in patients affected by immunodeficiencies (1) or autoimmune disorders (44–46). Recent studies from Scandinavia (47) and the United States (48) found no elevated risks of CLL associated with the broad categories of infectious disease and chronic inflammatory and allergic conditions. However, elevated risks were found to be associated with personal history of respiratory tract infections (pneumonia and chronic sinusitis), herpes viruses (simplex and zoster), chronic osteoarthritis, and prostatitis. It is possible that pneumonia or other infectious could be an early, prediagnostic sign of CLL because of the characteristic immunodeficiency. Nevertheless, two studies (47,48) reported that individuals with a previous history of chronic nonrheumatic valvular disease or chronic rheumatic heart disease had a 25% reduced risk of CLL, which might reflect decreased bacterial infections because of antibiotic prophylaxis in this patient group (49,50).

Interestingly, several biological, molecular, and functional evidences (see chaps.1,2, and 4) strongly support the possibility that an antigenic stimulation (either by self- or foreign antigens) might play a relevant role in the natural history of the disease. This may imply that chronic infectious or noninfectious prolonged self-antigenic stimulation is potentially relevant for the onset and progression of CLL.

Monoclonal B lymphocytes showing a CLL-like phenotype are frequently recognized in the peripheral blood of otherwise healthy individuals, thereby suggesting a potential etiological role in the pathogenesis of CLL. Detailed information on epidemiological patterns, biological features, and risk of clinical progression has recently been gathered, allowing a better understanding of the interrelationship between this entity and CLL.

DEFINITION OF MBL

NCI-IWCLL Guidelines

In the past, the clinical diagnosis of CLL required an absolute lymphocytosis with a lower threshold of greater than 5000 mature-appearing lymphocytes/μL in the peripheral blood (51). However, these guidelines were written at a time when relatively few laboratories would have been able to characterize CLL cells, unless they represented the majority of lymphocytes. As multiparameter flow cytometry has become more widely available, so it is more likely that CLL cells will be detected in individuals when they do not represent the majority of cells. Several studies have demonstrated that CLL-phenotype cells may be demonstrated at low level in the general population and in otherwise healthy first-degree relatives of CLL patients (52).

To ensure a uniformity in the classification of CLL and in particular to ensure that individuals with a very low level of CLL cells with a reactive T-cell lymphocytosis are not classified as having a hematological malignancy, the current National Cancer Institute - International Workshop on Chronic Lymphocytic Leukemia (NCI-IWCLL) guidelines propose that the threshold for diagnosis of CLL will require an absolute B-cell count above 5000/μL. It is recognized that CLL or SLL might be suspected in otherwise healthy adults who have an absolute increase in the clonal B lymphocytes, but who have less than 5000 B lymphocytes/μL blood. However, in the absence of lymphadenopathy, organomegaly, cytopenias, or disease-related symptoms, the presence of fewer than 5000 B lymphocytes per μL blood has to be defined as a distinct entity named monoclonal B-cell lymphocytosis (MBL) (53).

The diagnosis of MBL is based on the identification of a clonal lymphocyte population by immunophenotypic characterization. Different laboratories have used diverse approaches to identify minimal B-cell monoclonal lymphocytosis, making comparisons across geographical and ethnic and in different risk groups difficult. To standardize and facilitate future studies, Jerry Marti and colleagues proposed the following set of guidelines for the diagnostic characterization of a blood MBL (54).

Diagnostic Criteria

1. Detection of a monoclonal B-cell population in the peripheral blood with
   a. overall κ:λ ratio greater or less than 3:1, or
   b. greater than 25% of B cells lacking or expressing low-level surface immunoglobulin (sIg), or
   c. a disease-specific immunophenotype.
2. Repeat assessment should demonstrate that the monoclonal B-cell population is stable over a three-month period.

3. Exclusion criteria include
    a. lymphadenopathy and organomegaly, or
    b. associated autoimmune/infectious disease, or
    c. B-lymphocyte count greater than 5×10^9/L, or
    d. any other feature diagnostic of a B-LPD. However, a paraprotein may be present or associated with MBL and should be evaluated independently.
4. Subclassification:
    a. $CD5^+23^+$: together with low levels of CD20, CD79b, and sIg, represents the major subcategory and corresponds to a CLL immunophenotype (51).
    b. $CD5^+23^{+/-}$: with moderate level of CD20 and CD79b expression corresponds to an atypical CLL immunophenotype.
    c. $CD5^-$: corresponds to non-CLL LPD.

Figure 1 shows the phenotypic profiles with respect to CD20 and CD5.

Additional Comments

1. The detection of any B-cell monoclonal population by light chain restriction is a sufficient criterion. More than one set of κ/λ light chain reagents may be used to confirm the abnormal ratio. Confirmation with IgH-PCR (Immunoglobulin Heavy chain gene Polymerase Chain Reaction) may be helpful, but is not essential.
2. The monoclonal B-cell population may represent a minority of total B cells when identified by a disease-specific immunophenotype. These may be demonstrable even if the overall κ:λ ratio is normal, although clonality must be demonstrated within the cellular population identified by the disease-specific phenotype.
3. MBL lacking sIg is associated with $CD5^+CD23^+$ MBL.
4. A minimum of three colors (CD19 or CD20, antikappa, and antilambda) should be used to confirm clonality, although four or more colors are preferable.
5. The fluorescence intensity of sIg, CD20, and CD79b expression if moderately increased should be noted.
6. The number of cells analyzed should allow the formation of a cluster containing at least 50 events.
7. Repeat flow cytometric analysis is not necessary for research applications if monoclonality is confirmed by other approaches, e.g., fluorescence in situ hybridization or PCR, but may be useful for monitoring.
8. A disease-specific phenotype exists for hairy cell leukemia ($CD5^-CD103^+$ $CD11c^+CD25^{\pm}$), but it is probable that a full diagnosis of hairy cell leukemia will be made in the presence of any level of circulating disease.
9. Other subclassifications may be included if sufficiently specific tests with evidence of a clinical association can be confirmed.

MBL IN ANIMAL MODELS

Animal models have been extensively used to study LPDs, though in CLL their use has been limited because of the biological features of the disease, including latency of the onset and lack of known specific genetic abnormalities (55).

That notwithstanding, several genetic strains are frequently characterized by an increase in B-cell number and a progressive restriction of the Ig repertoire with the

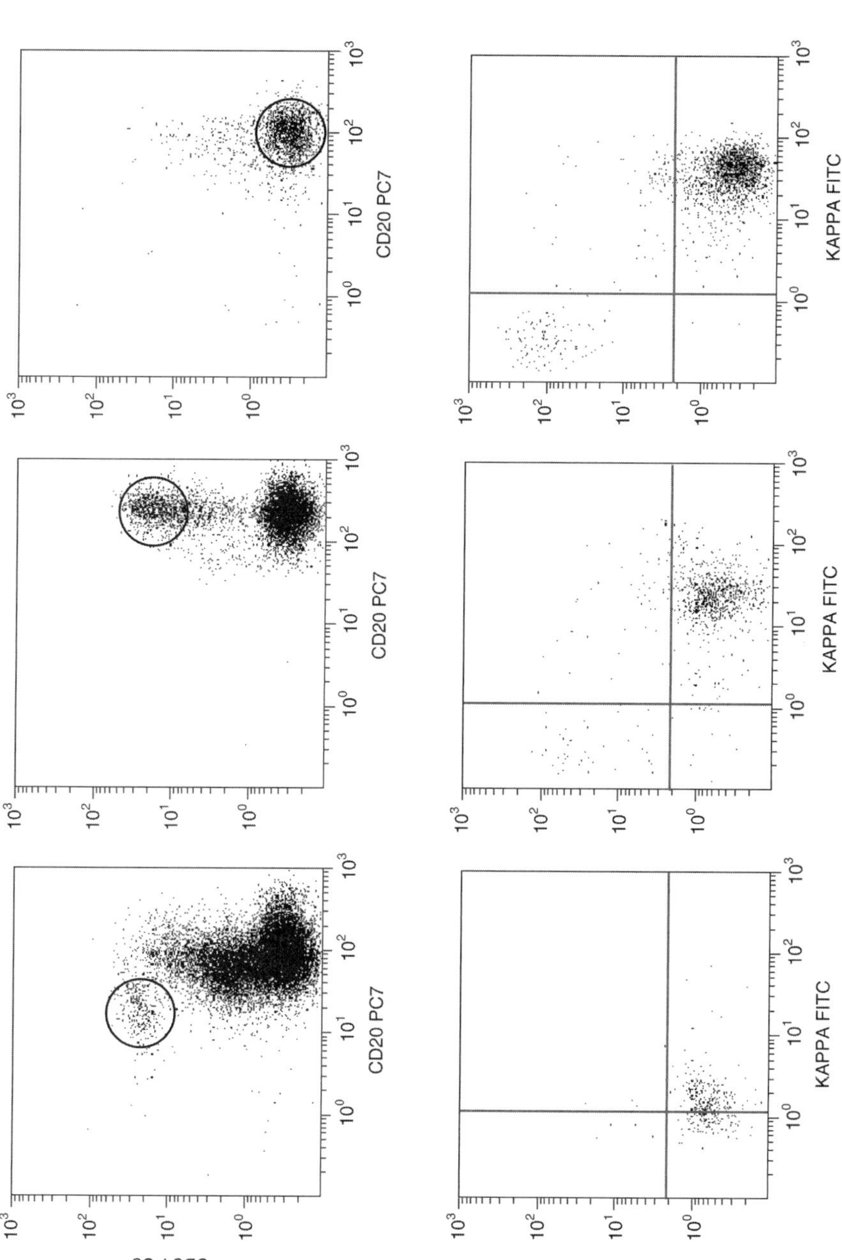

Figure 1 MBL are phenotypically heterogeneous and may express a CLL-like phenotype, being CD5[+] together with low levels of CD20 and Igs (*upper and lower left panels*), or an atypical CLL phenotype, being CD5[+] with normal levels of both CD20 and Ig (*upper and lower middle panels*). MBL can also lack completely CD5 expression (non-CLL phenotype, *upper and lower right panels*). *Abbreviations*: MBL, monoclonal B-cell lymphocytosis; CLL, chronic lymphocytic leukemia; Ig, immunoglobulin.

accumulation of oligo- and monoclonal B-cell populations with age, mainly $CD5^+$. This phenomenon closely resembles the MBL occurrence in aging humans, and, similarly, it shares several common features.

Typical examples are the New Zealand black (NZB) and the New Zealand white (NZW) mice. The NZB animal has been extensively studied as a model for autoimmune diseases such as systemic lupus erythematosus (SLE) (56,57), as it is characterized by autoimmunity early in life. In addition, aged NZB mice exhibit monoclonal lymphoproliferative expansions characterized by increased numbers of $CD5^+$ B cells (58), mainly detected in the spleen and peripheral blood (59), developing a frank leukemia usually after 9 to 12 months (60). Similarly, aged NZW mice also exhibit an expansion of $CD5^+$ B-1 cells and eventually develop a CLL-like disease with time (61).

These two strains are commonly used to produce the (NZB × NZW) F1 hybrid model that spontaneously develops an autoimmune disease similar to human SLE (62–64). These mice develop higher titres of anti-DNA autoantibodies, but have a lower incidence of B-cell malignancies as compared with the parental NZB and NZW strains.

Genetic studies have provided evidence that different major histocompatibility complex (MHC) haplotypes in these mice may be responsible for the development of an SLE- or CLL-like phenotype. H-2-congenic mice established from NZB, NZW, and (NZB × NZW) F1 mice showed that H-2d/z heterozygosity in all the three strains predisposed mice to develop an SLE-like disease (61,65). Contrary to this, H-2z/z homozygous mice developed CLL characterized by accumulation of $CD19^+CD5^+$ B-1 cells in peripheral blood and lymphoid organs (61,66).

The development of $CD5^+$ clonal populations is not a unique feature of B/W-related mice, but the occurrence of clonal $CD5^+$ B-cell populations appears to be a rather frequent phenomenon in mice, as it can be observed in all strains tested, though with a greater delay of onset. In normal strains, including BALB/c, C57BL/6, and CBA mice, B-cell monoclonal expansions can be detected only in senescent mice (>15 months). The age of onset of clonal development is the only major difference between normal mice strains and New Zealand-related mice, where the process seems to be accelerated. However, once present, the $CD5^+$ clones expand and migrate similarly in all strains (67,68).

Initially, all the B-cell clones that were detected in the unfractionated splenic B-cell populations of these animals were detected in the $CD5^+$, but not in the $CD5^-$-negative B-cell populations (67). A further analysis clearly demonstrated that stable monoclonal expansions can be observed in both $CD5^+$ and $CD5^-$ B lymphocytes (as well as in plasma cells) (69), as it occurs in human MBL, suggesting that this phenomenon might be a common event because of the normal aging of all B-cell compartments.

GENERAL POPULATION STUDIES IN HEALTHY ADULTS

Superfund Sites in the United States

A series of cross-sectional population-based studies were conducted in the United States to determine whether subclinical organ-system dysfunction associated with prior health conditions was more common in residents who lived near hazardous waste sites (target population) than in residents who lived in comparison areas. Target populations consisted of residents living in well-defined areas that were located close to hazardous waste sites. The selection of each target area was based on environmental sampling data that identified contaminated soil, groundwater, surface water, or sediment. The comparison areas were located in the same general region; they were more than five miles from the site of interest and were not near any other hazardous waste sites. The comparison area for each study was matched to the target area with regard to demographic factors, including style and age of housing, household income, and location in or near an urban population center. Typically, participants were required to have lived in the area for at least one full year to be eligible for the study.

The study protocol incorporated standardized medical test batteries that included an immune biomarker panel with basic immunophenotyping for the major lymphocyte lineages T cells, B cells, and natural killer (NK) cells and selected markers for lymphocyte subsets. This basic immunophenotyping panel did not include κ/λ analysis. All initial immunophenotyping was conducted at the U.S. Centers for Disease Control and Prevention (CDC) laboratory using two-color panels. Results were obtained from 4420 participants ranging in age from less than 1 to 78 years. Using this two-color panel, B-cell phenotypic patterns suggesting the presence of a monoclonal B-cell population were observed in 11 participants ranging in age from 47 to 72 years. All but one had a total B-cell count in the highly elevated range. Three of these participants were referred for further testing by κ/λ immunophenotyping at the U S Food and Drug Administration, and κ-restricted monoclonality was found in all of them (70).

Follow-up investigations were conducted in 1997 and 2003 to determine whether monoclonality could be confirmed in participants with suggestive phenotypes in the original studies and to determine whether monoclonal B-cell populations could be detected by κ/λ analysis in additional participants with high B-cell counts. The inclusion criteria were age above 40 years during the initial study and total B-cell counts, $CD5^+$ B-cell counts, or $CD5^+$ B-cell percentage of all B cells in the upper 2.5th percentile of the study population. All of the 11 persons with suggestive phenotypes met the eligibility criteria, but 2 of the 11 were excluded when they were found to have a diagnosed B-cell malignancy. Of the 74 eligible individuals, 59 participated in the first follow-up and 49 participated in the second follow-up. Of the original nine presumptive MBL cases, six participated in the first follow-up, and monoclonal B-cell populations were confirmed by κ/λ phenotyping and PCR immunoglobulin heavy chain (IGH) rearrangement in all of them. Two additional MBL cases were uncovered among the 53 participants with no previous findings, making a total of eight cases identified in the first follow-up. Four MBL cases had died by the second follow-up, and MBL was still present in the remaining four (71).

Detection of MBL in Hospital Outpatients

The U.K. Study

In the study from the United Kingdom, 910 EDTA (ethylenediaminetetraacetic acid) peripheral blood samples from 425 males and 485 females were selected. Samples had a normal leukocyte count and differential, normal platelet count, and normal hemoglobin level. Samples were chosen from GP referrals, ophthalmology, gynecology, cardiology, dermatology, orthopedic preop, or patients presenting to the emergency room with chest pain and shortness of breath or trauma and no previous or current record of malignancy. Samples were balanced to represent the age and sex distribution of the normal U.K. population.

Leukocytes were prepared from EDTA peripheral blood by ammonium chloride lysis and incubated with CD19 PE-Cy5 (CD19 phycoerythrin-Cy5) and CD5 APC (CD5 allophycocyanin) plus CD20 FITC (CD20 fluorescein isothiocyanate) and CD79b PE or antikappa FITC and antilambda PE as well as CD19 PE-Cy5 and CD5 APC. A minimum of 200,000 total leukocytes was acquired and cases were classified as having MBL if at least 50 B-cell events met the criteria for three CLL regions on the basis of protein expression and restricted light chain expression was confirmed. Cells with a CLL phenotype and evidence of light chain restriction were detected in 21 of 425 male and 11 of 485 female individuals, or 3.5% of total. The prevalence increased with age, from 2.1% in the individuals between the ages of 40 and 60 years to 5.0% for individuals over 60 years (chi-square $p = 0.01$). The highest prevalence was found in individuals aged 70 to 79 years, with 8.2% of males and 7.3% of females having a detectable CLL-phenotype population. The male predominance was consistent for all age groups, although least pronounced in the 70- to 79-year-old group. The absolute numbers of CLL-phenotype cells were low, with a median of 13 CLL-phenotype cells/µL, ranging from 3 to 1458 CLL-phenotype cells/µL. Furthermore, the CLL-phenotype cells represented a minor proportion of total B lymphocytes in most cases, at a median of 11%, ranging from 3% to 95% of total B lymphocytes. In addition, a $CD5^-$ MBL was detected because of a perturbation of κ:λ ratio in a further 9 (1%) of the 910 of individuals. These were mostly elderly individuals (median age 78 years, range 49–88 years) (72).

The Italian Study

The original Italian study (73) was conducted in a rural community, outside Turin metropolitan area, and was performed over a period of 20 months in order to exclude any potential seasonal bias. Five hundred individuals (269 females and 231 males) older than 65 years (mean age 73.7 years, the oldest being 98 years) were enrolled. They were outpatients from three different facilities and were referred for common routine blood test (e.g., blood glucose, blood lipids). Those who had a history or a suspicion of malignancy were excluded from the study. All individuals included in the study had a normal blood cell count, with no evidence of lymphocytosis at the routine blood test.

Peripheral blood was drawn and analyzed using two different flow-cytometric protocols: (*i*) CD19/CD5/κ/λ to detect unbalanced light chains ratio in both $CD5^-$ and $CD5^+$ B-lymphocyte populations, as a sign of monoclonality, and (*ii*) CD19/CD20/CD5/CD79b, which detects the CLL-specific phenotype (74). The light chain restriction method allowed to reveal 19 of 500 MBL cases, and an extended cytofluorograph analysis showed that they belonged to three different subtypes: CLL-like, atypical-CLL, and non-CLL, with the first being the most frequent (9/500; 1.8%). Monoclonality was also confirmed with an IGH rearrangement analysis by PCR. Using the more sensitive disease-specific protocol, additional CLL-like MBL could then be detected (13/350; 3.7%), giving rise to a cumulative frequency of 5.5%, in the overall population of individuals older than 65 years, closely resembling the 5% frequency reported among the elderly (>60 years) in the U.K. study (72). CLL-like MBL represented a negligible proportion of total $CD19^+$ B cells, with a mean of 1.8% (range 0.7–4%) of total B lymphocytes, the mean value of total $CD19^+$ B cells being 165/uL (range 85–264/uL) and representing 4% to 20% of all lymphocytes. The prevalence of monoclonal B cells increased with age, being higher in individuals older than 75 years. Also a male prevalence was manifest, especially among the latter age group.

It is interesting to note that beside the different geographical origin both the British and the Italian study (72,73) differed also in terms of selection (primary care vs. hospital outpatients), thereby excluding any potential ethnic or social bias and underscoring the widespread essence of MBL.

A more recent study from the same Italian group was carried out enrolling all individuals older than 18 years belonging to a rural community, outside the Milan metropolitan area, for a total of 1725 individuals. In this study, a more sensitive five-color cytometric technique has been used, and a higher number of events was acquired (1,000,000 vs. 200,000), allowing for the detection of an even higher number of MBL (128/1725; 7.4%). Again, the majority of the MBL detected showed a CLL-like phenotype (89/1725; 5.2%), indicating that the presence of monoclonal B lymphocytes are a very frequent and common phenomenon, and its actual prevalence in the normal population may be higher than previously reported, depending on the sensitivity of the technique used.

FAMILY STUDIES

The study of inherited susceptibility has been a highly informative area of clinical research over the last two decades. The identification of susceptibility genes provides a greater understanding of the mechanisms of disease pathogenesis, offering insight into potential targets for therapeutic intervention. Over 50 families showing distinct clustering of CLL have been reported in the literature (20). This evidence of inherited susceptibility, often termed "familial CLL," is potentially of major importance in identifying some of the events responsible for disease initiation.

Although it is often suggested that familial clusters of common malignancies can be ascribed to ascertainment bias, this is clearly not the case for CLL. A family with three siblings affected with CLL would be expected to occur by chance about every 1000 years in England. Hence, multiple case families provide very strong evidence for an increased familial risk. In addition, a number of large families have been reported, which suggest that predisposition to CLL and other LPDs may be caused by the inheritance of a dominantly acting gene (or genes) with incomplete penetrance and pleiotropic effects (20).

All epidemiological studies that have systematically examined the risk for the development of CLL and other LPDs in relatives of patients (13,18,75–78) have reported elevated risks of CLL in relatives. A study based on around 6000 CLL cases within the Swedish family cancer database demonstrated a sevenfold increase in risk of CLL in first-degree relatives. In addition, risks of other LPDs were also shown to be elevated (17).

Recently, a large scale international study of genomewide linkage in 206 CLL families using high-density single nucleotide polymorphism (SNP) array analysis identified several chromosomal areas of interest, including 2q21.2, 6p22.1, and 18q21.1 and associated candidate genes CXCR4, HLA alleles, and SMAD7, respectively. The results suggest that multiple genes are contributing to the risk of developing CLL in families, and each loci could be epistatic or acting independently (79). Although linkage analysis has proved to be one of the most successful strategies for identifying predisposition loci, the paucity of multiple case families than can be ascertained limits the power of such studies. Only a few families from the 206 pedigrees had been tested for MBL status, and it was noted that future mapping studies of high-risk families incorporating data on MBL status on all available family members would be desirable to better characterize the model.

The reason why MBL status may be so important is the very high prevalence of CLL-phenotype MBL in healthy first-degree relatives of affected individuals in CLL families. The overall relative risk for detection of CLL-phenotype MBL in CLL families is fourfold in comparison with the general population, but for young adults aged 16 to 40 years, the relative risk is 17-fold (80).

The increased relative risk in younger adults may argue for susceptibility in familial CLL, and indeed the average age of onset in familial CLL is approximately 10 to 20 years earlier than in sporadic CLL (20). However, large studies have demonstrated that anticipation is not significant (17), and suggest that, at least in a proportion of families, there is an inherited abnormality that increases susceptibility to development of CLL at a much earlier age than the general population, thus increasing the lifelong risk of developing a clinically apparent CLL clone within the family as a whole.

Analysis of familial CLL also provides strong evidence that the indolent and aggressive forms of CLL share a common oncogenic pathway because the distribution of poor and good risk prognostic factors, including IGHV mutation status, ZAP70, and CD38 expression, is similar between familial and sporadic cases and also segregates within individuals in CLL families (81,82). As the factors responsible for inherited susceptibility are independent of the factors responsible for disease prognosis, determining of the root cause of CLL will require identifying the genetic factors common to CLL-phenotype MBL, indolent CLL, and progressive CLL.

MBL AND SENESCENCE OF THE IMMUNE SYSTEM

Aging deeply affects the immune system in both mice and humans (83), as clearly indicated by the fact that the elderly are more susceptible to pathogens and show an increased morbidity and mortality because of infectious diseases (84), paralleled by a progressive decline in humoral immunity (85). However, B-cell generation continues unabated during adulthood (86–88), and the bone marrow microenvironment does not show any obvious abnormalities. For this reason, the decline in humoral immunity has been commonly attributed to changes in the T-cell compartment (89–91), as a consequence of the thymic involution occurring after puberty (92), in principle depending on an altered helper T-cell activity (67,93). Nevertheless, it is long known that aging individuals tend to produce less diverse antibodies because of limited IGHV gene usage and a lower incidence of somatic hypermutations leading to an antibody response of limited heterogeneity (94,95). Therefore, not only changes in the T-cell compartments but also changes in the B-cell compartments could account for the defects in the immune system observed in older individuals.

The presence of B-cell monoclonal expansions may also concur to this phenomenon. In the past, this was apparently limited to the occurrence of serum monoclonal Igs with age in the overall rare setting of monoclonal gammopathy of undetermined significance (MGUS) (96), but now appears to be a rather widespread event in the elderly, as indicated by the presence of MBL populations in both human (72,73) and mouse (67–69,97).

The fact that MBL clones show a rather heterogeneous phenotype of monoclonal B cells (73), being both CD5$^+$ and CD5$^-$, but also with different levels of CD20 expression (Fig. 1), indicates that this event cannot be disregarded as only belonging to a "curios" B-cell population, but as a more generalized phenomenon, maybe merely reflecting a physiological aspect of immune senescence.

It is well known that aging mice and humans also show decreased diversity of the T-cell repertoire associated to the progressive occurrence of oligoclonal or monoclonal T-cell expansions (98,99), predominantly affecting the CD8$^+$ subset (99–101). In addition, mature CD4$^+$CD8$^+$ double-positive (DP) T cells (2–3% of all circulating T cells) also show the presence of monoclonality in greater than 50% of the individuals older than 65 years (102–104), with a phenotype similar to that of the rare T-cell large granular lymphocyte leukemias, another usually clinically indolent disease.

CD8$^+$ monoclonal expansions have been associated with CMV (Cytomegalovirus) chronic infection (105,106), and DP T lymphocytes have recently been demonstrated to take part in the adaptive immune response against infectious pathogens and in particular against self-limited and latent (e.g., EBV, CMV) viral infections (107). Taking this into account, it can be hypothesized that age-related appearance of monoclonality may be a mere epiphenomenon of a long exposure to chronic antigenic stimulation leading over time to the progressive expansion of the activated clone, thereby becoming manifest especially at an advanced age (108). The hypothesis of an infectious nature of immune-senescence is now well accepted at least in the case of CD8$^+$ T-cell clones.

Though no similar antilatent viral infection has so far been demonstrated for expanding MBL clones, this evidence for DP T cells makes it intriguing to hypothesize that similarly the age-related occurrence of MBL might be dependent on some sort of persistent antigenic stimulus. In the case of B lymphocytes, one may potentially take into consideration also the action of self-antigens. Along the same line of reasoning, the idea of a persistent/ongoing chronic stimulation in the natural history of at least a portion of CLL cases has been repeatedly proposed and supported by experimental evidences (109). Therefore, if this will be confirmed, it may help to draw a scenario suggesting that chronic and relentless activation may then be the prerequisite for the progression to overt malignancy, following a nondispensable oncogenic hit (110).

BIOLOGICAL ASSOCIATION BETWEEN MBL AND CLL

There is a debate in the CLL community about whether MBL cells are genuinely neoplastic or may reflect a normal counterpart of CLL. For this reason, there are several studies which have aimed to identify the extent of any biological relationship between CLL and MBL. Experimental approaches, including phenotypic characterization and cell purification with molecular and cytogenetic analyses, have been recently performed, which helped to shed some light.

Phenotype

The majority of MBL cases show the same expression pattern for the routine diagnostic markers CD5, CD20, CD23, and CD79b as typical CLL. However, in some respects this is a circular argument because the cells are being defined as CLL-like on the basis of these markers. In the original studies, the antigens CD10, CD11a, CD22, CD27, and FMC7 were also assessed, and the monoclonal cells present in these otherwise normal individuals were phenotypically identical to clinical CLL in all cases studied. To assess the protein expression profile in more detail, 18 markers were studied on CD5$^+$23$^+$ MBL cells identified in hospital outpatients with normal blood counts ($n = 11$) and were compared with CLL cells ($n = 9$), normal mature B cells and B-progenitors cells ($n = 7$), and other B-LPDs ($n = 26$). The markers were CD10, CD21, CD22, CD24, CD25, CD27, CD31, CD37, CD39, CD40, CD69, CD81, CD82, CCR6, CCR7, CXCR4, CXCR5, and LAIR-1 with routine diagnostic markers CD5, CD20, CD23, and CD79b excluded to minimize bias. Unsupervised k-means clustering analysis identified two major groups using the dChip analysis program as reported previously (111). The first cluster contained 21 cases, of which 19 of 21 were CLL or MBL, with other disorders including one mantle cell lymphoma and one marginal zone lymphoma. The second cluster contained the normal B cells and the remaining 25 cases, of which only one case was CLL, and no cases of MBL were included. This demonstrates an extremely close association in the extended protein expression profile of CD5$^+$23$^+$ MBL from individuals with a normal blood count and CLL (112), confirming the close biological relationship between the two entities.

Microarray Profiling

Similar evidences were obtained by Brian McCarthy and colleagues using microarray analysis. They previously identified a selected panel of genes comprising FMOD, CKAP4, PI3Kc2b, LEF1, PFTK1, Bcl2 and GPM6a in order of receiver operating characteristic (ROC) concordance. The panel was then used to categorize and predict the relationship of RNA expression between normal donors, MBL cases, and CLL patients. Using this approach, the group could readily distinguish MBL from normal B cells, and the results suggest that LEF1 is a common feature of CLL at all stages of disease (113).

IGHV Gene Usage in MBL

Two recent studies addressed the question of the potential relationship between MBL and CLL, by analyzing the IGHV gene repertoire used in CLL-like MBL cases identified through scientific studies of individuals with normal blood counts and no overt symptoms of a hematological malignancy. In addition, a second group of individuals who had been referred to hematology clinic for investigation of a current or prior mild lymphocytosis and have identifiable CLL-phenotype cells but with a count still below 5000/µL and no other symptoms were also investigated (114–116). There were no significant differences in IGHV gene use between CLL-like MBL cases with a normal blood count and those with an absolute lymphocytosis. Overall, the majority of CLL-like MBL (80–85% of the cases) used mutated IGHV gene, though few unmutated cases could be consistently observed, with some being 100% homologous to the corresponding germ line gene. The mutated cases used predominantly are IGHV3-07, IGHV3-23, IGHV3-30 or IGHV4-34, and IGHV4-59/61 genes, which are also frequently expressed by mutated CLL cases and rarely by unmutated CLL (117). This is shown in Figure 2. These genes belong to the IGHV3 and IGHV4 gene families, which are also the most frequently used families in the normal repertoire. Studies of the normal repertoire have investigated a limited number of

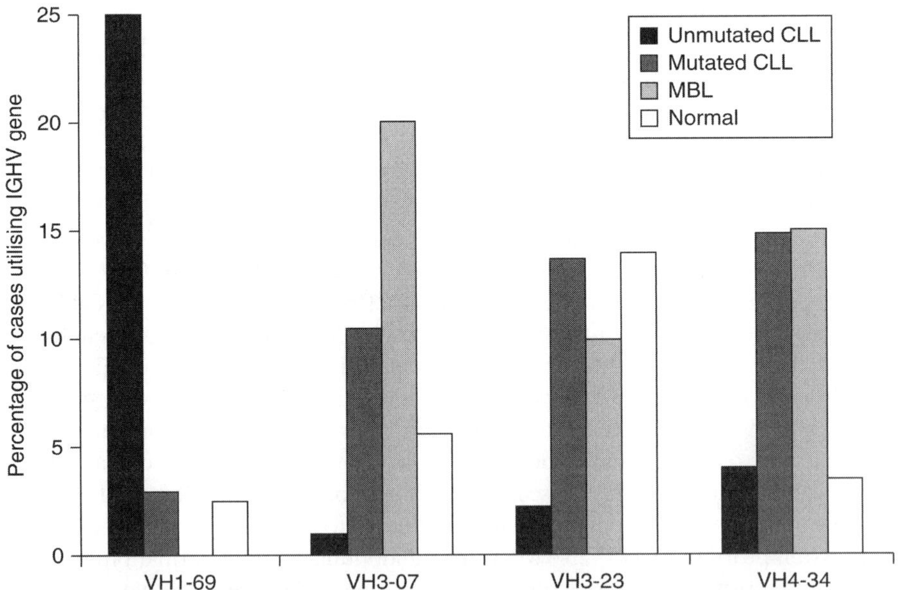

Figure 2 The IGHV gene usage in CLL-phenotype MBL cells is similar to that of mutated CLL and different from unmutated CLL and normal B cells. The four IGHV genes that are most differentially used between CLL, MBL, and normal B cells are shown. The data for CLL-type MBL are from Rawstron et al. (116), for CLL is from Stamatopoulos et al. (117), and for normal B-cells from Fais et al. (129). *Abbreviations*: IGHV, immunoglobulin heavy chain; MBL, monoclonal B-cell lymphocytosis; CLL, chronic lymphocytic leukemia.

normal donors; therefore, it is difficult to determine normal IGHV use, especially in the elderly population. Therefore, one may conclude that the CLL-phenotype MBL show the same biased usage of IGHV genes that are the hallmark of indolent CLL, but this might represent the overall usage of IG genes seen in normal B lymphocytes from elderly donors.

Clonal Selection Vs. Clonal Diversification

Intraclonal heterogeneity in the IGHV genes occurs in approximately half of MGUS patients, but is not present in multiple myeloma (MM) (118). The majority of MGUS patients that progress to MM lack intraclonal variation at the MGUS stage, suggesting that clonal selection is a critical pathway for disease progression in myeloma (119,120). To determine whether clonal selection is also important in MBL and CLL, we compared the degree of IGHV intraclonal heterogeneity in clinic MBL patients with that in CLL patients with progressive disease immediately prior to treatment.

Intraclonal variation was observed in both groups of patients: the median number of unique clones was 2 of 10 (range 0–7/10) in MBL patients and 3 of 10 (range 0–5/10) in CLL patients. Intraclonal variation was generally restricted to 1- or 2-point mutations in each sequence, and for the IGHV gene, the replacement:silent (R:S) ratio of mutations was 1.7 in the framework regions and 3.3 in the complementarity-determining regions. Independent of disease category, unmutated CLL/MBL had a higher degree of intraclonal variation than mutated CLL. The results demonstrate that intraclonal heterogeneity is a frequent occurrence in both MBL and CLL. Clonal heterogeneity is either independent of, or inversely related to, the Ig mutation status, demonstrating that both mutated and unmutated CLL have undergone (or are continuing to undergo) somatic hypermutation. The mechanisms of disease progression in MBL/CLL are clearly biologically distinct from MGUS/myeloma, and these data provide strong evidence for an antigen-driven selection process in CLL (121).

FISH

There is no specific chromosomal translocation associated with CLL, but a 13q deletion is detected in the leukemic cells from over 50% of CLL patients (122). Unlike deletions in other disorders, which often affect the whole of 13q (123), only the 13q14 region is commonly deleted in CLL (124). As a sole abnormality, deletion of 13q14 is associated with a good prognosis. Trisomy 12 and deletion of 11q and/or 17p are also common in CLL; the latter two abnormalities confer a poor prognosis (122). In a recent study, Rawstron et al. performed interphase fluorescent in situ hybridization (FISH) analysis on CD19-selected cells from 38 CLL-type MBL cases with normal blood counts and 33 CLL-type MBL cases with a lymphocytosis. The proportion of cases with a deletion of 13q14 was similar in all groups, detectable in 39% (15/38) of CLL-type MBL with a normal blood count and 58% (19/33) CLL-type MBL cases with a lymphocytosis, compared with the detection rate of 55% (178/325) in CLL (122). Markers associated with poor prognosis (deletion of ATM or P53) were not detected or rarely detected in MBL, and then only in cases with a lymphocytosis. When detected in CLL-type MBL with a lymphocytosis (2/33 ATM deletion and 1/33 P53 deletion), the abnormalities were present in less than 20% of the MBL cells. The proportion of cells with a deletion of 13q14 in the outpatient normal-count MBL group was 5% to 90% of total B cells (115,116). The results demonstrate that the chromosomal abnormality most closely associated with CLL is readily detectable in the CLL-phenotype MBL cells found in individuals with a normal blood count. The presence of poor prognosis markers (ATM deletion and P53 deletion) in MBL questions the real essence of this entity, suggesting a more close resemblance to fully-fledged CLL, and calling for caution when using these cases to study MBL biology.

Clinical Association Between MBL and CLL

Outcome data on MBL patients are limited, partly because the diagnostic criteria have only recently been published and partly because multiparameter flow cytometry was not generally used for diagnosis in the previous century.

Sarah Fung and colleagues recently reported on the outcome for patients with MBL compared to those with stage A CLL (125). The key findings of this paper are that MBL patients have a low probability of early progression, with no patients requiring treatment or dying of CLL-related causes after a median 2.5-year follow-up. There was a trend toward improved progression-free survival compared to Rai stage 0 CLL, but overall survival was very similar between MBL and stage 0 CLL.

A study from the Mayo Clinic has demonstrated that the time to treatment from diagnosis in cases with a total lymphocyte count above 5000 cells/μL was not significantly different if the total B-cell count was higher or lower than 5000 cells/μL, although again there were fewer than 50 MBL cases (126). In a more recent multicenter study, sequential monitoring was performed in 185 CLL-phenotype MBL cases presenting with a lymphocytosis with a median follow-up of 6.7 years (range 0.2–11.8 years). The commonly used cut-point of 5000 lymphocytes/μL was not predictive of outcome. Progressive lymphocytosis, defined as the development of a lymphocyte count that was more than double the presentation level and that increased further at subsequent assessments, was demonstrated in 51 cases (27.5%). The presentation CLL cell count was the only significant independent factor predicting progressive lymphocytosis, whether assessed using cut-points or as a continuous variable. Cases with a count below 1900 CLL cells/μL showed little or no change in total lymphocyte count during follow-up. The hazard ratio was 1.46 (95% confidence interval, 1.12–1.91) for each 1000 CLL cell/μL increase in presentation count (Cox proportional hazard model $p = 0.005$).

Of the 51 cases with a progressive lymphocytosis, 28 of 51 (55%) proceeded to develop further objective evidence of disease progression with a confirmed increase in CLL count above 5000 cells/μL in combination with development of progressive lymphadenopathy/splenomegaly (17/28), and/or anemia or thrombocytopenia (4/28), and/or a lymphocyte doubling time of less than six months (6/28), and/or a substantially increased CLL count above 50,000 cells/μL associated with drenching night sweats or persistent infections (5/28). Thirteen of these patients required chemotherapy for CLL. The estimated rate of progression to CLL requiring treatment is 1.1% per year (95% confidence interval, 0.7–1.9%). None of the factors assessed predicted for the risk of disease progression or requiring treatment. Seven of thirteen treated patients remain alive with a median 1.9 years (range 0–8.6 years) follow-up from initiation of treatment.

The age and hemoglobin concentration at diagnosis were the only independent factors for overall survival. By definition, anemia at diagnosis was not associated with the CLL-phenotype cells. Of 62 deaths, 13 of 62 had documented evidence of disease progression, and the potential causes of death were noted to include CLL in only 4 of 13. Therefore, there is no evidence that MBL has a significant effect on mortality, although progression to CLL may contribute to mortality in a small proportion of cases (115,116).

Predicting outcome in MBL patients is unlikely to be possible using conventional prognostic markers. Lymphocyte doubling time is uninformative because CLL-phenotype cells usually do not represent the majority of lymphocytes. CLL cell CD38 expression does not predict outcome, and initial data suggest that most patients with progressive disease have mutated IGHV genes (127). The reason for the lack of prognostic power is not clear and requires further study, particularly as some patients show an aggressive disease course.

There are many parallels with MGUS: the rate of progression to a stage requiring treatment of 1% per year is similar; the Kaplan–Meier curves of disease progression show no plateau over time, indicating that, as with MGUS, indefinite periodic monitoring may be indicated; and the majority of deaths are due to unrelated causes, even in patients showing evidence of disease progression, although there may be underlying associations that have not yet been identified.

CONCLUSIONS

Monoclonal expansions of B lymphocytes (now defined MBL) (54) may be detected in an increasing number of otherwise healthy individuals (72,73), depending on the progressive improvements in the flow-cytometric technique used to detect them. Of interest, the majority of MBL cells originate from the $CD5^+$ B-cell pool (128), which, in contrast, accounts for a minority of circulating B lymphocytes in humans. An extended phenotype together with microarray analyses of this major MBL subset clearly indicates a close resemblance to CLL, the most common leukemia in aging adults (72,73).

This phenotypic similarity, together with the presence of monoclonality and the increased frequency among the male population, promptly suggests the possibility that MBL may be considered in some respect a preleukemic phase of CLL, similarl to the relationship between MGUS and MM.

That notwithstanding, the prevalence of MBL in the population is at least 100-fold higher than that of CLL, and monoclonality may be just a sign of the senescence process of the normal immune system, thereby indicating the possibility that MBL may be a sort of normal counterpart of CLL, for which neoplastic transformation is not the inevitable fate but rather a quite rare event.

Several biological studies have been performed and more are needed to answer to this critical question, i.e., whether a biological relationship between MBL and CLL exists and to which extent, as no final conclusion can be drawn. The first clinical studies with longer follow-ups are coming out and demonstrating a yearly progression to CLL requiring chemotherapy of approximately 1%. Though this is a strong evidence of a close association similar to the association between MGUS and MM, at the same time it witnesses the rarity of the evolution into a life-threatening disease. Further biological studies are needed to clearly identify those cases that are at higher risk of progression, thereby needing a periodic monitoring, and to avoid lengthy and expensive follow-ups for the enormous number of people carrying MBL in the general population, who will never develop any leukemic disease.

REFERENCES

1. Rozman C, Montserrat E. Chronic lymphocytic leukemia. N Engl J Med 1995; 333(16):1052–1057.
2. Herrinton LJ. Epidemiology of the revised European-American lymphoma classification subtypes. Epidemiol Rev 1998; 20(2):187–203.
3. Turesson I, Linet MS, Bjorkholm M, et al. Ascertainment and diagnostic accuracy for hematopoietic lymphoproliferative malignancies in Sweden 1964-2003. Int J Cancer 2007; 121(10):2260–2266.

4. Ries LA, Wingo PA, Miller DS, et al. The annual report to the nation on the status of cancer, 1973–1997, with a special section on colorectal cancer. Cancer 2000; 88(10):2398–2424.

5. de Lima M, O'Brien S, Lerner S, et al. Chronic lymphocytic leukemia in the young patient. Semin Oncol 1998; 25(1):107–116.

6. Dores GM, Anderson WF, Curtis RE, et al. Chronic lymphocytic leukemia and small lymphocytic lymphoma: overview of the descriptive epidemiology. Br J Haematol 2007; 139(5): 809–819.

7. Cartwright RA, Gurney KA, Moorman AV. Sex ratios and the risks of hematological malignancies. Br J Haematol 2002; 118(4):1071–1077.

8. Morton LM, Wang SS, Devesa SS, et al. Lymphoma incidence patterns by WHO subtype in the United States, 1992–2001. Blood 2006; 107(1):265–276.

9. Boggs DR, Chen SC, Zhang ZN, et al. Chronic lymphocytic leukemia in China. Am J Hematol 1987; 25(3):349–354.

10. Harris NL, Jaffe ES, Stein H, et al. A revised European-American classification of lymphoid neoplasms: a proposal from the International Lymphoma Study Group. Blood 1994; 84(5): 1361–1392.

11. Weiss NS. Geographical variation in the incidence of the leukemias and lymphomas. Natl Cancer Inst Monogr 1979; (53):139–142.

12. Zent CS, Kyasa MJ, Evans R, et al. Chronic lymphocytic leukemia incidence is substantially higher than estimated from tumor registry data. Cancer 2001; 92(5):1325–1330.

13. Linet MS, Van Natta ML, Brookmeyer R, et al. Familial cancer history and chronic lymphocytic leukemia. A case-control study. Am J Epidemiol 1989; 130(4):655–664.

14. Gale RP, Cozen W, Goodman MT, et al. Decreased chronic lymphocytic leukemia incidence in Asians in Los Angeles County. Leuk Res 2000; 24(8):665–669.

15. Herrinton LJ, Goldoft M, Schwartz SM, et al. The incidence of non-Hodgkin's lymphoma and its histologic subtypes in Asian migrants to the United States and their descendants. Cancer Causes Control 1996; 7(2):224–230.

16. Pan JW, Cook LS, Schwartz SM, et al. Incidence of leukemia in Asian migrants to the United States and their descendants. Cancer Causes Control 2002; 13(9):791–795.

17. Goldin LR, Pfeiffer RM, Li X, et al. Familial risk of lymphoproliferative tumors in families of patients with chronic lymphocytic leukemia: results from the Swedish Family-Cancer Database. Blood 2004; 104(6):1850–1854.

18. Gunz FW, Gunz JP, Veale AM, et al. Familial leukemia: a study of 909 families. Scand J Haematol 1975; 15(2):117–131.

19. Neuland CY, Blattner WA, Mann DL, et al. Familial chronic lymphocytic leukemia. J Natl Cancer Inst 1983; 71(6):1143–1150.

20. Yuille MR, Matutes E, Marossy A, et al. Familial chronic lymphocytic leukemia: a survey and review of published studies. Br J Haematol 2000; 109(4):794–799.

21. Capalbo S, Trerotoli P, Ciancio A, et al. Increased risk of lymphoproliferative disorders in relatives of patients with B-cell chronic lymphocytic leukemia: relevance of the degree of familial linkage. Eur J Haematol 2000; 65(2):114–117.

22. Goldin LR, Sgambati M, Marti GE, et al. Anticipation in familial chronic lymphocytic leukemia. Am J Hum Genet 1999; 65(1):265–269.

23. Horwitz M, Goode EL, Jarvik GP. Anticipation in familial leukemia. Am J Hum Genet 1996; 59(5):990–998.

24. Wiernik PH, Ashwin M, Hu XP, et al. Anticipation in familial chronic lymphocytic leukemia. Br J Haematol 2001; 113(2):407–414.

25. Finch SC, Linet MS. Chronic leukaemias. Baillieres Clin Haematol 1992; 5(1):27–56.

26. Linet MS, Schubauer-Berigan MK, Weisenburger DD, et al. Chronic lymphocytic leukemia: an overview of aetiology in light of recent developments in classification and pathogenesis. Br J Haematol 2007; 139(5):672–686.

27. Preston DL, Kusumi S, Tomonaga M, et al. Cancer incidence in atomic bomb survivors. Part III. Leukemia, lymphoma and multiple myeloma, 1950–1987. Radiat Res 1994; 137(suppl 2):S68–S97.

28. Preston DL, Pierce DA, Shimizu Y, et al. Effect of recent changes in atomic bomb survivor dosimetry on cancer mortality risk estimates. Radiat Res 2004; 162(4):377–389.

29. Darby SC, Reeves G, Key T, et al. Mortality in a cohort of women given X-ray therapy for metropathia haemorrhagica. Int J Cancer 1994; 56(6):793–801.

30. Hall P, Boice JD, Jr., Berg G, et al. Leukemia incidence after iodine-131 exposure. Lancet 1992; 340(8810):1–4.

31. Muirhead CR, Bingham D, Haylock RG, et al. Follow up of mortality and incidence of cancer 1952-98 in men from the UK who participated in the UK's atmospheric nuclear weapon tests and experimental programmes. Occup Environ Med 2003; 60(3):165–172.

32. Rericha V, Kulich M, Rericha R, et al. Incidence of leukemia, lymphoma, and multiple myeloma in Czech uranium miners: a case-cohort study. Environ Health Perspect 2006; 114(6):818–822.

33. Smith BJ, Zhang L, Field RW. Iowa radon leukemia study: a hierarchical population risk model for spatially correlated exposure measured with error. Stat Med 2007; 26(25):4619–4642.

34. Blair A, Purdue MP, Weisenburger DD, et al. Chemical exposures and risk of chronic lymphocytic leukemia. Br J Haematol 2007; 139(5):753–761.

35. Blair A, White DW. Leukemia cell types and agricultural practices in Nebraska. Arch Environ Health 1985; 40(4):211–214.

36. Brown LM, Blair A, Gibson R, et al. Pesticide exposures and other agricultural risk factors for leukemia among men in Iowa and Minnesota. Cancer Res 1990; 50(20):6585–6591.

37. Burmeister LF, Van Lier SF, Isacson P. Leukemia and farm practices in Iowa. Am J Epidemiol 1982; 115(5):720–728.

38. Miligi L, Costantini AS, Bolejack V, et al. Non-Hodgkin's lymphoma, leukemia, and exposures in agriculture: results from the Italian multicenter case-control study. Am J Ind Med 2003; 44(6):627–636.

39. Zheng T, Blair A, Zhang Y, et al. Occupation and risk of non-Hodgkin's lymphoma and chronic lymphocytic leukemia. J Occup Environ Med 2002; 44(5):469–474.

40. Nanni O, Amadori D, Lugaresi C, et al. Chronic lymphocytic leukaemias and non-Hodgkin's lymphomas by histological type in farming-animal breeding workers: a population case-control study based on a priori exposure matrices. Occup Environ Med 1996; 53(10):652–657.

41. Wolf PH, Andjelkovich D, Smith A, et al. A case-control study of leukemia in the U.S. rubber industry. J Occup Med 1981; 23(2):103–108.

42. Kogevinas M, Sala M, Boffetta P, et al. Cancer risk in the rubber industry: a review of the recent epidemiological evidence. Occup Environ Med 1998; 55(1):1–12.

43. Glass DC, Gray CN, Jolley DJ, et al. Leukemia risk associated with low-level benzene exposure. Epidemiology 2003; 14(5):569–577.

44. Landgren O, Engels EA, Caporaso NE, et al. Patterns of autoimmunity and subsequent chronic lymphocytic leukemia in Nordic countries. Blood 2006; 108(1):292–296.

45. Linet MS, McCaffrey LD, Humphrey RL, et al. Chronic lymphocytic leukemia and acquired disorders affecting the immune system: a case-control study. J Natl Cancer Inst 1986; 77(2): 371–378.

46. Rosenblatt KA, Koepsell TD, Daling JR, et al. Antigenic stimulation and the occurrence of chronic lymphocytic leukemia. Am J Epidemiol 1991; 134(1):22–28.

47. Landgren O, Rapkin JS, Caporaso NE, et al. Respiratory tract infections and subsequent risk of chronic lymphocytic leukemia. Blood 2007; 109(5):2198–2201.

48. Landgren O, Gridley G, Check D, et al. Acquired immune-related and inflammatory conditions and subsequent chronic lymphocytic leukemia. Br J Haematol 2007; 139(5):791–798.

49. Carapetis JR, McDonald M, Wilson NJ. Acute rheumatic fever. Lancet 2005; 366(9480): 155–168.

50. Sirois DA, Fatahzadeh M. Valvular heart disease. Oral Surg Oral Med Oral Pathol Oral Radiol Endod 2001; 91(1):15–19.

51. Cheson BD, Bennett JM, Grever M, et al. National Cancer Institute-sponsored Working Group guidelines for chronic lymphocytic leukemia: revised guidelines for diagnosis and treatment. Blood 1996; 87(12):4990–4997.

52. Marti G, Abbasi F, Raveche E, et al. Overview of monoclonal B-cell lymphocytosis. Br J Haematol 2007; 139(5):701–708.

53. Hallek M, Cheson BD, Catovsky D, et al. Guidelines for the diagnosis and treatment of chronic lymphocytic leukemia: a report from the International Workshop on Chronic Lymphocytic Leukemia (IWCLL) updating the National Cancer Institute-Working Group (NCI-WG) 1996 guidelines. Blood 2008; 111(12):5446–5456.

54. Marti GE, Rawstron AC, Ghia P, et al. Diagnostic criteria for monoclonal B-cell lymphocytosis. Br J Haematol 2005; 130(3):325–332.

55. Dennis C. Cancer: off by a whisker. Nature 2006; 442(7104):739–741.

56. Raveche ES, Steinberg AD. Lymphocytes and lymphocyte functions in systemic lupus erythematosus. Semin Hematol 1979; 16(4):344–370.

57. Theofilopoulos AN. Genetics of systemic autoimmunity. J Autoimmun 1996; 9(2):207–210.

58. Raveche ES. Possible immunoregulatory role for CD5 + B cells. Clin Immunol Immunopathol 1990; 56(2):135–150.

59. Seldin MF, Conroy J, Steinberg AD, et al. Clonal expansion of abnormal B cells in old NZB mice. J Exp Med 1987; 166(5):1585–1590.

60. Phillips JA, Mehta K, Fernandez C, et al. The NZB mouse as a model for chronic lymphocytic leukemia. Cancer Res 1992; 52(2):437–443.

61. Hamano Y, Hirose S, Ida A, et al. Susceptibility alleles for aberrant B-1 cell proliferation involved in spontaneously occurring B-cell chronic lymphocytic leukemia in a model of New Zealand white mice. Blood 1998; 92(10):3772–3779.

62. Helyer BJ, Howie JB. Renal disease associated with positive lupus erythematosus tests in a cross-bred strain of mice. Nature 1963; 197:197.

63. Theofilopoulos AN, Dixon FJ. Murine models of systemic lupus erythematosus. Adv Immunol 1985; 37:269–390.

64. Tokado H, Yumura W, Shiota J, et al. Lupus nephritis in autoimmune-prone NZB × NZW F1 mice and mechanisms of transition of the glomerular lesions. Acta Pathol Jpn 1991; 41(1):1–11.

65. Hirose S, Kinoshita K, Nozawa S, et al. Effects of major histocompatibility complex on autoimmune disease of H-2-congenic New Zealand mice. Int Immunol 1990; 2(11):1091–1095.

66. Okamoto H, Nishimura H, Shinozaki A, et al. H-2z homozygous New Zealand mice as a model for B-cell chronic lymphocytic leukemia: elevated bcl-2 expression in CD5 B cells at premalignant and malignant stages. Jpn J Cancer Res 1993; 84(12):1273–1278.

67. LeMaoult J, Delassus S, Dyall R, et al. Clonal expansions of B lymphocytes in old mice. J Immunol 1997; 159(8):3866–3874.

68. Stall AM, Farinas MC, Tarlinton DM, et al. Ly-1 B-cell clones similar to human chronic lymphocytic leukemias routinely develop in older normal mice and young autoimmune (New Zealand Black-related) animals. Proc Natl Acad Sci U S A 1988; 85(19):7312–7316.

69. LeMaoult J, Manavalan JS, Dyall R, et al. Cellular basis of B cell clonal populations in old mice. J Immunol 1999; 162(11):6384–6391.

70. Vogt RF, Shim YK, Middleton DC, et al. Monoclonal B-cell lymphocytosis as a biomarker in environmental health studies. Br J Haematol 2007; 139(5):690–700.

71. Shim YK, Vogt RF, Middleton D, et al. Prevalence and natural history of monoclonal and polyclonal B-cell lymphocytosis in a residential adult population. Cytometry B Clin Cytom 2007; 72(5):344–353.

72. Rawstron AC, Green MJ, Kuzmicki A, et al. Monoclonal B lymphocytes with the characteristics of "indolent" chronic lymphocytic leukemia are present in 3.5% of adults with normal blood counts. Blood 2002; 100(2):635–639.

73. Ghia P, Prato G, Scielzo C, et al. Monoclonal CD5+ and CD5− B-lymphocyte expansions are frequent in the peripheral blood of the elderly. Blood 2004; 103(6):2337–2342.

74. Rawstron AC, Kennedy B, Evans PA, et al. Quantitation of minimal disease levels in chronic lymphocytic leukemia using a sensitive flow cytometric assay improves the prediction of outcome and can be used to optimize therapy. Blood 2001; 98(1):29–35.

75. Cartwright RA, Bernard SM, Bird CC, et al. Chronic lymphocytic leukemia: case control epidemiological study in Yorkshire. Br J Cancer 1987; 56(1):79–82.

76. Giles GG, Lickiss JN, Baikie MJ, et al. Myeloproliferative and lymphoproliferative disorders in Tasmania, 1972-80: occupational and familial aspects. J Natl Cancer Inst 1984; 72(6):1233–1240.

77. Goldgar DE, Easton DF, Cannon-Albright LA, et al. Systematic population-based assessment of cancer risk in first-degree relatives of cancer probands. J Natl Cancer Inst 1994; 86(21): 1600–1608.

78. Pottern LM, Linet M, Blair A, et al. Familial cancers associated with subtypes of leukemia and non-Hodgkin's lymphoma. Leuk Res 1991; 15(5):305–314.

79. Sellick GS, Goldin LR, Wild RW, et al. A high-density SNP genome-wide linkage search of 206 families identifies susceptibility loci for chronic lymphocytic leukemia. Blood 2007; 110(9): 3326–3333.

80. de Tute R, Yuille M, Catovsky D, et al. Monoclonal B-cell lymphocytosis (MBL) in CLL families: substantial increase in relative risk for young adults. Leukemia 2006; 20(4): 728–729.

81. Aoun P, Zhou G, Chan WC, et al. Familial B-cell chronic lymphocytic leukemia: analysis of cytogenetic abnormalities, immunophenotypic profiles, and immunoglobulin heavy chain gene usage. Am J Clin Pathol 2007; 127(1):31–38.

82. Sakai A, Marti GE, Caporaso N, et al. Analysis of expressed immunoglobulin heavy chain genes in familial B-CLL. Blood 2000; 95(4):1413–1419.

83. Hodes RJ. Aging and the immune system. Immunol Rev 1997; 160:5–8.

84. Wick G, Grubeck-Loebenstein B. The aging immune system: primary and secondary alterations of immune reactivity in the elderly. Exp Gerontol 1997; 32(4–5):401–413.

85. Ben-Yehuda A, Weksler ME. Host resistance and the immune system. Clin Geriatr Med 1992; 8(4):701–711.

86. Ghia P, Melchers F, Rolink AG. Age-dependent changes in B lymphocyte development in man and mouse. Exp Gerontol 2000; 35(2):159–165.

87. Ghia P, ten Boekel E, Sanz E, et al. Ordering of human bone marrow B lymphocyte precursors by single-cell polymerase chain reaction analyses of the rearrangement status of the immunoglobulin H and L chain gene loci. J Exp Med 1996; 184(6):2217–2229.

88. Nunez C, Nishimoto N, Gartland GL, et al. B cells are generated throughout life in humans. J Immunol 1996; 156(2):866–872.

89. Ben-Yehuda A, Szabo P, Dyall R, et al. Bone marrow declines as a site of B-cell precursor differentiation with age: relationship to thymus involution. Proc Natl Acad Sci U S A 1994; 91(25): 11988–11992.

90. Song H, Price PW, Cerny J. Age-related changes in antibody repertoire: contribution from T cells. Immunol Rev 1997; 160:55–62.

91. Yan XJ, Albesiano E, Zanesi N, et al. B cell receptors in TCL1 transgenic mice resemble those of aggressive, treatment-resistant human chronic lymphocytic leukemia. Proc Natl Acad Sci U S A 2006; 103(31):11713–1178.

92. Weksler ME, Hutteroth TH. Impaired lymphocyte function in aged humans. J Clin Invest 1974; 53(1):99–104.

93. Szabo P, Zhao K, Kirman I, et al. Maturation of B cell precursors is impaired in thymic-deprived nude and old mice. J Immunol 1998; 161(5):2248–2253.

94. Klinman NR, Kline GH. The B-cell biology of aging. Immunol Rev 1997; 160:103–114.

95. LeMaoult J, Szabo P, Weksler ME. Effect of age on humoral immunity, selection of the B-cell repertoire and B-cell development. Immunol Rev 1997; 160:115–126.

96. Kyle RA, Therneau TM, Rajkumar SV, et al. Prevalence of monoclonal gammopathy of undetermined significance. N Engl J Med 2006; 354(13):1362–1369.

97. Ben-Yehuda A, Szabo P, LeMaoult J, et al. Increased VH 11 and VH Q52 gene use by splenic B cells in old mice associated with oligoclonal expansions of CD5 + B cells. Mech Ageing Dev 1998; 103(2):111–121.

98. Grunewald J, Jeddi-Tehrani M, Dersimonian H, et al. A persistent T cell expansion in the peripheral blood of a normal adult male: a new clinical entity? Clin Exp Immunol 1992; 89(2): 279–284.

99. Posnett DN, Sinha R, Kabak S, et al. Clonal populations of T cells in normal elderly humans: the T cell equivalent to "benign monoclonal gammapathy." J Exp Med 1994; 179(2):609–618.

100. Hingorani R, Choi IH, Akolkar P, et al. Clonal predominance of T cell receptors within the CD8+ CD45RO+ subset in normal human subjects. J Immunol 1993; 151(10):5762–5769.

101. Wack A, Cossarizza A, Heltai S, et al. Age-related modifications of the human alphabeta T cell repertoire due to different clonal expansions in the CD4+ and CD8+ subsets. Int Immunol 1998; 10(9):1281–1288.

102. Colombatti A, Doliana R, Schiappacassi M, et al. Age-related persistent clonal expansions of CD28(−) cells: phenotypic and molecular TCR analysis reveals both CD4(+) and CD4(+)CD8(+) cells with identical CDR3 sequences. Clin Immunol Immunopathol 1998; 89(1):61–70.

103. Richards SJ, Sivakumaran M, Parapia LA, et al. A distinct large granular lymphocyte (LGL)/ NK-associated (NKa) abnormality characterized by membrane CD4 and CD8 coexpression. The Yorkshire Leukemia Group. Br J Haematol 1992; 82(3):494–501.

104. Ghia P, Prato G, Stella S, et al. Age-dependent accumulation of monoclonal CD4+CD8+ double positive T lymphocytes in the peripheral blood of the elderly. Br J Haematol 2007; 139(5):780–790.

105. Khan N, Shariff N, Cobbold M, et al. Cytomegalovirus seropositivity drives the CD8 T cell repertoire toward greater clonality in healthy elderly individuals. J Immunol 2002; 169(4): 1984–1992.

106. Ouyang Q, Wagner WM, Wikby A, et al. Large numbers of dysfunctional CD8+ T lymphocytes bearing receptors for a single dominant CMV epitope in the very old. J Clin Immunol 2003; 23(4):247–257.

107. Nascimbeni M, Shin EC, Chiriboga L, et al. Peripheral CD4(+)CD8(+) T cells are differentiated effector memory cells with antiviral functions. Blood 2004; 104(2):478–486.

108. Pawelec G, Akbar A, Caruso C, et al. Human immunosenescence: is it infectious? Immunol Rev 2005; 205:257–268.

109. Ghia P, Caligaris-Cappio F. The origin of B-cell chronic lymphocytic leukemia. Semin Oncol 2006; 33(2):150–156.

110. Rawstron AC, Yuille MR, Fuller J, et al. Inherited predisposition to CLL is detectable as subclinical monoclonal B-lymphocyte expansion. Blood 2002; 100(7):2289–2290.

111. Rawstron AC, de Tute R, Jack AS, et al. Flow cytometric protein expression profiling as a systematic approach for developing disease-specific assays: identification of a chronic lymphocytic leukemia-specific assay for use in rituximab-containing regimens. Leukemia 2006; 20(12):2102–2110.

112. Rawstron AC, Bennett F, Hillmen P. The biological and clinical relationship between CD5+23+ monoclonal B-cell lymphocytosis and chronic lymphocytic leukemia. Br J Haematol 2007; 139(5):724–729.

113. McCarthy B, Wang XP, Paul S, et al. Gene expression profiling can distinguish physiologic B-cell chronic lymphocytic leukemia clonal expansions from preleukemic and leukemic clones. J Investig Med 2006; 54(2):S386–S386.

114. Ghia P, Dagklis A, Fazi C, et al. How does MBL relate to CLL pathogenesis? A perspective from the Immunoglobulin gene repertoire analysis. Haematologica 2008; 93(S1):28.

115. Rawstron AC, Bennet FL, O'Connor SJ, et al. Monoclonal B-cell lymphocytosis and chronic lymphocytic leukemia. N Engl J Med 2008; 359(6):575–583.

116. Rawstron AC, Bennett FL, O'Connor SJM, et al. Monoclonal B-cell lymphocytosis (MBL) is a precursor state for chronic lymphocytic leukemia (CLL) with 1% progression per year. Blood 2007; 110(11):230A–231A.

117. Stamatopoulos K, Belessi C, Moreno C, et al. Over 20% of patients with chronic lymphocytic leukemia carry stereotyped receptors: Pathogenetic implications and clinical correlations. Blood 2007; 109(1):259–270.

118. Sahota SS, Leo R, Hamblin TJ, et al. Ig V-H gene mutational patterns indicate different tumor cell status in human myeloma and monoclonal gammopathy of undetermined significance. Blood 1996; 87(2):746–755.

119. Zojer N, Ludwig H, Fiegl M, et al. Patterns of somatic mutations in V-H genes reveal pathways of clonal transformation from MGUS to multiple myeloma. Blood 2002; 100(11): 103A–103A.

120. Zojer N, Ludwig H, Fiegl M, et al. Patterns of somatic mutations in V-H genes reveal pathways of clonal transformation from MGUS to multiple myeloma. Blood 2003; 101(10): 4137–4139.

121. Rawstron AC, Fenton JAL, Plummer M, et al. Monoclonal B-cell lymphocytosis (MBL) and CLL show intraclonal variation: cases classified as "unmutated" have the greatest clonal diversity. Blood 2006; 108(11):13A–13A.

122. Dohner H, Stilgenbauer S, Benner A, et al. Genomic aberrations and survival in chronic lymphocytic leukemia. N Engl J Med 2000; 343(26):1910–1916.

123. Fonseca R, Oken MM, Harrington D, et al. Deletions of chromosome 13 in multiple myeloma identified by interphase FISH usually denote large deletions of the q arm or monosomy. Leukemia 2001; 15(6):981–986.

124. Calin GA, Dumitru CD, Shimizu M, et al. Frequent deletions and down-regulation of micro-RNA genes miR15 and miR16 at 13q14 in chronic lymphocytic leukemia. Proc Natl Acad Sci U S A 2002; 99(24):15524–15529.

125. Fung SS, Hillier KL, Leger CS, et al. Clinical progression and outcome of patients with monoclonal B-cell lymphocytosis. Leuk Lymphoma 2007; 48(6):1087–1091.

126. Shanafelt TD, Kay NE, Call TG, et al. MBL or CLL: Which classification best categorizes the clinical course of patients with an absolute lymphocyte count $>/=5 \times 10(9)L(-1)$ but a B-cell lymphocyte count $<5 \times 10(9)L(-1)$? Leuk Res 2008.

127. Bennett FL, Fenton JAL, O'Connor SJM, et al. Disease progression in monoclonal B-Cell lymphocytosis is independent of VH mutation status. Blood 2006; 108(11):13A–13A.

128. Kantor A. A new nomenclature for B cells. Immunol Today 1991; 12(11):388.

129. Fais F, Ghiotto F, Hashimoto S, et al. Chronic lymphocytic leukemia B cells express restricted sets of mutated and unmutated antigen receptors. J Clin Invest 1998; 102(8):1515–1525.

6

Apoptosis Dysregulation in CLL

Victoria Del Gaizo Moore and Anthony Letai
Medical Oncology, Dana-Farber Cancer Institute, Boston, Massachusetts, U.S.A.

INTRODUCTION TO APOPTOSIS

Apoptosis, a type of programmed cell death, is a genetically encoded process that is engaged when a cell detects the existence of sufficient damage or derangement. Examples of insults that trigger programmed cell death include oncogene activation, genomic instability, growth factor withdrawal, DNA damage, and anoikis. Most or all cancer cells endure many of these insults and thus need to circumvent apoptosis to survive. Chronic lymphocytic leukemia (CLL) cells, characterized by a low rate of proliferation and prolonged life span, are often considered to have a defect in their apoptosis pathways rather then aberrant cell cycle progression (1,2). Therefore, CLL is often described as malignancy of failed apoptosis (3), seemingly implying that the apoptotic pathway is broken. However, CLL cells are very sensitive to agents that induce apoptosis (4). This observation suggests that apoptosis signaling in CLL cells is not irreparably broken, but rather reversibly blocked in CLL. While the molecular alterations that circumvent apoptosis can potentially occur at many different levels, it is becoming increasingly clear that the mitochondrion is a key place in the apoptotic pathway for these blocks to occur in CLL. The major proteins involved in apoptotic signaling at the mitochondrion are BCL-2 family members.

The Intrinsic Apoptosis Pathway

The BCL-2 family of proteins contains three main groups of proteins categorized by function and homology: multidomain pro-apoptotic proteins, multidomain anti-apoptotic proteins, and BH3-only pro-apoptotic proteins. BAX, BAK, and BOK are members of the multidomain pro-apoptotic group and share homology in three of the BCL-2 homology (BH) domains, the BH1, 2, and 3 regions (5). Expression of BOK is generally restricted to reproductive tissues; thus it plays an insignificant role in most other tissues (6). Multidomain anti-apoptotic proteins, such as BCL-2, MCL-1, BFL-1, BCL-XL, and BCL-W, share homology in BH1, 2, 3, and 4 domains. BH3-only members share homology with the rest of the family only in possessing a BH3 domain. This BH3 domain is a roughly 20-amino acid amphipathic alpha-helix. The sequence varies considerably among different proteins, with amino acids at only two positions being strictly conserved. This makes an informatic screen of the genome for BH3-only genes very difficult. It may well be that many proteins with a functional BH3 domain remain to be discovered.

In response to death and derangement signals, BH3-only proteins are upregulated and activated by myriad means, including increased transcription, proteins stabilization, posttranslational modification, and translocation to the mitochondrion (7–9) (Fig. 1). Once at the mitochondrion, BH3-only proteins can exert their pro-death function in two distinct ways. Activator BH3-only proteins, such as BID and BIM, can activate BAX or BAK, inducing their allosteric change and oligomerization (9–11). Sensitizer BH3-only

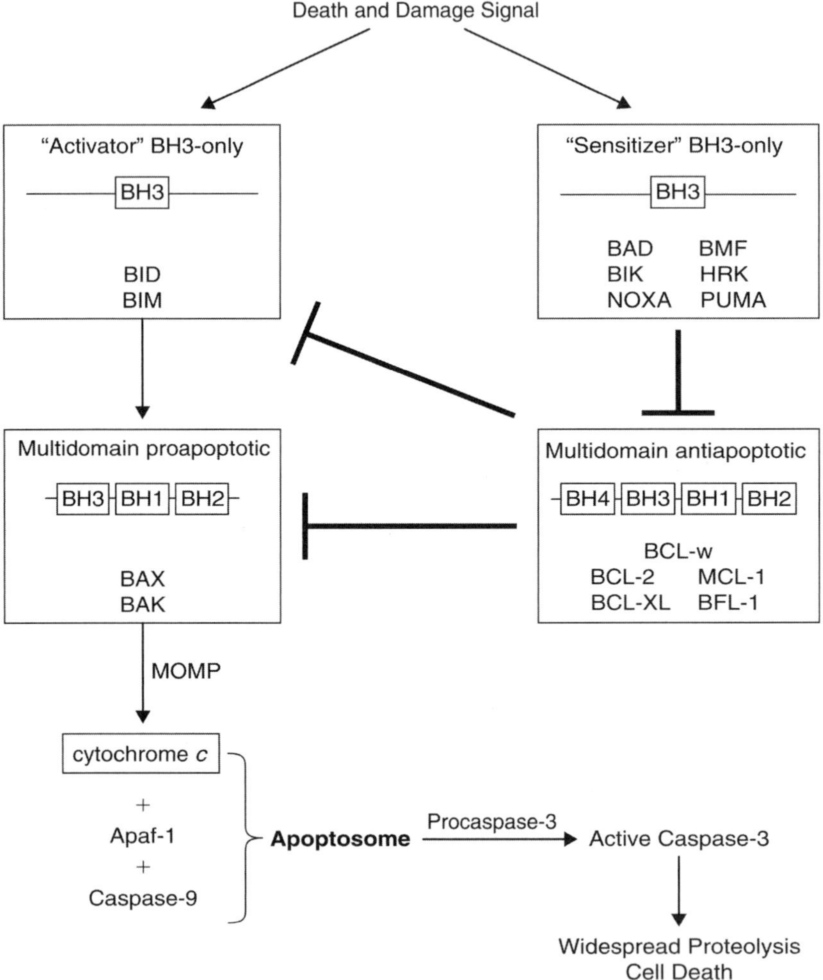

Figure 1 A schematic representation of the control of the intrinsic (or mitochondrial) pathway of apoptosis by the BCL-2 protein family. Activator BH3-only proteins are upregulated by diverse cellular derangements. Activators then activate BAX or BAK, inducing their oligomerization, which in turn induces MOMP. Pro-apoptotic factors are released, including cytochrome c, which cooperate in forming the apoptosome to activate effector caspases. BCL-2 and related anti-apoptotic proteins inhibit apoptosis by binding and sequestering activators to prevent their activation of BAX or BAK. Alternatively, they may also bind monomeric BAX and BAK to prevent their oligomerization. Sensitizer BH3-only proteins bind BCL-2 and related anti-apoptotic proteins to displace activators and provoke apoptosis. *Abbreviation*: MOMP, mitochondrial outer membrane permeabilization.

proteins, such as BAD, BIK, NOXA, PUMA, BMF, and HRK, cannot directly engage BAX or BAK but instead bind to anti-apoptotic proteins (10–12). By competing for the BH3 domain-binding site, senstizer proteins can induce cell death by displacing activator BH3-only proteins. If few activator proteins are present, the binding of a large amount of sensitizer BH3-only proteins lowers the threshold for apoptosis. Once they are activated, BAX and BAK oligomers cooperate in the formation of a pore in the outer mitochondrial membrane, causing mitochondrial outer membrane permeabilization (MOMP) (13–15). For most purposes, MOMP may be considered the point of commitment to program cell death from which a cell will rarely recover. MOMP allows pro-apoptotic factors, including cytochrome c and second mitochondria-derived activator of caspases (SMAC), or direct inhibitor of apoptosis-binding protein of low isoelectric point (DIABLO), from mitochondria to be released into the cytosol (16). Once released, cytochrome c forms a holenzyme complex with APAF-1 and the initiator caspase, Caspase-9 (17,18). In the presence of ATP, this complex, known as the apoptosome, cleaves procaspase 3, into the effector caspase 3, resulting in widespread proteolysis, leading to cellular dysfunction and death (16).

The Extrinsic Apoptotic Pathway

Apoptosis can also be initiated through death receptor pathway through signaling at the cell membrane. This extrinsic pathway is engaged when ligands such as TNF, CD95/FAS ligand, or TRAIL bind to cell surface receptors. Binding of ligands causes changes in the intracellular domains of the receptors, leading to formation of a death-inducing signaling complex (DISC) that includes procaspase 8 molecules. Perhaps via "induced proximity," the procaspase 8 molecules are autoproteolytically cleaved into active caspase 8 [reviewed in (19)]. This process can be blocked by the protein c-FLIP. In certain cells, called "type I" cells, caspase 8 can cleave and activate sufficient quantities of effector caspases 3 and 7 to commit the cell to an apoptotic death. In other, "type II," cells, mitochondrial amplification of the death signal is required. This is effected via cleavage of the BH3-only protein BID by caspase 8. Cleaved BID then engages BAX or BAK, inducing their oligomerization, MOMP, and apoptosome formation. Even though initiation of the intrinsic and extrinsic apoptotic pathways is different, both converge at the activation of downstream effector caspases 3 and 7 allowing cleavage of a variety of proteins as well as amplification of the death signaling.

Apoptosis is not readily induced via ligation of cell surface death receptors and the extrinsic apoptotic pathway in CLL (20–23). Indeed, in contrast with the response of many other cancers, addition of TRAIL ligand to CLL cells has little effect, which may be explained by low surface expression of TRAIL receptors or a high ratio of c-FLIP to caspase-8 that prevents caspase-8 activation (24). An alternative model holds that the relative insensitivity of CLL cells to TRAIL is due to their preferential signaling via the TRAIL-R1 receptor, while TRAIL preferentially signals via TRAIL-R2 (25,26). A recent study, however, found that pretreatment of CLL cells with valproic acid (VPA) sensitizes them to TRAIL (24). The cause of this sensitization was found to be that VPA decreases c-FLIP expression in a dose-dependent manner in CLL cells. Since TRAIL fails to induce apoptosis in most nontransformed cells (27), it has the potential to be an effective therapy for many cancers (28). TRAIL kills normal B cells poorly, suggesting that methods of improving CLL sensitivity to TRAIL, like pretreatment of CLL cells with VPA, may yet provide selective toxicity to leukemic cells. A phase Ib/II clinical trial evaluating Apo2L/TRAIL in combination with rituximab for follicular lymphoma is ongoing.

THE CONTROL OF MITOCHONDRIAL APOPTOSIS IN CLL
BY THE BCL-2 FAMILY OF PROTEINS

BCL-2

BCL-2 was identified at the break point of t(14;18) translocation common in follicular lymphoma (29–31). Despite the presence of a t(14;18) in fewer than 5% of B-CLL patients (32), BCL-2 is found to be expressed at high levels in nearly all CLL cells compared with peripheral blood lymphocytes (33,34). In fact, BCL-2 protein levels in CLL cells are comparable to those founding follicular lymphoma cells that bear the t(14;18) (34). Since chromosomal or genetic alterations of the *bcl-2* gene locus are rare in CLL cells (33,35), an early explanation for BCL-2 protein overexpression was *bcl-2* gene hypomethylation (33). However, methylation status alone did not fully correlate with the amount of protein present in patient cells. More recently, another chromosomal abnormality, deletion at 13q14.3, which occurs in roughly 50% of CLL cases, has been linked to BCL-2 protein expression dysregulation (36). This region encodes for two micro-RNAs (miR), miR-15 and miR-16, which keep BCL-2 levels in check in healthy cells posttranslationally. However, it has been found that both miRs are downregulated in as many as 65% of B-CLL patients (37). Furthermore, if normal levels of miR-15 and miR-16 are restored in leukemia cell lines, BCL-2 levels decrease and apoptosis is initiated, lending support to this hypothesis. Of course, there remains a significant portion of CLL cases, probably greater than a third, in which miR-15 and miR-16 levels are not reduced, and no t(14;18) is present, for which the mechanism of BCL-2 upregulation remains obscure. BCL-2 protein is readily detectable in most if not all CLL patient samples (34,38), and some have correlated higher BCL-2 expression with inferior outcome and progressive disease clinically (39–41).

While it is clear that BCL-2 is widely, perhaps universally, expressed at high levels in CLL, it was less clear how BCL-2 functions in CLL. In an early study of BCL-2 levels in CLL, it was found that BCL-2 levels did not correlate with response to chemotherapy (42). A recent larger study encompassing 235 patients found no relation between BCL-2 expression levels and progression-free survival or clinical response to either fludarabine or fludarabine plus cyclophosphamide (43). It is safe to say that BCL-2 expression level has not emerged as a useful prognostic parameter in the clinic.

This is not to say, however, that BCL-2 plays a biologically unimportant role in CLL biology. We have recently examined whether CLL cells require BCL-2 function to maintain survival (34). BH3 profiling is an assay that can be used to detect apoptotic blocks in cancer cells. In one application, it can be used to detect cellular dependence on BCL-2 function (10,44). When we applied BH3 profiling to a series of CLL cells from previously untreated patients, we found that the cells were uniformly dependent on BCL-2. To test this dependence, we measured in vitro sensitivity to the small molecule antagonist of BCL-2 (as well as BCL-XL and BCL-W), ABT-737, made by Abbott Laboratories. ABT-737 belongs to a class of drugs called "BH3 mimetics" because they behave like BH3 domains, competing with them for binding to anti-apoptotic proteins like BCL-2. We found that all of the dozens of primary CLL samples tested were exquisitely sensitive to ABT-737, with an EC50 < 10 nM. Intriguingly, death could be seen in as little as four hours, suggesting that the CLL cells were already "primed" for death. We found that the basis for this priming was the fact that CLL cells express large amounts of the activator BH3-only protein BIM, almost all of which is sequestered by BCL-2. We describe BCL-2 in this state as being primed by an activator. When BCL-2 function is abrogated by ABT-737, BIM is released to induce BAX and BAK oligomerization and death (Fig. 2). Thus,

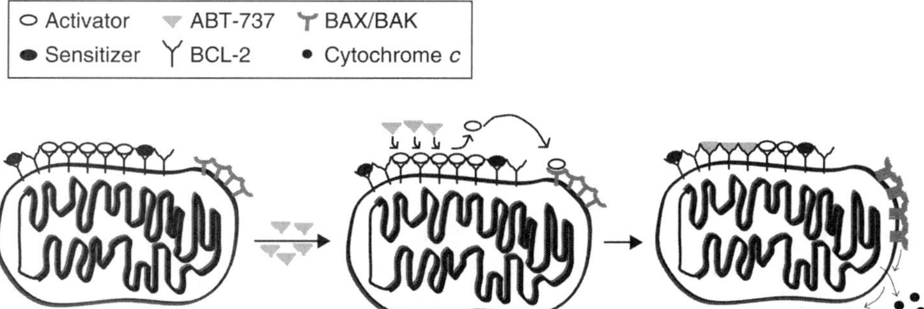

Figure 2 BH3 mimetics displace BIM from BCL-2 in CLL to cause apoptosis. Large amounts of BIM are sequestered by BCL-2 in CLL (*top*). BH3 mimetics that target BCL-2 displace BIM (*middle*), which in turn induces BAX or BAK oligomerization, MOMP, and cell death (*bottom*). *Abbreviations:* CLL, chronic lymphocytic leukemia; MOMP, mitochondrial outer membrane permeabilization.

untreated CLL appears to be generally "addicted" to BCL-2 function, due to the requirement that large amounts of BIM be tonically sequestered by BCL-2.

The selectivity of this strategy for malignant cells over normal cells likely rests on the fact that malignant cells like CLL are more likely to possess BCL-2 (or BCL-XL or BCL-W) primed by an activator, a requirement for sensitivity to the drug. The priming apparently requires the type of cellular dysfunction frequently encountered in cancer, but rarely in normal cells. However, certain normal tissues may indeed be primed, as evidenced by the thrombocytopenia and lymphopenia that consistently were found in preclinical animal testing of ABT-737 (45–47). Such side effects were shown to be due to drug contacting the appropriate target and appeared likely to be tolerable. As of this writing, an orally available derivative of ABT-737, ABT-263, is in phase I clinical trials for small cell lung cancer, lymphoma, and CLL. In addition, Ascenta and Gemin X have BH3 mimetic small molecule drugs directed at BCL-2 and related proteins in phase I clinical trials that include CLL patients.

Oblimersen (Genasense), made by Genta, is a phosphorothioated antisense DNA compound targeting BCL-2. Preclinical studies found that antisense inhibition of *bcl-2* levels could induce death in cancer cell lines (48). Preclinical studies showed reduction of BCL-2 in certain cells. However, numerous clinical studies in many diseases, including CLL, failed to reach their designated clinical endpoints. More recently, however, in a study of CLL, evidence emerged indicating that an improvement in response rate could be observed in relapsed CLL patients when oblimersen was added to fludarabine and cyclophosphamide (49). Nonetheless, the overall performance of the drug in CLL has been disappointing. Sufficient questions remain, however, regarding the ability of this drug to effectively reduce BCL-2 levels in vivo, so that clinical testing of this agent should not be considered a true proof of the principle of targeting BCL-2 in CLL.

Most are quite familiar with BCL-2 acting as an inhibitor of cell death due to chemotherapy. For the targeted agent ABT-737, in contrast, BCL-2 expression is a requirement for sensitivity. However, we have shown that sensitivity depends not only on expression of BCL-2 but also on the simultaneous priming of BCL-2 by an activator BH3-only protein like BIM (10,34,44). Thus, it is the primed BCL-2 that confers sensitivity to BCL-2 antagonism.

It is worth extending this discussion to consideration of sensitivity to conventional chemotherapy. CLL is generally much more sensitive to conventional chemotherapy than most cancers. At the same time, CLL expresses more BCL-2 than most cancers. Yet thousands of in vitro studies over twenty years have convincingly demonstrated that BCL-2 provides protection against numerous toxins, including most types of chemotherapy. An explanation of this apparent paradox can be found in a comparison of the source and condition of BCL-2 in the in vitro and cancer cases. The function of BCL-2 as an anti-apoptotic protein has been tested most commonly in models in which BCL-2 was overexpressed in an established cell line. Thus, a cell line that already had a favorable balance of anti-apoptotic to pro-apoptotic signaling was provided with yet more BCL-2. This extra, unoccupied BCL-2 provided an additional anti-apoptotic reserve that could absorb additional death signaling provoked by chemotherapy treatment. In literally thousands of studies, when a number of toxic agents were subsequently applied, it has consistently been found that the BCL-2-expressing cells were much less likely to die than parental cells.

In the case of cancer cells, however, there is no possibility of adding exogenous BCL-2. Increases in BCL-2 expression arise as a result of selection. The selection pressure is generated by increased death signaling, likely due to the numerous aberrancies inherent to the cancer phenotype. These death signals are ultimately conducted to BCL-2 via conversion to activator pro-death BH3-only proteins. Thus, in cancer cells that select for BCL-2, the BCL-2 is largely occupied by pro-apoptotic BH3-only proteins. Not only does this prevent the BCL-2 from providing extra anti-apoptotic reserve to endure chemotherapy treatment, it actually primes the cell for death, as ample activators are present on the BCL-2 protein. In such a situation, generation of modest quantities of either activator or sensitizer proteins is sufficient to free activator proteins from BCL-2 so they can interact with BAX and BAK and commit the cell to death. Thus, in some cases, expression of BCL-2, if it is primed with activator proteins, can contribute to and correlate with chemosensitivity. The essential difference between the cancer situation and the in vitro situation is that in cancer, the BCL-2 is more likely to be "full," whereas in the in vitro situation, the BCL-2 is more likely to be "empty."

Other Anti-Apoptotic Proteins

It is important to consider the role of the other known anti-apoptotic proteins in CLL. Since activator proteins can bind to all anti-apoptotic proteins (10,11), having an excess of any or more than one anti-apoptotic protein could influence the cancer cell's biology as well as response to targeted therapy. For instance, if a cell were to overexpress two different anti-apoptotics, that cell would be able to tolerate more stress since more binding sites would be available for sequestering activator and therefore preventing BAX/BAK activation. Furthermore, displacing bound activator from one anti-apoptotic could be less effective at inducing apoptosis. Once released from one anti-apoptotic protein, the displaced activator would have another place to hide, the second anti-apoptotic protein. In CLL, BCL-XL and BCL-W protein levels have not been thoroughly examined, but one study showed that BCL-XL levels are minimal, and BCL-W protein was not detectable (34). Another recent study confirmed low BCL-W gene expression, and both gene and protein expression of BCL-XL was detectable (50). BFL-1 has been linked to a block in apoptosis in CLL. Higher than normal mRNA expression of BFL-1 is thought to contribute to apoptosis resistance, since fludarabine-resistant B-CLL samples have higher expression in in vitro (51). One explanation for this observation is that BFL-1 may provide protection in different cells to death receptor–induced apoptosis (52) or that BFL-1 can cooperate with the oncogene E1A. However, excess BFL-1 could also be a safe haven for upregulated BID or BIM, just as BCL-2 can. The absence of reliable antibodies for detecting human BFL-1 on immunoblot has hampered studies of protein levels in CLL.

MCL-1 protein levels have been better studied in the context of CLL. Untreated patients can have low and somewhat variable MCL-1 protein levels in primary CLL cells (42). Recently, MCL-1 protein levels were shown to be low in untreated patients, as much as 10-fold lower than BCL-2 protein (34). In general, higher MCL-1 expression has been found to correlate with decreased sensitivity to chemotherapy. An elevated MCL-1/BAX ratio was found to correlate with inferior clinical response to rituximab (53). A correlation between MCL-1 levels and response to chemotherapy has been investigated where higher MCL-1 protein was found in nonresponders or partial responders compared with complete responders (42,54). Saxena et al. also found that higher MCL-1 protein expression was associated with patients who failed to achieve a complete response to chemotherapy (54). A 6- or 18-nucleotide insertion was found in the MCL-1 promoter of 17 of 58 patients. Presence of the insertion correlated with increased MCL-1 expression and inferior clinical response (55). An in vitro study of the influence of environment on CLL cell survival found that the inhibition of apoptosis in cultured CLL cells by a follicular dendritic cell line was dependent upon CD44-dependent induction of MCL-1 (56). In summary, while untreated CLL cells appear to be tonically dependent on BCL-2 for survival, expression of MCL-1 may contribute to chemoresistance and inferior clinical outcome. It is worth noting that ABT-737 does not target MCL-1, so that overexpression of MCL-1 is a potential mode of resistance in CLL cells that are initially sensitive to treatment (57–61).

BH3-ONLY PROTEINS

While activator BIM upregulation is important in the apoptotic block found in CLL, changes in sensitizer BH3-only proteins have also been observed. Sensitizer upregulation, especially in the context of a CLL cell's response to chemotherapeutic agents, can impact a drug's effect on anti-apoptotic proteins not only because sensitizer can occupy their binding pockets but also because sensitizers interact with other proteins within the cell. In one study, both mRNA and protein expression of BMF and NOXA were found to be significantly higher in CLL cells as compared with tonsil B cells (62). A recent study confirmed that NOXA gene and protein expression is detectable in CLL, but variable (50). Furthermore, treating CLL cells with proteasome inhibitors upregulated NOXA and increased apoptosis in CLL cells. This finding should be taken with some caution; however, as proteasome inhibitors cause changes in protein levels of many different targets. During fludarabine treatment of primary CLL cells, PUMA protein is induced (62). Furthermore, the degree of Puma upregulation correlated with IgVH mutation status (mutated had higher PUMA induction) and was absent in samples with p53 mutations. The fact that death in CLL cells frequently occurs via the intrinsic apoptotic pathway implies that BH3-only proteins are required for conducting death signals, but we are far from a comprehensive knowledge of their participation.

BAX and BAK

Since BAX and BAK are the effector molecules in the signaling cascade in the mitochondrial pathway of apoptosis, protein expression and proper functioning of these proteins are important. Not only would low or no expression of BAX//BAK in a cell be a mechanism to initially avoid apoptosis but also a way to escape chemotherapy-induced death (63). For example, certain lymphoma cells have been found to lack expression of BAX and BAK (44). These cells do not need to overexpress any anti-apoptotic proteins to sequester activator proteins. Rather they avoid apoptosis by not being able to respond to death insults because they have lost the ability to cause cytochrome c release, which is necessary for MOMP. As a consequence, these same cells are resistant to targeted therapy such as treatment with ABT-737 or conventional chemotherapeutics such as Vincristine and Etoposide. At the DNA level, a single nucleotide polymorphism, G(-248)A, was identified in the BAX promoter of CLL cells (64) and was shown to decrease transcription levels and subsequently protein levels. Initially, it appeared that there was a correlation between this polymorphism and disease progression and treatment response. However, a larger cohort study of CLL patients and healthy controls revealed that there is no significant difference between the two groups (65). At the protein level, consistent BAX and variable but detectable BAK protein has been observed (34,42). Many other studies have focused on BCL-2/BAX protein ratios. Some groups have identified BCL-2/BAX ratio as important is assessing apoptosis regulation in CLL and treatment response (54,66–68), while others provide evidence to the contrary (42,69). Whether the protein ratios are of significance or not, it is important that there is presence of functional BAX or BAK to permit apoptosis via the mitochondrial pathway. A loss of BAX or BAK protein or function has not been described thus far for CLL.

Inhibitors of Apoptosis

Caspase activation can be further modulated by the influence of a family of proteins known as Inhibitors of Apoptosis (IAPs) proteins. IAPs are a family of regulating proteins that modulate caspase activity, at least in part by binding directly to caspases (70). IAPs share conserved domains, each containing one to three baculovirus IAP domains and bind to caspases via these domains. For example, XIAP binds to and inhibits caspase 3, 7, and 9 (71,72). It is hypothesized that IAPs could be working constitutively in the cell to prevent small numbers of active caspases from accidentally triggering a full-blown apoptotic cascade. In mammals, the protein SMAC acts as a competitive antagonist of the IAP-caspase interaction. SMAC competes for the binding site in IAPs that binds caspases. SMAC function is largely controlled by its subcellular localization in the mitochondrial intermembrane space in healthy cells. In the event of MOMP, SMAC is released into the cytosol (73). IAPs become overwhelmed by SMAC's inhibitory function, which allows release of the caspases and restoration of proteolytic activity (74,75).

It should be noted, however, that while certain IAPs do appear to inhibit caspase activity, their anti-apoptotic function may extend beyond mere interaction with caspases. In fact, recent reports on the utility of small molecule SMAC mimetics in cancer may be based more on their ability to provoke NFκB-dependent production of TNF-α than on their ability to induce caspase activity directly (76,77). Genentech currently has a small molecule SMAC mimetic in phase I clinical trials in cancer. However, it is not clear whether this strategy will find a foothold in the treatment of CLL.

There has been relatively little study of the function of the IAP axis in CLL. Some have reported high constituitive expression of IAPs in both normal and CLL lymphocytes (78). When specific IAP family members were compared among lymphoid malignancies, CLL cells were shown to have high mRNA expression of C-IAP2 and low expression of Survivin (79). In fact, when a cluster analysis was performed with CIAP1 and 2, Survivin, and BCL-2, it was found that CLL samples tightly clustered and can be distinguished from acute lymphocytic leukemia, non-Hodgkins lymphoma, and control samples. Furthermore, CIAP-2/Survivin ratio was significantly higher in CLL than in any other lymphoid malignancies studied, presumably because individual expression levels were high and low (52). One group found that though XIAP is expressed in CLL, it appears to play an insignificant role in inhibiting an apoptotic response in CLL (80). In summary, several IAP proteins have been observed to be expressed in CLL cells. The biological role of these proteins has yet to be determined.

CONCLUSION

While CLL is often described as a disease of failed apoptosis, it would probably be more accurate to describe it as a disease of blocked or suspended apoptosis. Like most, if not all, cancers, CLL cells select for a block in apoptosis to survive the death signaling that accompanies the aberrations of oncogenesis. In CLL, BCL-2 overexpression and sequestration of BIM play a critical role in blocking apoptosis, rendering it quite sensitive to antagonism of BCL-2 function. Likely due to its primed state, the high levels of BCL-2 expression in BCL-2 CLL do not seem to confer chemoresistance. In fact, it is relatively easy to trigger apoptosis in CLL, both in vitro and in vivo. While CLL cells are sensitive to current chemotherapies routinely used to treat the disease, CLL is not curable. Studies focusing on the apoptotic pathway of relapsed and refractory CLL are lacking. Such studies will be necessary to understand why an initially chemosensitive cancer ultimately becomes resistant. Several agents targeting BCL-2 in clinical trials are attempting to improve the clinical course of CLL. The outcome of these clinical trials is of great significance to those who hope, as we do, that targeting apoptosis directly can yield significant clinical benefits.

REFERENCES

1. Reed JC. Molecular biology of chronic lymphocytic leukemia: implications for therapy. Semin Hematol 1998; 35:3–13.
2. Caligaris-Cappio F, Hamblin TJ. B-cell chronic lymphocytic leukemia: a bird of a different feather. J Clin Oncol 1999; 17:399–408.
3. Packham G, Stevenson FK. Bodyguards and assassins: Bcl-2 family proteins and apoptosis control in chronic lymphocytic leukaemia. Immunology 2005; 114:441–449.
4. Keating MJ, O'Brien S, Albitar M, et al. Early results of a chemoimmunotherapy regimen of fludarabine, cyclophosphamide, and rituximab as initial therapy for chronic lymphocytic leukemia. J Clin Oncol 2005; 23:4079–4088.
5. Gross A, McDonnell JM, Korsmeyer SJ. BCL-2 family members and the mitochondria in apoptosis. Genes Dev 1999; 13:1899–1911.
6. Hsu SY, Kaipia A, McGee E, et al. Bok is a pro-apoptotic Bcl-2 protein with restricted expression in reproductive tissues and heterodimerizes with selective anti-apoptotic Bcl-2 family members. Proc Natl Acad Sci U S A 1997; 94:12401–12406.
7. Huang DC, Strasser A. BH3-only proteins—essential initiators of apoptotic cell death. Cell 2000; 103:839–842.
8. Kelekar A, Thompson CB. Bcl-2-family proteins: the role of the BH3 domain in apoptosis. Trends Cell Biol 1998; 8:324–330.
9. Wei MC, Lindsten T, Mootha VK, et al. tBID, a membrane-targeted death ligand, oligomerizes BAK to release cytochrome c. Genes Dev 2000; 14:2060–2071.
10. Certo M, Del Gaizo, Moore V, Nishino M, et al. Mitochondria primed by death signals determine cellular addiction to antiapoptotic BCL-2 family members. Cancer Cell 2006; 9:351–365.
11. Letai A, Bassik MC, Walensky LD, et al. Distinct BH3 domains either sensitize or activate mitochondrial apoptosis, serving as prototype cancer therapeutics. Cancer Cell 2002; 2:183–192.
12. Kuwana T, Bouchier-Hayes L, Chipuk JE, et al. BH3 domains of BH3-only proteins differentially regulate Bax-mediated mitochondrial membrane permeabilization both directly and indirectly. Mol Cell 2005; 17:525–535.

13. Cheng EH, Wei MC, Weiler S, et al. BCL-2, BCL-X(L) sequester BH3 domain-only molecules preventing BAX- and BAK-mediated mitochondrial apoptosis. Mol Cell 2001; 8:705–711.
14. Wolter KG, Hsu YT, Smith CL, et al. Movement of Bax from the cytosol to mitochondria during apoptosis. J Cell Biol 1997; 139:1281–1292.
15. Gross A, Jockel J, Wei MC, et al. Enforced dimerization of BAX results in its translocation, mitochondrial dysfunction and apoptosis. EMBO J 1998; 17:3878–3885.
16. Wang X. The expanding role of mitochondria in apoptosis. Genes Dev 2001; 15:2922–2933.
17. Zou H, Li Y, Liu X, et al. An APAF-1.cytochrome c multimeric complex is a functional apoptosome that activates procaspase-9. J Biol Chem 1999; 274:11549–11556.
18. Bratton SB, Walker G, Srinivasula SM, et al. Recruitment, activation and retention of caspases-9 and -3 by Apaf-1 apoptosome and associated XIAP complexes. EMBO J 2001; 20:998–1009.
19. Danial NN, Korsmeyer SJ. Cell death: critical control points. Cell 2004; 116:205–219.
20. Romano C, De Fanis U, Sellitto A, et al. Induction of CD95 upregulation does not render chronic lymphocytic leukemia B-cells susceptible to CD95-mediated apoptosis. Immunol Lett 2005; 97:131–139.
21. Kang J, Kisenge RR, Toyoda H, et al. Chemical sensitization and regulation of TRAIL-induced apoptosis in a panel of B-lymphocytic leukaemia cell lines. Br J Haematol 2003; 123:921–932.
22. Cheng J, Hylander BL, Baer MR, et al. Multiple mechanisms underlie resistance of leukemia cells to Apo2 Ligand/TRAIL. Molecular cancer therapeutics 2006; 5:1844–1853.
23. MacFarlane M, Harper N, Snowden RT, et al. Mechanisms of resistance to TRAIL-induced apoptosis in primary B cell chronic lymphocytic leukaemia. Oncogene 2002; 21:6809–6818.
24. Lagneaux L, Gillet N, Stamatopoulos B, et al. Valproic acid induces apoptosis in chronic lymphocytic leukemia cells through activation of the death receptor pathway and potentiates TRAIL response. Exp Hematol 2007; 35:1527–1537.
25. MacFarlane M, Inoue S, Kohlhaas SL, et al. Chronic lymphocytic leukemic cells exhibit apoptotic signaling via TRAIL-R1. Cell Death Differ 2005; 12:773–782.
26. Natoni A, MacFarlane M, Inoue S, et al. TRAIL signals to apoptosis in chronic lymphocytic leukaemia cells primarily through TRAIL-R1 whereas cross-linked agonistic TRAIL-R2 antibodies facilitate signalling via TRAIL-R2. Br J Haematol 2007; 139:568–577.
27. Yagita H, Takeda K, Hayakawa Y, et al. TRAIL and its receptors as targets for cancer therapy. Cancer Sci 2004; 95:777–783.
28. Kelley SK, Ashkenazi A. Targeting death receptors in cancer with Apo2L/TRAIL. Curr Opin Pharmacol 2004; 4:333–339.
29. Tsujimoto Y, Gorham J, Cossman J, et al. The t(14;18) chromosome translocations involved in B-cell neoplasms result from mistakes in VDJ joining. Science 1985; 229:1390–1393.
30. Cleary ML, Sklar J. Nucleotide sequence of a t(14;18) chromosomal breakpoint in follicular lymphoma and demonstration of a breakpoint-cluster region near a transcriptionally active locus on chromosome 18. Proc Natl Acad Sci U S A 1985; 82:7439–7443.
31. Bakhshi A, Jensen JP, Goldman P, et al. Cloning the chromosomal breakpoint of t(14;18) human lymphomas: clustering around JH on chromosome 14 and near a transcriptional unit on 18. Cell 1985; 41:899–906.
32. Adachi M, Tefferi A, Greipp PR, et al. Preferential linkage of bcl-2 to immunoglobulin light chain gene in chronic lymphocytic leukemia. J Exp Med 1990; 171:559–564.
33. Hanada M, Delia D, Aiello A, et al. bcl-2 gene hypomethylation and high-level expression in B-cell chronic lymphocytic leukemia. Blood 1993; 82:1820–1828.
34. Del Gaizo Moore V, Brown JR, Certo M, et al. Chronic lymphocytic leukemia requires BCL2 to sequester prodeath BIM, explaining sensitivity to BCL2 antagonist ABT-737. J Clin Invest 2007; 117:112–121.
35. Mariano MT, Moretti L, Donelli A, et al. bcl-2 gene expression in hematopoietic cell differentiation. Blood 1992; 80:768–775.
36. Dohner H, Stilgenbauer S, Benner A, et al. Genomic aberrations and survival in chronic lymphocytic leukemia. N Engl J Med 2000; 343:1910–1916.

37. Calin GA, Dumitru CD, Shimizu M, et al. Frequent deletions and down-regulation of micro-RNA genes miR15 and miR16 at 13q14 in chronic lymphocytic leukemia. Proc Natl Acad Sci U S A 2002; 99:15524–15529.
38. Schena M, Larsson LG, Gottardi D, et al. Growth- and differentiation-associated expression of bcl-2 in B-chronic lymphocytic leukemia cells. Blood 1992; 79:2981–2989.
39. Faderl S, Keating MJ, Do KA, et al. Expression profile of 11 proteins and their prognostic significance in patients with chronic lymphocytic leukemia (CLL). Leukemia 2002; 16:1045–1052.
40. Robertson LE, Plunkett W, McConnell K, et al. Bcl-2 expression in chronic lymphocytic leukemia and its correlation with the induction of apoptosis and clinical outcome. Leukemia 1996; 10:456–459.
41. Marschitz I, Tinhofer I, Hittmair A, et al. Analysis of Bcl-2 protein expression in chronic lymphocytic leukemia. A comparison of three semiquantitation techniques. Am J Clin Pathol 2000; 113:219–229.
42. Kitada S, Andersen J, Akar S, et al. Expression of apoptosis-regulating proteins in chronic lymphocytic leukemia: correlations with in vitro and in vivo chemoresponses. Blood 1998; 91:3379–3389.
43. Grever MR, Lucas DM, Dewald GW, et al. Comprehensive assessment of genetic and molecular features predicting outcome in patients with chronic lymphocytic leukemia: results from the US Intergroup Phase III Trial E2997. J Clin Oncol 2007; 25:799–804.
44. Deng J, Carlson N, Takeyama K, et al. BH3 profiling identifies three distinct classes of apoptotic blocks to predict response to ABT-737 and conventional chemotherapeutic agents. Cancer Cell 2007; 12:171–185.
45. Mason KD, Carpinelli MR, Fletcher JI, et al. Programmed anuclear cell death delimits platelet life span. Cell 2007; 128:1173–1186.
46. Oltersdorf T, Elmore SW, Shoemaker AR, et al. An inhibitor of Bcl-2 family proteins induces regression of solid tumors. Nature 2005; 435:677–681.
47. Zhang H, Nimmer PM, Tahir SK, et al. Bcl-2 family proteins are essential for platelet survival. Cell Death Differ 2007; 14:943–951.
48. Jansen B, Schlagbauer-Wadl H, Brown BD, et al. bcl-2 antisense therapy chemosensitizes human melanoma in SCID mice. Nat Med 1998; 4:232–234.
49. O'Brien S, Moore JO, Boyd TE, et al. Randomized phase III trial of fludarabine plus cyclophosphamide with or without oblimersen sodium (Bcl-2 antisense) in patients with relapsed or refractory chronic lymphocytic leukemia. J Clin Oncol 2007; 25:1114–1120.
50. Smit LA, Hallaert DY, Spijker R, et al. Differential Noxa/Mcl-1 balance in peripheral versus lymph node chronic lymphocytic leukemia cells correlates with survival capacity. Blood 2007; 109:1660–1668.
51. Morales AA, Olsson A, Celsing F, et al. High expression of bfl-1 contributes to the apoptosis resistant phenotype in B-cell chronic lymphocytic leukemia. Int J Cancer 2005; 113:730–737.
52. Karsan A, Yee E, Kaushansky K, et al. Cloning of human Bcl-2 homologue: inflammatory cytokines induce human A1 in cultured endothelial cells. Blood 1996; 87:3089–3096.
53. Bannerji R, Kitada S, Flinn IW, et al. Apoptotic-regulatory and complement-protecting protein expression in chronic lymphocytic leukemia: relationship to in vivo rituximab resistance. J Clin Oncol 2003; 21:1466–1471.
54. Saxena A, Viswanathan S, Moshynska O, et al. Mcl-1 and Bcl-2/Bax ratio are associated with treatment response but not with Rai stage in B-cell chronic lymphocytic leukemia. Am J Hematol 2004; 75:22–33.
55. Moshynska O, Sankaran K, Pahwa P, et al. Prognostic significance of a short sequence insertion in the MCL-1 promoter in chronic lymphocytic leukemia. J Natl Cancer Inst 2004; 96:673–682.
56. Pedersen IM, Kitada S, Leoni LM, et al. Protection of CLL B cells by a follicular dendritic cell line is dependent on induction of Mcl-1. Blood 2002; 100:1795–1801.
57. Chen S, Dai Y, Harada H, et al. Mcl-1 down-regulation potentiates ABT-737 lethality by cooperatively inducing Bak activation and Bax translocation. Cancer Res 2007; 67:782–791.
58. Dai Y, Grant S. Targeting multiple arms of the apoptotic regulatory machinery. Cancer Res 2007; 67:2908–2911.

59. Konopleva M, Contractor R, Tsao T, et al. Mechanisms of apoptosis sensitivity and resistance to the BH3 mimetic ABT-737 in acute myeloid leukemia. Cancer Cell 2006; 10:375–388.

60. Tahir SK, Yang X, Anderson MG, et al. Influence of Bcl-2 family members on the cellular response of small-cell lung cancer cell lines to ABT-737. Cancer Res 2007; 67:1176–1183.

61. van Delft MF, Wei AH, Mason KD, et al. The BH3 mimetic ABT-737 targets selective Bcl-2 proteins and efficiently induces apoptosis via Bak/Bax if Mcl-1 is neutralized. Cancer Cell 2006; 10:389–399.

62. Mackus WJ, Kater AP, Grummels A, et al. Chronic lymphocytic leukemia cells display p53-dependent drug-induced Puma upregulation. Leukemia 2005; 19:427–434.

63. Wei MC, Zong WX, Cheng EH, et al. Proapoptotic BAX and BAK: a requisite gateway to mitochondrial dysfunction and death. Science 2001; 292:727–730.

64. Saxena A, Moshynska O, Sankaran K, et al. Association of a novel single nucleotide polymorphism, G(-248)A, in the 5′-UTR of BAX gene in chronic lymphocytic leukemia with disease progression and treatment resistance. Cancer Lett 2002; 187:199–205.

65. Skogsberg S, Tobin G, Krober A, et al. The G(-248)A polymorphism in the promoter region of the Bax gene does not correlate with prognostic markers or overall survival in chronic lymphocytic leukemia. Leukemia 2006; 20:77–81.

66. Thomas A, El Rouby S, Reed JC, et al. Drug-induced apoptosis in B-cell chronic lymphocytic leukemia: relationship between p53 gene mutation and bcl-2/bax proteins in drug resistance. Oncogene 1996; 12:1055–1062.

67. Pepper C, Bentley P, Hoy T. Regulation of clinical chemoresistance by bcl-2 and bax oncoproteins in B-cell chronic lymphocytic leukaemia. Br J Haematol 1996; 95:513–517.

68. Pepper C, Hoy T, Bentley DP. Bcl-2/Bax ratios in chronic lymphocytic leukaemia and their correlation with in vitro apoptosis and clinical resistance. Br J Cancer 1997; 76:935–938.

69. Johnston JB, Daeninck P, Verburg L, et al. P53, MDM-2, BAX and BCL-2 and drug resistance in chronic lymphocytic leukemia. Leuk Lymphoma 1997; 26:435–449.

70. Liston P, Fong WG, Korneluk RG. The inhibitors of apoptosis: there is more to life than Bcl2. Oncogene 2003; 22:8568–8580.

71. Silke J, Ekert PG, Day CL, et al. Direct inhibition of caspase 3 is dispensable for the anti-apoptotic activity of XIAP. EMBO J 2001; 20:3114–3123.

72. Suzuki Y, Nakabayashi Y, Nakata K, et al. X-linked inhibitor of apoptosis protein (XIAP) inhibits caspase-3 and -7 in distinct modes. J Biol Chem 2001; 276:27058–27063.

73. Vaux DL, Silke J. Mammalian mitochondrial IAP binding proteins. Biochem Biophys Res Commun 2003; 304:499–504.

74. Du C, Fang M, Li Y, et al. Smac, a mitochondrial protein that promotes cytochrome c-dependent caspase activation by eliminating IAP inhibition. Cell 2000; 102:33–42.

75. Verhagen AM, Ekert PG, Pakusch M, et al. Identification of DIABLO, a mammalian protein that promotes apoptosis by binding to and antagonizing IAP proteins. Cell 2000; 102:43–53.

76. Varfolomeev E, Blankenship JW, Wayson SM, et al. IAP antagonists induce autoubiquitination of c-IAPs, NF-kappaB activation, and TNFalpha-dependent apoptosis. Cell 2007; 131:669–681.

77. Vince JE, Wong WW, Khan N, et al. IAP antagonists target cIAP1 to induce TNFalpha-dependent apoptosis. Cell 2007; 131:682–693.

78. Munzert G, Kirchner D, Stobbe H, et al. Tumor necrosis factor receptor-associated factor 1 gene overexpression in B-cell chronic lymphocytic leukemia: analysis of NF-kappa B/Rel-regulated inhibitors of apoptosis. Blood 2002; 100:3749–3756.

79. de Graaf AO, van Krieken JH, Tonnissen E, et al. Expression of C-IAP1, C-IAP2 and SURVIVIN discriminates different types of lymphoid malignancies. Br J Haematol 2005; 130:852–859.

80. Schliep S, Decker T, Schneller F, et al. Functional evaluation of the role of inhibitor of apoptosis proteins in chronic lymphocytic leukemia. Exp Hematol 2004; 32:556–562.

7
Differential Diagnosis, Staging, and Prognostic Factors

Thorsten Zenz, Hartmut Döhner, and Stephan Stilgenbauer
Department of Internal Medicine III, University of Ulm, Ulm, Germany

INTRODUCTION

Chronic lymphocytic leukemia (CLL) is a chronic lymphoproliferative disorder of B lymphocytes (mature B-cell neoplasm). Small lymphocytic lymphoma (SLL) is considered the same disease in a nonleukemic form (1,2). The progressive accumulation of monoclonal B lymphocytes leads to leukocytosis, lymphadenopathy, hepatosplenomegaly, and bone marrow failure and is sometimes associated with autoimmune disease.

The differential diagnosis, staging, and various ways of assessing prognosis will be reviewed in this chapter.

DIAGNOSIS AND DIFFERENTIAL DIAGNOSIS

The most noteworthy abnormality among laboratory findings in CLL is lymphocytosis in the peripheral blood (and bone marrow). In fact, nowadays most patients are diagnosed while asymptomatic because of abnormal blood counts. Although the absolute blood lymphocyte threshold for diagnosing CLL has been placed at >5000 to 10,000/μL, a large majority of patients present with counts as high as 200,000/μL. CLL is the most common leukemia in the western world and will therefore head the list of the differential diagnosis of lymphocytosis. The availability of phenotypic markers makes it possible to distinguish other lymphoproliferative diseases from CLL (see below). The morphology and immunophenotype usually allow the diagnosis of CLL with relative ease, but in atypical cases, cytogenetic analysis or histology may be needed.

Various groups have recommended that the threshold for the diagnosis of CLL should be an absolute lymphocyte count of >10,000/μL or >5000/μL (3,4). The International Workshop on CLL (IWCLL) addressed minimum diagnostic requirements for the diagnosis of CLL and recommended a threshold of >10,000/μL (4). The National Cancer Institute Working Group on CLL defined eligibility criteria for entering prospective protocol studies (3). If the blood lymphocyte phenotype is clearly that of typical B-CLL, the Working Group and the current revision state that CLL can be diagnosed if the blood lymphocyte count is >5000/μL, below this value in asymptomatic patients, a diagnosis of monoclonal B lymphocytosis (MBL) should be made (5).

Anemia and thrombocytopenia may be observed at the time of initial diagnosis. Low hemoglobin (<11 or 10 g/dL) and/or platelet levels (<100,000/μL) are observed at the time of diagnosis in about 20% of patients, are a sign of more advanced disease, and predict for poorer prognosis.

Autoimmune hemolytic anemia (AHA) is a common complication in CLL. The direct antiglobulin test (DAT, Coombs' test) may be positive at some time during the course of the disease in up to 35% of cases; overt AHA occurs in 11% percent of cases (6). In a recent analysis within the United Kingdom, CLL4 trial, the pretreatment incidence of a positive DAT was 14%. Ten percent developed AHA. The DAT correctly predicted the development, or not, of AHA after therapy in 83% of cases; however, only 28% of DAT+ patients developed AHA. AHA, or a positive DAT, independently predicted for reduced overall survival (7).

Autoimmune thrombocytopenia is most often diagnosed on the basis of the presence of adequate numbers of megakaryocytes in the bone marrow with an abnormally low platelet count in the peripheral blood. This complication occurs in 2% to 3% of patients with CLL (6).

Agranulocytosis may be encountered in CLL, but is rare in the absence of therapy (approximately 0.5%). In patients with total white blood cell counts >100,000/μL, the absolute neutrophil count may be normal (i.e., >1500/μL) in spite of a neutrophil percentage of 1% or 2%.

Significant degrees of hypogammaglobulinemia and neutropenia may result in increased predisposition of patients with CLL to major bacterial infections. In addition, the use of purine analogs as treatment for CLL has resulted in an increased incidence of opportunistic infections (e.g., tuberculosis, candida, pneumocystis) (8).

Morphology

The malignant cell in B-CLL has the appearance of a normal, mature, small lymphocyte. There are uniform populations of small lymphocytes (2,9). The nucleus almost fills the entire cell. The nuclear chromatin is clumped, and a nucleolus is usually not discernible and inconspicuous (Fig. 1). In addition to the typical small cells, a small proportion of cells may consist of larger lymphocytes with a wider cytoplasm, a larger, somewhat notched nucleus, lacy-appearing nuclear chromatin and a visible nucleolus. These "prolymphocytes" may account for a minority of the overall population of lymphocytes in B-CLL, usually less than 10%. Most of the other conditions associated with blood lymphocytosis, such as leukemic mantle cell lymphoma, prolymphocytic leukemia (PLL), or hairy cell leukemia (HCL) have their own characteristic morphological features distinct from CLL. The diagnosis can usually be made by the peripheral blood smear, where the mature-appearing small lymphocytes may account for 50% to 100% of the leukocytes and should be confirmed by immunophenotyping. Commonly flattened or smudged cells are found (Gumprecht's phenomenon).

The characteristic findings on the bone marrow aspirate smear include increased cellularity, with lymphocytes accounting for >30% of all nucleated cells. A bone marrow biopsy examination is not required for establishing a diagnosis of CLL, but it is warranted to clarify the reason for cytopenias, has some prognostic value, and is needed for remission assessment (3–5,10).

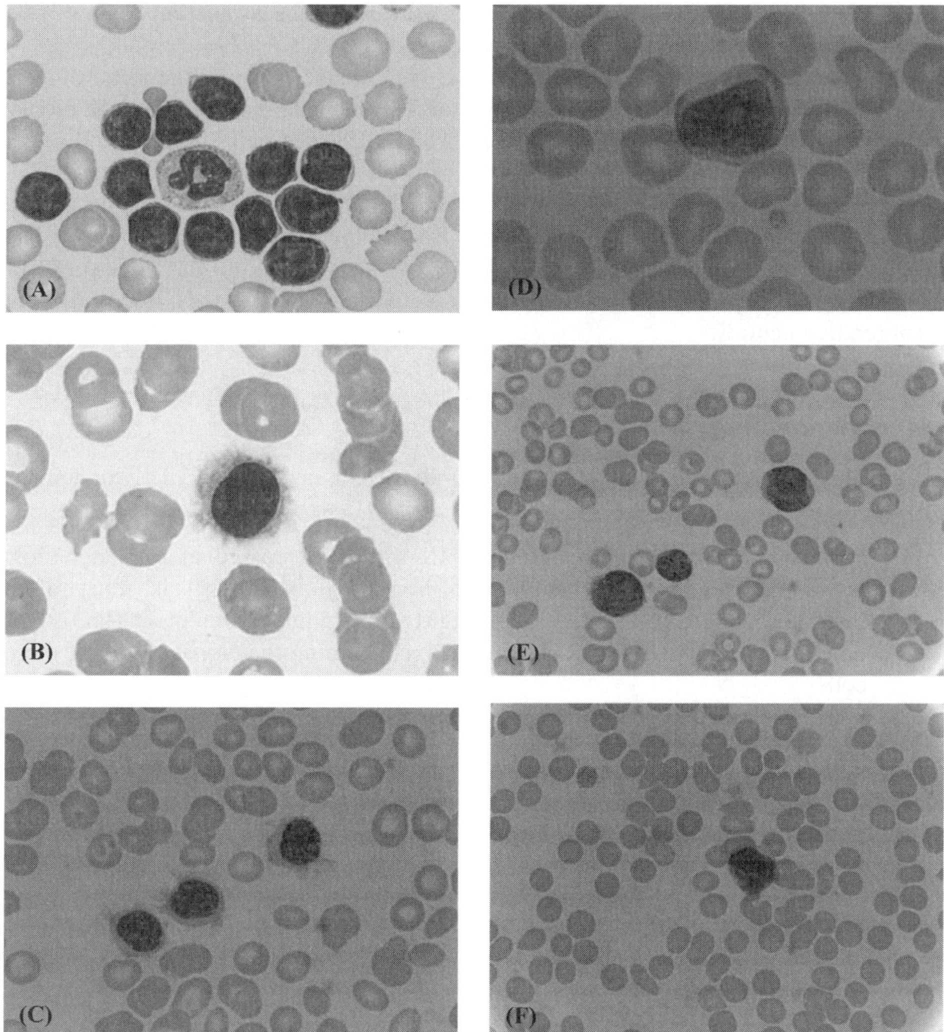

Figure 1 Morphology of lymphocytes in CLL, different lymphoid leukemias (A: CLL, B: HCL, C: SMZL with villous lymphocytes, D: B-PLL, E: leukemic MCL, F: Sezary cell). *Abbreviations*: CLL, chronic lymphocytic leukaemia; HCL, hairy cell leukaemia; SMZL, splenic marginal zone lymphoma; B-PLL, B-prolymphocytic leukemia; MCL, mantle cell lymphoma. *Source*: Courtesy of Dr. M. Bommer (*See Color Insert*).

Histology

In addition to an increased percentage of mature-appearing lymphocytes in the smears of the bone marrow aspirate, there are three types of infiltrative patterns of lymphocytes, which are recognized in trephine biopsy specimens of the bone marrow: nodular, interstitial, and diffuse. Sometimes in a biopsy sample one may see a mixture of nodular and interstitial or nodular and diffuse infiltrative patterns. Patients with diffuse infiltration tend to have advanced disease and relatively poorer outlook, whereas for prognostic purposes, nodular and interstitial patterns may be grouped together and termed "nondiffuse" (nodular partial remission); this latter pattern is associated with less advanced disease and a better prognosis (10,11). However, this association has not been observed in a recent trial in Binet stage A patients (12).

As was noted above, B-cell CLL and SLL are considered to be the same disease with different manifestations (2). The diagnosis of SLL is made via a lymph node biopsy in a patient without peripheral lymphocytosis, while CLL is usually diagnosed through examination of the peripheral blood and bone marrow in patients with lymphocytosis. The histopathologic lymph node findings in SLL and CLL are identical and consist of a diffusely effaced nodal architecture with few residual germinal centers (13,14) The infiltrate is mostly mature-appearing, small lymphocytes, with an admixture of prolymphocytes and paraimmunoblasts. Mitotic activity is usually very low, but there are proliferative centres.

Immunophenotyping

There are three major aspects of phenotypic findings classical of B-CLL lymphocytes (15,16):

1. Surface membrane immunoglobulin (SmIg) is expressed at extremely low levels in CLL (SmIg weak). The immunoglobulin (Ig) is most often immunoglobulin M (IgM) or both IgM and immunoglobulin D (IgD), and only a single Ig light chain is expressed, confirming the clonal nature of these cells.
2. Expression of the B-cell-associated antigens CD23 and CD19 and CD20.
3. Coexpression of CD5, a T-cell associated antigen, together with the B-cell markers.

In addition, CLL cells are negative for cyclin D1 and CD10. FMC7, CD22, and CD79b are usually negative or weakly expressed (17). Cases with unmutated VH mutation status have been reported to be CD38+, although the correlation is imperfect (18,19). A scoring system for differentiating CLL from other B-cell lymphoproliferative diseases has been devised on the basis of the above immunophenotypic findings. Each of the following cellular characteristics is scored with one point (16):

- Staining for surface Ig is weakly positive
- CD5+
- CD23+
- CD79b or CD22 is weakly positive
- FMC7−

A score of 4 or 5 had an accuracy of 97% for the diagnosis of CLL, while most of the other non-CLL B-cell lymphoproliferative diseases had scores of 0 to 2.

Differential Diagnosis

There are several malignant lymphoproliferative disorders, which may be similar to CLL in its clinical presentation, particularly leukemic mantle cell lymphoma (MCL), follicular, and other non-Hodgkin's lymphoma (17,20). In contrast to the phenotypic features of CLL, however, the amount of SmIg is abundant in most lymphomas, and with the exception of MCL, the lymphocytes are usually CD5 negative. Features distinguishing these conditions from CLL are summarized below.

Mantle Cell Lymphoma

Small lymphocytes with irregular or cleaved nuclei are seen in MCL and share positivity for CD5 and CD20 with B-CLL (Fig. 1). Accordingly, MCL in a leukemic phase can mimic B-CLL. However, unlike B-CLL, cells in MCL stain strongly for cyclin D1 and SmIg and are negative for CD23 (2,21). In addition, MCL carries the typical cytogenetic abnormality t(11;14)(q13;q32). Because of the poor prognosis and different treatment approaches, the differentiation of leukemic MCL from CLL is of particular importance.

Lymphoplasmacytic Lymphoma

Lymphoplasmacytic lymphoma is a malignancy in which the malignant B cells show variable degrees of maturation toward plasma cells. Such cells may display positivity for cytoplasmic Ig, PCA1 (a finding, which is not present in CLL), and CD38 (which can be present in patients with CLL). The cells are mostly negative for CD5 and CD23. Many cases show the typical IgM paraproteinemia of Waldenströms macroglobulinemia (2). While malignant lymphocytes can be present in the peripheral blood, leukocyte counts are typically lower than in CLL.

Hairy Cell Leukemia

HCL is usually associated with cytopenia (leucocyte counts rarely exeeding 10×10^9/L except in HCL variant), but in cases with an elevated lymphocyte count in the peripheral blood, the distinction from CLL is usually possible because of the typical morphological features of hairy cells with cytoplasmic projections (Fig. 1). A bone marrow biopsy will show diffuse infiltration with hairy cells in a characteristic loose fashion, with a well-defined rim of cytoplasm leaving a clear zone around the cells. HCL shows a moderately strong acid phosphatase reaction, not inhibited by tartaric acid [tartaric acid–resistant acid phosphatase test (TRAP+)]. In addition, the cells in HCL are always positive for B-cell markers (CD19, CD20, CD22), and unlike CLL, CD5, and CD23 negative, and positive for CD25, CD11c, and CD103 (2,22).

Splenic Marginal Zone Lymphoma with Villous Lymphocytes

Splenic marginal zone lymphoma (SMZL) with villous lymphocytes is a rare disorder comprising less than 1% of lymphoid neoplasms. SMZL should be thought of in cases of unclassifiable chronic lymphoid leukemias that are CD5–. The cells of SMZL are small with a condensed chromatin and no nucleolus and show polar vili (villous lymphocytes) (Fig. 1). The immunophenotype shows a low CLL score with no or little CD23 expression, strong surface Ig, CD79b and FMC7 expression, which help to differentiate it from CLL.

Prolymphocytic Leukemia

The main feature distinguishing PLL from CLL is the morphology of blood lymphocytes: large cells with somewhat immature-appearing nuclear chromatin, a prominent central nucleolus, and a relatively small amount of cytoplasm (2,23–25). While there are some immunophenotypic features that may help to diagnose B-PLL, the differentiation from CLL is a cytological one (Fig. 1). The differentiation of T-PLL from B-PLL will be obvious from the immunophenotype (see below).

Marked splenomegaly and rapidly rising lymphocyte counts are typical features of the disease. While, very high WBC count, splenomegaly, and bone marrow involvement are common in both B-cell PLL and T-cell PLL, a distinguishing feature can be the presence of skin lesions (25%–27%) and serous effusions, especially pleural effusion (15%), in T-PLL (24,25). Phenotypically, prolymphocytes may be either B cells or T cells and are distinct from CLL lymphocytes.

The B-cell variant of PLL (B-PLL) is usually CD19+, CD20+, CD22+, CD79a+, and FMC7+ (2,23). Prolymphocytes must exceed 55%, and cases of transformed CLL are excluded. B-PLL is rare, accounting for about 1% of lymphocytic leukemias. Marked splenomegaly and rapidly rising lymphocyte counts are typical features of the disease. Many cases of B-PLL have been shown to harbor translocations involving 14q32 and particularly t(11;14)(q13;q32), which is characteristic of MCL (see above), suggesting that these cases may in fact be leukemic MCL.

T-PLL is derived from peripheral T cells negative for TDT and CD1a. Different profiles regarding CD4 and CD8 can be found: CD4+/CD8– (60%), CD4+/CD8+ (25%) (almost unique to T-PLL), or CD4–/CD8+ (15%). The cells are usually also positive for CD2, CD3, CD5, CD7, and CD45 (RO) (24–26). The peripheral blood films show small to medium cells with round, oval, or sometimes irregular nucleus and a visible nucleolus. A typical feature is cytoplasmic protusions.

The small cell variant of T-PLL comprises about 20% of all cases of T-PLL and may be misdiagnosed when using morphology alone.

Large Granular Lymphocyte Leukemia

Large granular lymphocyte (LGL) leukemia, or T-cell granular lymphocytic leukemia, is characterized by the presence of large mononuclear cells with slightly eccentrically placed nuclei and moderately abundant cytoplasm with fine azurophilic granules. The disease is heterogenous, but lymphocytosis is usually mild ($<20 \times 10^9$/L), and neutropenia is a frequent feature. The lymphocytes are T/NK-cells and express a mature postthymic phenotype: CD3+, CD4–, CD8+, CD57+ (80%). Rarer variants may be CD4+, CD8–; show $\gamma \delta$ TCR; or may be double positive (CD4+, CD8+). Many cases originally diagnosed as "T-CLL" have been reclassified as either the small cell variant of T-cell prolymphocytic leukemia (T-PLL, see above), or more often as T-cell LGL leukemia (22,26). As a result, it has been suggested that the diagnosis of T-CLL should be discarded in favor of these other diagnoses.

Sezary Syndrome

In the leukemic manifestation of cutaneous T-cell lymphoma (CTCL), the lymphocytes have a cerebriform nucleus (Sezary cells), which is usually CD4+, CD8–, leading to an increased CD4/8 ratio with increased CD4+/CD7– cells (Fig. 1). This differential diagnosis usually poses no difficulty due to the predominant and typical skin involvement.

Adult T-Cell Lymphoma/Leukemia

Adult T-cell lymphoma/leukemia (ATLL) has a unique incidence in certain parts of the world (Japan and the Caribbean) and in immigrants from those regions (22,26). ATLL cells are highly pleomorphic and have a characteristic nucleus with clumped chromatin and polylobulated nucleus (flower cells). The presence of antibodies to human T-lymphotropic virus type I infection is characteristic of this disease, which is also associated with lesions of skin, bone, and liver, and hypercalcemia.

STAGING

Historically the staging for patients with CLL has been based on thorough clinical examination and complete blood count. In cases with cytopenia of uncertain origin, bone marrow examination should be performed. This workup was supplemented by clinical chemistry and in some cases a Coombs test to investigate hemolysis. With the advent of more intensive treatment regimens, including the use of monoclonal antibodies, serology for viruses should also be investigated if treatment is planned (e.g., hepatitis). Ultrasound has been widely used, but is not needed to ascertain clinical stage according to the Binet and Rai staging systems. An overview of the updated guidelines for the diagnosis and pretreatment evaluation has recently summarized the current workup in CLL (5).

The Rai system is based upon a hierachical grouping of disease manifestations of blood and bone marrow (lymphocytosis/Rai 0), enlarged lymph nodes (lymphadenopathy Rai I), spleen and liver (Rai II), and bone marrow failure [anemia (Rai III) and thrombocytopenia (Rai IV)] (27). The median survival times from the time of diagnosis in the series of patients studied by Rai et al. were 150 months for stage 0, 101 months for stage I, 71 months for stage II, and only 9 months in stages III and IV.

As there were only three distinct actuarial survival patterns (stage O, stages I and II combined, and stages III and IV combined), the Rai staging, similarly to the Binet system, was modified to consist of three groups (28):

- Low risk—Rai stage O
- Intermediate risk—Rai stages I and II combined
- High risk—Rai stages III and IV combined

The Binet staging system takes into consideration five potential sites of involvement: cervical, axillary, and inguinal lymph nodes (whether unilateral or bilateral, each area is counted as one), spleen, and liver. Patients are classified according to the number of involved sites plus the presence of anemia (hemoglobin <10 g/dL) and/or thrombocytopenia (platelets $<100,000/\mu L$) (29):

- Stage A—fewer than three involved lymphoid sites
- Stage B—three or more involved lymphoid sites
- Stage C—presence of anemia and/or thrombocytopenia.

This system is of great value in stratifying patients with survival curves corresponding to the Rai low-risk, intermediate-risk, and high-risk groups, respectively.

The International Workshop Group on CLL (IWCLL) recommended that, in practice, an integrated system using both methods should be used (4). According to this recommendation, each Binet stage is to be further identified by the appropriate Rai stage (e.g., A0, AI, AII, BI, BII, CIII, CIV). However, this integrated system has not been widely accepted, and most clinicians use either the Rai (North America) or Binet (Europe) method for patient management and therapeutic investigation.

Radiological Assessment

The use of CT scans has entered the scene of staging in CLL similar to non-Hodgkins lymphoma, and the advantages of a precise lymph node assessment appear self-evident. This is particularly important if a patient is entered into a clinical trial, where computed tomography (CT) of the abdomen, pelvis, and chest are recommended as baseline studies. Such studies provide a measure of the size of the liver, spleen, and retroperitoneal nodes for comparison with subsequent reexaminations to determine the level of clinical response

Table 1 Overview of the Current Guidelines for the Diagnosis and Assessment of CLL Patients According to the Updated NCI Guidelines (modified)

Diagnosis of CLL	General practice	Clinical trial
Complete blood count and differential count	+	+
Immunophenotyping of lymphocytes	+	+
Assessment prior to treatment		
History and physical performance status	+	+
Complete blood count and differential	+	+
Marrow aspirate and biopsy	+	+
Serum chemistry	+	+
Serum Ig	+	+
DAT	+	+
Chest radiograph	+	+
History/workup of infection	+	+
Cytogenetics (FISH) for del(13q), del(11q), del(17p), add(12), del(6q)	(+)	+
IgV$_H$ mutational status, ZAP-70, and CD38	(+)	+
CT scan of chest, abdomen, and pelvis	−	+
MRI, Lymphangiogram, gallium scan, PET scans	−	−
Abdominal ultrasound	(+/−)	+

Abbreviations: CLL, chronic lymphocytic leukaemia; NCI, National Cancer Institute; DAT, direct antiglobulin test; FISH, fluorescence in situ hybridization; CT, computed tomography; MRI, magnetic resonance imaging; PET, positron emission tomographic; Ig, immunoglobulin.
Source: From Ref. 5.

on protocol-based therapy. A recent report detailed the results of abdominal CT performed in 140 patients consecutively diagnosed with CLL in Rai stage 0 disease. An abnormal abdominal CT was found in 27% of patients and correlated with increased bone marrow infiltration, high lymphocyte count, increased ZAP-70 expression, and short lymphocyte doubling time. Patients with abnormal CT progressed more frequently and had a shorter time to progression than those with normal CT (median, 3.5 years vs. not reached, respectively; $p < 0.001$) and required earlier treatment intervention. In a multivariate analysis, only high ZAP-70 expression (RR = 3.60) and an abnormal abdominal CT (RR = 2.71) correlated with disease progression (30). The recent update on the guidelines for the diagnosis and treatment of CLL suggests using CT scans for response assessment in clinical trials (5) (Table 1).

Positron emission tomographic (PET) scanning is generally of no value in CLL, but it might be helpful when transformation of CLL into a more aggressive lymphoma variant (Richter's transformation) is thought to have occurred.

PROGNOSIS

While the diagnosis of CLL is relatively simple to make, the disease is characterized by a highly variable clinical course. Some patients have no or minimal symptoms and may have a normal life expectancy, while others progress early and may die of their disease. Treatment has traditionally been used for advanced stage or symptomatic disease. Over recent years, highly effective and potentially curative approaches such as the combination of antibodies with chemotherapy and allogeneic stem cell transplantation have been developed and used in CLL. In recent years, molecular and cellular markers have been

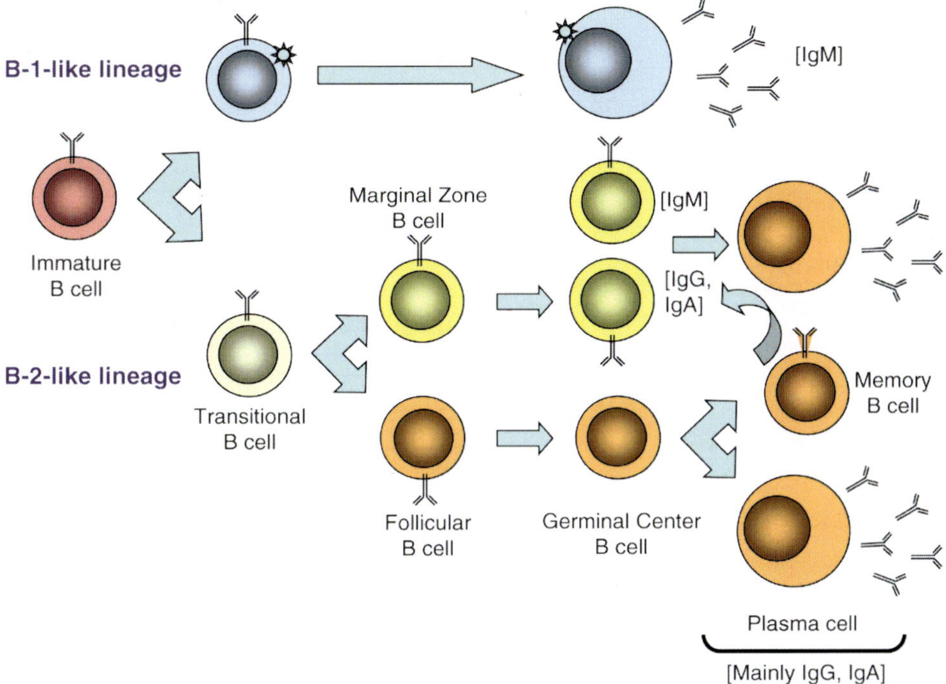

Figure 1.1 Maturation pathways that normal B lymphocytes could follow. This schema is based primarily on studies carried out in mice. The relationship of some of the proposed pathways to human B cells has not been defined (e.g., B-1 cell differentiation pathway) (*see page 2*).

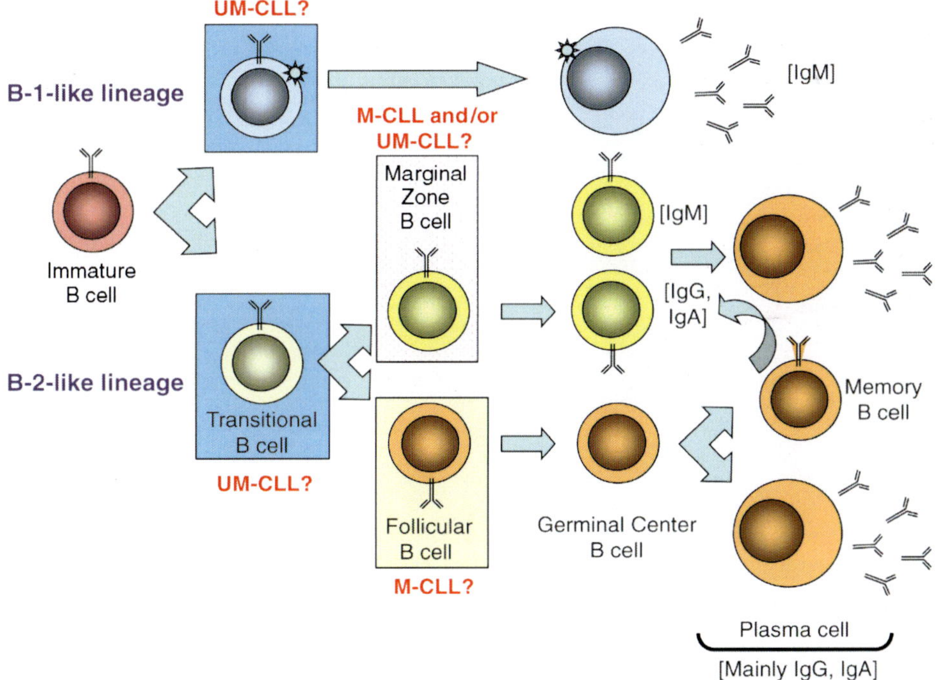

Figure 1.2 Stages of maturation at which U-CLL and M-CLL cells might emerge (see Figure 1). Boxes indicate potential cell types that could give rise to U-CLL and/or M-CLL. *Abbreviations*: U-CLL, unmutated CLL; M-CLL, mutated CLL (*see page 11*).

Generation of gene expression data by DNA microarray hybridization

Unsupervised analysis	**Supervised analysis**
Identification of cell types that have not been classified a priori	Identification of expression differences btw. samples that have been defined a priori

Unsupervised hierarchical clustering algorithms to cluster... *Supervised pattern discovery algorithms to compare...*

IgV mutated and unmutated CLL
• no differences btw. the two subtypes

IgV mutated vs. unmutated CLL
• identification of a small set of differentially expressed genes
• generation of a classifier

CLL together with other transformed B-cells
• CLL show a distinct GEP
• CLL form a subcluster w/ mantle cell lymphoma and hairy cell leukemia

DLBCL BL   FL DLBCL   CLL   MCL   HCL

CLL vs. normal and transformed B-cells
• identification of the CLL signature

CLL vs. specific signature of normal B-cells
• identification of the cellular origin

CLL, untreated vs. treated w/ drug/receptor stimulation
• identification of a drug or activation-induced signature

Figure 2.1 GEP-based strategies for the identification of CLL subtypes and differentially expressed genes between CLL subtypes. Gene expression data generated by DNA microarray hybridization are analyzed by unsupervised or supervised analysis methods, depending on the particular question (indicated in the boxes). The dendrogram resulting from unsupervised hierarchical clustering of samples representing various types of mature B-cell malignancies (*bottom left*). *Abbreviation*: CLL, chronic lymphocytic leukemia (*see page 21*).

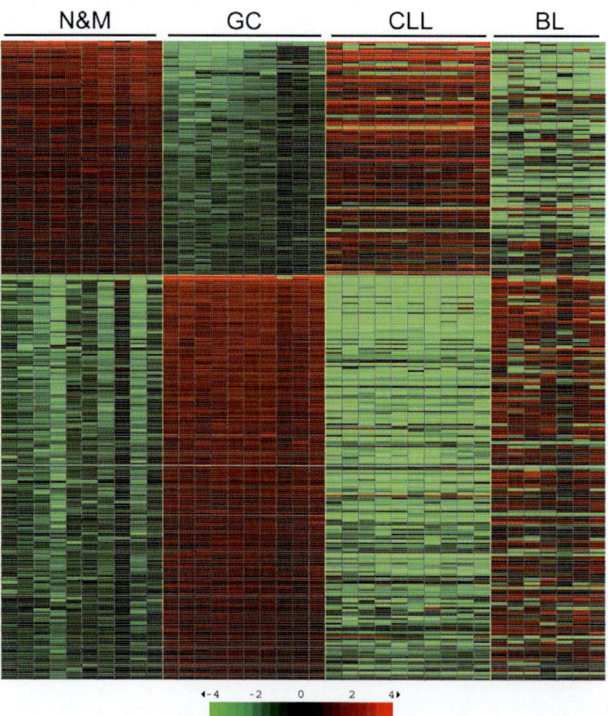

Figure 2.2 Visualization of the histological derivation of CLL and Burkitt lymphoma by GEP. Genes differentially expressed between naïve and memory B cells (N&M) on the one hand and GC B cells (GC B) on the other were identified by supervised pattern discovery analysis. The expression level of the respective genes in CLL and Burkitt lymphoma (BL) is shown along with the differentially expressed genes. The relatedness of the tumor cases to either the GC B cells or the non-GC B cells is visible from the expression values coded in shades of gray and can be quantitatively expressed by statistical analysis (not shown). Upregulated and downregulated genes are identified by darker and lighter gray tones, respectively. *Abbreviations*: CLL, chronic lymphocytic leukemia; GC, germinal center (*see page 26*).

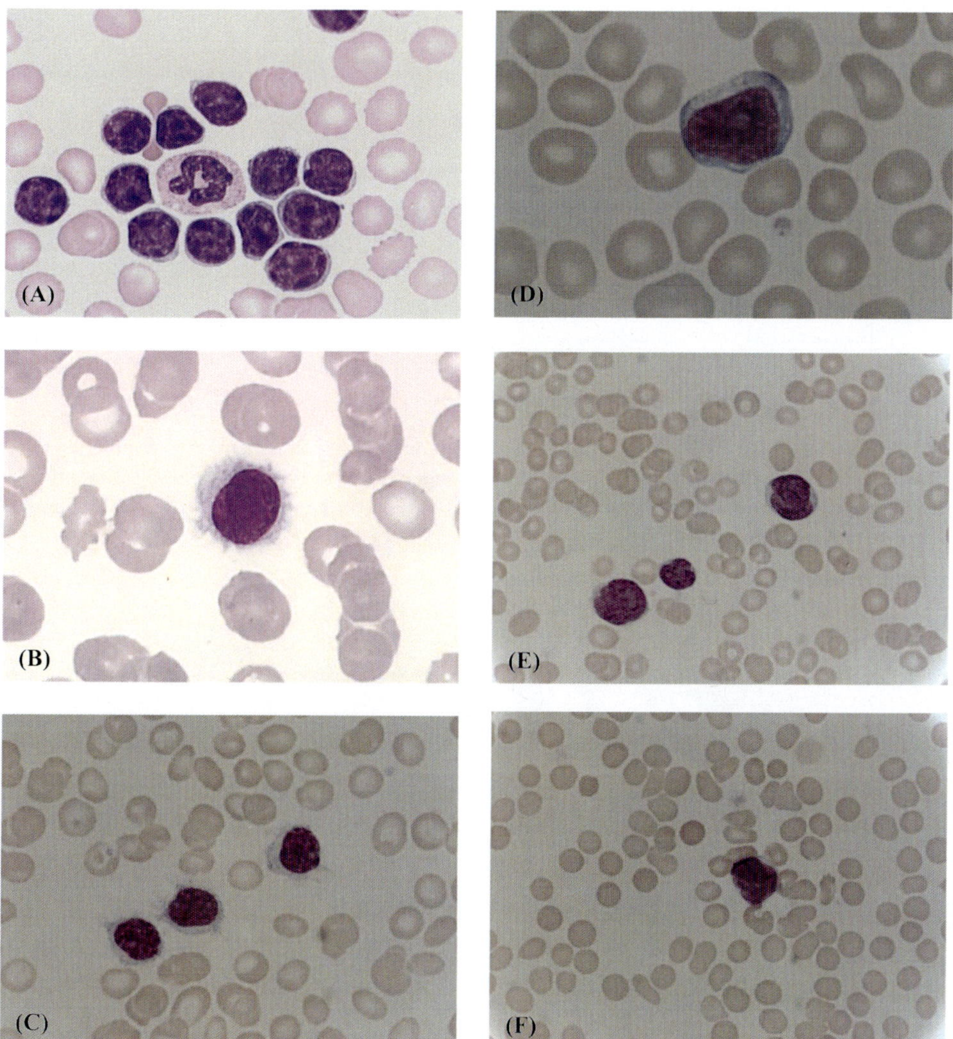

Figure 7.1 Morphology of lymphocytes in CLL, different lymphoid leukemias (A: CLL, B: HCL, C: SMZL with villous lymphocytes, D: B-PLL, E: leukemic MCL, F: Sezary cell). *Abbreviations*: CLL, chronic lymphocytic leukaemia; HCL, hairy cell leukaemia; SMZL, splenic marginal zone lymphoma; B-PLL, B-prolymphocytic leukemia; MCL, mantle cell lymphoma. *Source*: Courtesy of Dr. M. Bommer (*see page 105*).

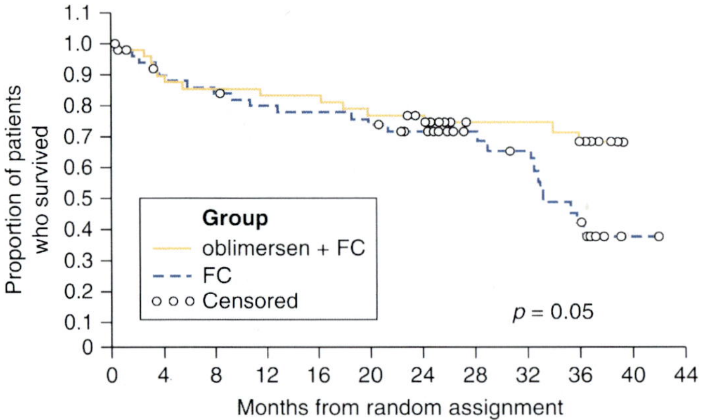

Figure 9.3 Kaplan-Meier survival curves for fludarabine-sensitive patients by treatment group. Median overall survival not reached for the oblimersen sodium and FC arm versus 33.2 months for the FC-only arm (hazard ratio = 0.53, p = 0.05). *Abbreviation*: FC, fludarabine and cyclophosphamide. *Source*: From Ref. 82 (*see page 159*).

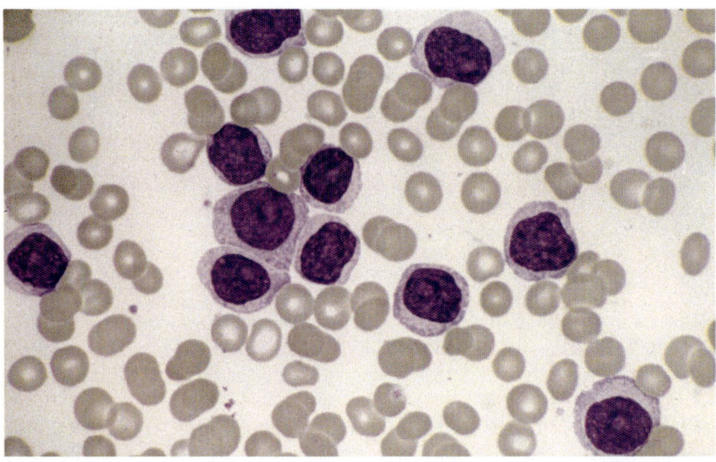

Figure 13.1 May-Grumwald-Giemsa stained peripheral blood film from a patient with B-PLL showing prolymphocytes with a regular nuclear outline, single nucleolus, and a relatively abundant pale cytoplasm. *Abbreviation*: B-PLL, B-cell prolymphocytic leukaemia (*see page 219*).

discovered, and some of these are now used to stratify patients to different treatment options. The following will summarize the important molecular techniques used to study CLL cells and will relate to the clinical consequences and prognostic value.

Clinical Stage According to Binet and Rai

The standard clinical procedures to estimate prognosis in CLL are the staging systems developed by Rai and Binet (27,29). These systems rely solely on physical examination and a blood count. The prognostic impact of these staging systems was confirmed in many independent series of patients. However, there is heterogeneity in the course of the disease between individual patients within a single stage group. More importantly, biologic risk factors such as the VH mutation status and genomic aberrations may have the power to identify subgroups of patients with poor prognosis among early stage patients. Both parameters have been shown in multivariate analysis to provide prognostic information independently of the clinical stage (19).

Markers of Tumor Burden: Lymphocyte Count, Lymphocyte Doubling Time, Serum Lactate Dehydrogenase and Bone Marrow Infiltration Pattern

Apart from the clinical staging systems, other easily assessable parameters of disease activity and tumor burden such as the lymphocyte count, the lymphocyte doubling time, the serum lactate dehydrogenase (LDH) level, and the bone marrow infiltration pattern have been shown to be of prognostic relevance in CLL. Elevated LDH levels and high lymphocyte counts are associated with disease activity. In multivariate analyses including clinical (age, stage, etc.) and genetic (VH status, genomic aberrations, etc.) variables, these parameters were independent prognostic factors (19,31). Although partially correlated with clinical stage, the lymphocyte doubling time was shown to have a clear prognostic significance by itself: whereas a doubling time of 12 months or less identified a population of patients with poor prognosis, a doubling time longer than 12 months was indicative of good prognosis as substantiated by a long treatment-free period and survival. In addition, a short lymphocyte doubling time predicts rapid disease progression in patients in the early clinical stages (12,32). Another marker for tumor burden, the bone marrow histology pattern, has been evaluated for prognostic reasons. Several studies showed that cases with diffuse bone marrow infiltration had a poor prognosis as compared with cases presenting with a nodular pattern (10,33). There is a strong association of the bone marrow infiltration pattern with clinical stage and absolute lymphocyte counts. In a recent analysis from the German CLL Study Group (GCLLSG), bone marrow infiltration pattern was associated with progression-free survival but not overall survival and was not an independent prognostic factor (12).

Serum Parameters: β2-microglobulin, Thymidine Kinase, and Soluble CD23

A number of serologic parameters such as β2-microglobulin (β2-MG), thymidine kinase (TK), and soluble CD23 (sCD23) have been shown to provide information about patients' outcome.

TK is a cellular enzyme known to be involved in a "salvage pathway" for DNA synthesis and is probably related to the number of dividing neoplastic cells, reflecting tumor mass and the rate of tumor cell proliferation. It was shown that TK levels correlate with the proliferative activity of CLL cells and that elevated levels predict disease progression in CLL (34). In a recent study, TK appeared to detect a subgroup of patients with early, nonsmoldering CLL at risk for rapid disease progression and provided independent prognostic information on progression-free survival (35). In the prospective CLL1 trial of the GCLLSG, elevated serum TK was a strong predictor for rapid disease progression among Binet stage A patients (12).

CD23 is a functionally relevant surface molecule on B-CLL cells. High levels of sCD23 at initial diagnosis were linked with disease progression in early stage B-CLL. Furthermore, sCD23 was associated with a diffuse bone marrow infiltration pattern, a short lymphocyte doubling time, and elevated serum TK levels.

β2-MG is an extracellular protein that is noncovalently associated with the class I major histocompatibility complex. Serum levels show a correlation with the clinical staging systems according to Binet and Rai. β2-MG is associated with adverse prognostic features at presentation, and higher values have been found in CLL patients with a shorter survival (12,36). Response to chemotherapy seems to be worse in patients with high β2-MG levels. Recently, a prognostic nomogram based on a retrospective analysis from the M. D. Anderson Cancer Center (MDACC) has been developed including age, β2-MG, absolute lymphocyte count, sex, Rai stage, and number of involved lymph node groups (37).

VH Mutational Status

One of the most important molecular genetic parameters to dissect pathogenic and prognostic subgroups of CLL is the mutation status of the VH genes (18,38). Patients with CLL can be divided into two groups: one with unmutated VH genes, assumed to originate from pregerminal center cells, and another with mutated VH genes, thought to originate from postgerminal center cells. Of note, the definition of VH mutated or unmutated CLL relies on an arbitrarily defined threshold of 98% homology to the most similar germ line gene. Importantly, it could be demonstrated that the VH mutation status is clinically highly relevant (18,38). While CLL with unmutated VH follows an unfavorable course with rapid progression, CLL with mutated VH often shows slow progression and long survival. Figure 2 depicts the survival curves for patients distributed over all stages ($N = 300$) and separately for patients diagnosed with Binet stage A disease ($N = 189$) from our single-center cohort (17). Furthermore, independent of the mutation status, the usage of specific VH genes such as V3-21 is associated with an inferior outcome (39). In addition, patients with a rearranged V3-21 show certain molecular characteristics with shorter than average complementarity determining regions (CDRs) (HCDR3) and almost identical HCDR3 sequences with a conserved amino acid motif and a highly restricted usage of the λ V2-14 gene in most cases (39). Considering that the CDRs of both the heavy- and light-chain V region comprise the antigen-binding site of the Ig molecule, these findings indicate striking similarities in the B-cell receptors (BCRs) of V3-21 using CLL cases and suggest a stimulatory influence of an unknown antigen in the disease development. In addition, other frequently used and highly restricted VDJ combinations have been identified (40).

"Surrogate" Markers for VH Status

As the determination of VH mutation status is technically demanding, a search for "surrogate markers," i.e., parameters that are strongly correlated with VH mutation status, was performed. Among these surrogate markers, ZAP-70, a molecule usually involved in T-cell receptor signalling, was identified in gene expression profiling studies and showed

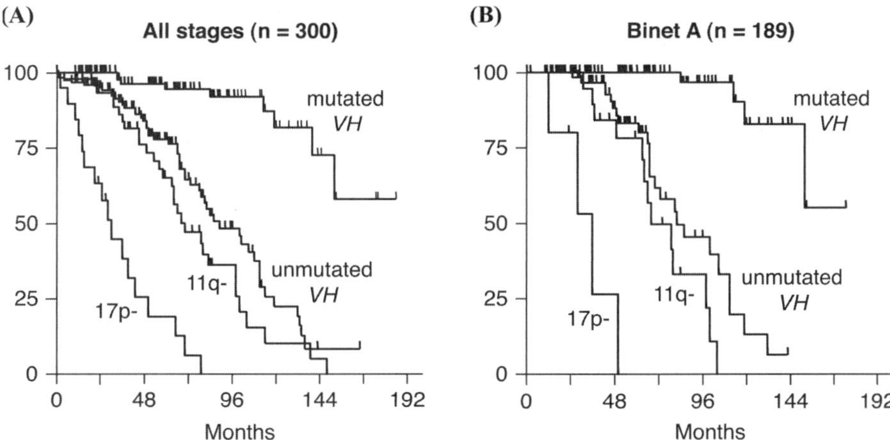

Figure 2 Prognostic relevance of genomic aberrations in CLL and VH mutation status in CLL. Survival probabilities among patients in the following genetic categories: 17p– (17p deletion irrespective of VH mutation status), 11q– (11q deletion irrespective of VH mutation status), unmutated VH (homology $\geq$98% and no 17p or 11q deletion), and mutated VH (homology <98% and no 17p or 11q deletion). (**A**) Among all 300 patients estimated, median survival times were 17p– 30 months, 11q– 70 months, VH $\geq$ 98% 89 months, and VH <98% not reached (54% survival at 152 months); (**B**) In Binet A patients only ($N = 189$), estimated median survival times were 17p– 36 months, 11q– 68 months, VH $\geq$ 98% 86 months, and VH < 98% not reached (52% survival at 152 months). *Abbreviation*: CLL, chronic lymphocytic leukaemia.

promise. The measurement of ZAP-70 levels by fluorescence-activated cell sorting (FACS) can separate distinct prognostic groups of Binet stage A CLL patients (41). In all patients in whom at least 20% of the leukemic cells were positive for ZAP-70, IgVH was unmutated, whereas IgVH mutations were found in 21 of 24 patients in whom less than 20% of the leukemic cells were positive for ZAP-70.

As is the case with any prognostic marker, the relationship of new prognostic markers must be correlated with other markers known to impact outcome. In a recent study, the association and the prognostic impact of ZAP-70 expression, the VH mutation status, and additional genetic high-risk factors such as V3-21 usage (associated with poor prognosis) and genomic aberrations were analysed (42). In agreement with previous reports, a strong association of high ZAP-70 expression and unmutated VH genes was confirmed (42–44). However, discordance of ZAP-70 expression and VH mutation status occurred in 25% of cases. The proportion of discordant cases was particularly high in the distinct subgroups with V3-21 usage and 17p or 11q deletion (39%). In a multivariate analysis, the VH mutation status, V3-21 usage, the presence of high-risk genomic aberrations, but not ZAP-70 expression, were identified as independent prognostic factors. However, the association of ZAP-70 and the VH mutation status was strong in cases without additional genetic high-risk features, and the majority of V3-21 cases showed high ZAP-70 expression irrespective of the VH mutation status. If high-risk genomic aberrations are present, it is important to consider this in addition to the prognostic impact of the VH status and ZAP-70 status for the prediction of the clinical course. In the absence of high-risk genomic aberrations, the VH status and ZAP-70 status may have similar prognostic impact and might therefore be alternatively applied. In addition to the prognostic consequences, the data provided evidence for a theoretical model of ZAP-70 expression in the pathogenesis of CLL, in which active BCR signaling stimulates the malignant clone. A survival advantage for CLL cells as a result of the BCR-related interaction with unknown antigens could explain the signs of antigen selection pressure, such as restricted VH gene usage. In contrast, 17p or 11q deletions, affecting critical cancer genes, may lead to an inherent survival advantage independent of ZAP-70 or BCR-mediated effects in CLL cells.

A problem concerning ZAP-70 determination in clinical practice is that there remain some challenges in the standardization of a FACS assay for its measurement. Before ZAP-70 determination can reliably be used outside specialized laboratories, this issue needs to be solved (45).

In the gene expression studies, a number of other genes have been identified with differential expression in the VH mutated and unmutated subgroups, suggesting that expression levels of these genes may be used to simplify VH mutational assessment by use of "surrogate marker(s)" (46). In a recent study, 10 genes were tested by real-time quantitative polymerase chain reaction (RQ-PCR) in unpurified samples from 130 CLL patients (47). In multivariate logistic regression analysis, expression levels of LPL, ZAP-70, ADAM29, and SEPT10 were the most predictive for IgVH mutational status. In univariate analysis, the expression of LPL was the best predictor, and in a multivariate analysis, LPL expression remained a significant predictor. These results supported the earlier findings showing a strong correlation between LPL and VH-mutation status and a prognostic impact of LPL expression levels (43,48).

While the study of the VH mutational status has greatly enhanced our understanding of the disease and increased our ability to separate prognostic subgroups in CLL, the role of the VH mutational status in guiding therapy is currently unresolved, and treatment decisions should not be based on this outside clinical trials.

Genomic Aberrations and CLL

Fluorescence in situ hybridization (FISH) allows the detection of chromosomal aberrations not only in dividing cells but also in interphase nuclei, an approach referred to as interphase cytogenetics. Genomic aberrations can be identified in about 80% of CLL cases by FISH with a disease-specific comprehensive probe set (31). The most common recurrent chromosomal abnormalities are deletions 13q, 11q, 17p, 6q, and trisomy 12 (31). Moreover, the rate of disease progression and the overall survival time of CLL subgroups as defined by specific genomic aberrations are significantly different (Fig. 2). Five prognostic categories have been defined in a statistical model showing poor survival in patients with 17p deletion, and 11q deletion (median survival 32 and 79 months) and better survival for patients with 12q trisomy, normal karyotype, and 13q deletion as the sole abnormality (114, 111, and 133 months, respectively). These observations have been reproduced in prospective clinical trials with very similar results (49). Specific genomic aberrations have provided some insights into the pathogenesis of the disease by pointing to candidate genes (17p13: TP53, 11q22–q23: ATM, and most likely other candidate genes), while for other loci (e.g., 13q), the precise role of possible tumor suppressors has not been fully elucidated. In addition, specific genomic aberrations have been associated with disease characteristics such as marked lymphadenopathy (11q deletion), and resistance to treatment with conventional chemotherapy (17p deletion) further documenting the importance of chromosomal aberrations on the course of CLL (50,51). Although the group of patients with deletion 17p is quite small in early stages and at first-line treatment (Table 2), the detection of this chromosome aberration is of importance because these patients are unlikely to respond to chemotherapy. This

Table 2 Incidence of Genomic Aberrations and VH Mutation Status in a Large Single-Center FISH Study Compared with Preliminary Results from Prospective Multicenter Trials of the German CLL Study Group for Different Clinical Situations

Study	13q–	13q– single	11q–	+12q	17p–	6q–	VH unmutated	VH mutated
Single-center[a]	55%	36%	18%	16%	7%	7%	56%	44%
CLL1[b]	59%	40%	10%	13%	4%	2%	41%	59%
CLL4[c]	53%	34%	21%	11%	3%	9%	69%	31%
CLL3[d]	52%	27%	22%	12%	3%	6%	68%	32%
CLL2H[e]	48%	14%	32%	18%	27%	9%	81%	19%

[a]Single-center cohort of CLL patients distributed over all stages.
[b]CLL1 trial of the GCLLSG for untreated Binet A patients with no classical indication for treatment.
[c]CLL4 trial (randomized F vs. FC) of the GCLLSG for untreated Binet B/C patients up to 65 years of age with treatment indication.
[d]CLL3 trial (early myeloablative radiochemotherapy and autologous stem cell transplantation) of the GCLLSG for Binet B/C patients up to 60 years of age with no or one line of prior therapy.
[e]CLL2H trial (subcutaneous alemtuzumab) of the GCLLSG for fludarabine-refractory patients with indication for treatment.
Abbreviations: CLL, chronic lymphocytic leukaemia; FISH, fluorescence in situ hybridization.

subgroup's poor prognosis has been confirmed in clinical trials; they have a significantly inferior outcome with regard to overall survival after first-line therapy with alkylating agents and purine analogs (49,51). As a result, the 17p– abnormality is the first biological marker to become incorporated in risk-stratified first-line treatment approaches in CLL (U.K. CAM-PRED study, German CLL2O study). There is a growing consensus that cytogenetics by FISH should be obtained (at least for 17p–) in every patient before therapy is given. Cases with 17p deletion account for a large proportion of the fludarabine-refractory cases. Nonetheless, not all cases of fludarabine-refractory CLL show high-risk cytogenetics, suggesting that the development of new markers predicting F-refractory disease could advance patient management. The outcome of fludarabine-refractory CLL even after treatment with p53-independent agents such as alemtuzumab is still poor, owing to the fact that the majority of patients do not achieve a remission and that the average duration of remission is short (52,53). The logical consequence of the central role of 17p deletion in refractory disease is a growing interest in therapies that act independently of p53. While this concept stems from the experience with F-refractory CLL, where response to chemotherapy has been particularly poor, it is likely to gain significance also for frontline therapies. It seems likely that certain subgroups of patients in addition to 17p– cases (e.g., ATM deficient) will benefit from therapies acting independent of the DNA-damage response.

Table 2 gives a summary of the incidences of genomic aberrations and the VH mutation status observed in a single-center cohort of patients distributed over all stage groups and from several multicenter trials of the GCLLSG. It is important to note that there are some differences with regard to the occurrence of high-risk (17p–, 11q–, unmutated VH) and low-risk (13q– single, mutated VH) markers indicating the distinct biological background of the patient cohorts enrolled in various studies and encountered in different clinical situations. High-risk cytogenetic aberrations are more likely to be found in more advanced disease and after therapy, suggesting that reassessment of chromosomal abnormalities may be useful during the course of disease (54).

Genomic Aberrations and VH Mutation Status

With the genomic aberrations and the VH mutation status, two separate genetic parameters of prognostic relevance are available, and they appear to be correlated. Unfavorable aberrations (11q–, 17p–) occur more frequently in VH unmutated, and favorable aberrations (13q– single) occur more frequently in the VH mutated subgroup (19,55,56). This unbalanced distribution of genomic aberrations emphasizes the different biological background of the CLL subgroups with mutated or unmutated VH but only partly explains their different clinical course. About two-thirds of the VH unmutated CLL cases show no unfavorable genomic aberrations indicating a differential influence of these factors.

To examine the individual prognostic value of genomic aberrations, the VH mutation status, and other clinical and laboratory features, we performed a multivariate analysis (17). The VH mutation status, 17p deletion, 11q deletion, age, leukocyte count, and LDH were identified as independent prognostic factors regarding overall survival. When the VH mutation status, 11q, and 17p aberrations were included in the model, the clinical stage of disease according to the systems of Rai or Binet was not identified as an independent prognostic factor (19). Similar results demonstrating a strong prognostic and independent impact of the VH mutation status and genomic aberrations were found in other series (55,56). Therefore, four subgroups of CLL with markedly differing survival probabilities can be defined by the VH mutation status, 11q deletion, and 17p deletion. On the basis of these studies, it appears that VH mutation status and genomic aberrations are among the strongest currently available parameters and are of independent value to predict outcome in CLL (Fig. 2).

In recent years, molecular and cellular markers have helped to elucidate major pathogenic aspects of CLL. More importantly for the treatment of patients, molecular genetics has helped to predict the prognosis of CLL. The development of molecular genetic techniques has proven pivotal in helping to subdivide CLL into distinct clinical subgroups and identify patients with specific clinical manifestations, e.g., rapid disease progression (unmutated VH), massive lymphadenopathy (11q–) or resistance to therapy (17p–). Patients with these genetic abnormalities may be candidates for clinical trials investigating alternative treatments and allogeneic stem cell transplantation. The near future is likely to bring greater insight into the prognosis and molecular basis of CLL as new techniques such as high-resolution single nucleotide polymorphism (SNP)-arrays, genomewide methylation, and miRNA profiling methods are investigated in extended patient cohorts.

ACKNOWLEDGMENTS

Drs. Alexander Kröber, Dirk Kienle, Dirk Winkler, Christof Schneider, and Andreas Bühler, Mrs Brückle, and Mrs Konrad are gratefully acknowledged for contributing to the genetic analyses. We thank Dr. M. Bommer for providing the photographic images.

REFERENCES

1. Harris NL, Jaffe ES, Diebold J, et al. World Health Organization Classification of neoplastic diseases of the hematopoietic and lymphoid tissues: report of the Clinical Advisory Committee Meeting-Airlie House, Virginia, November 1997. J Clin Oncol 1999; 17:3835.
2. Jaffe ES, Harris NL, Stein H, et al. eds. World Health Organization classification of tumours. Pathology and Genetics of Tumours of Haematopoietic and Lymphoid Tissues. Lyon: IARC Press, 2001.

3. Cheson BD, Bennett JM, Rai KR, et al. Guidelines for clinical protocols for chronic lymphocytic leukemia (CLL). Recommendations of the NCI-Sponsored Working Group. Am J Hematol 1988; 29:152–163.

4. Chronic lymphocytic leukemia: recommendations for diagnosis, staging, and response criteria. International Workshop on Chronic Lymphocytic Leukemia. Ann Intern Med 1989; 110:236–238.

5. Hallek M, Cheson BD, Catovsky D, et al. Guidelines for the diagnosis and treatment of chronic lymphocytic leukemia: a report from the International Workshop on Chronic Lymphocytic Leukemia (IWCLL) updating the National Cancer Institute-Working Group (NCI-WG) 1996 guidelines. Blood 2008; [Epub ahead of print].

6. Diehl LF, Ketchum LH. Autoimmune disease and chronic lymphocytic leukemia: autoimmune hemolytic anemia, pure red cell aplasia, and autoimmune thrombocytopenia. Semin Oncol 1998; 25:80–97.

7. Dearden C, Wade R, Else M, et al. The prognostic significance of a positive direct antiglobulin test in chronic lymphocytic leukaemia—a beneficial effect of the combination of fludarabine and cyclophosphamide on the incidence of hemolytic anemia. Blood 2008; 111(4):1820–1826. [Epub 2007, Nov 30].

8. Morrison VA. Management of infectious complications in patients with chronic lymphocytic leukemia. Hematology Am Soc Hematol Educ Program 2007; 2007:332–338.

9. Melo JV, Wardle J, Chetty M, et al. The relationship between chronic lymphocytic leukaemia and prolymphocytic leukaemia. III. Evaluation of cell size by morphology and volume measurements. Br J Haematol 1986; 64:469–478.

10. Rozman C, Montserrat E, Rodríguez-Fernández JM, et al. Bone marrow histologic pattern—the best single prognostic parameter in chronic lymphocytic leukemia: a multivariate survival analysis of 329 cases. Blood 1984; 64(3):642–648.

11. Lipshutz MD, Mir R, Rai KR, et al. Bone marrow biopsy and clinical staging in chronic lymphocytic leukemia. Cancer 1980; 46:1422–1427.

12. Bergmann MA, Eichhorst B, Busch R, et al. Prospective evaluation of prognostic parameters in early stage Chronic Lymphocytic Leukemia (CLL): results of the CLL1-Protocol of the German CLL Study Group (GCLLSG). Blood (ASH Annual Meeting Abstracts), 2007; 110:625.

13. Dick FR, Maca RD. The lymph node in chronic lymphocytic leukemia. Cancer 1978; 41:283–292.

14. Müller-Hermelink HK, Catovsky D, Montserrat E, et al. Chronic lymphocytic leukaemia/small lymphocytic lymphoma. In: Jaffe ES, Harris NL, Stein H, et al. eds. World Health Organization Classification of Tumours. Pathology and Genetics of Tumours of Haematopoietic and Lymphoid Tissues. Lyon: IARC Press, 2001.

15. Matutes E, Owusu-Ankomah K, Morilla R, et al. The immunological profile of B-cell disorders and a proposal of a scoring system for the diagnosis of CLL. Leukemia 1994; 8:1640–1645.

16. Moreau EJ, Matutes E, A'Hern RP, et al. Improvement of the chronic lymphocytic leukemia scoring system with the monoclonal antibody SN8 (CD79b). Am J Clin Pathol 1997; 108:378–382.

17. Oscier D, Fegan C, Hillmen P, et al. Guidelines on the diagnosis and management of chronic lymphocytic leukaemia. Br J Haematol 2004; 125:294–317.

18. Damle RN, Wasil T, Fais F, et al. Ig V gene mutation status and CD38 expression as novel prognostic indicators in chronic lymphocytic leukemia. Blood 1999; 94:1840–1847.

19. Kröber A, Seiler T, Benner A, et al. V(H) mutation status, CD38 expression level, genomic aberrations, and survival in chronic lymphocytic leukemia. Blood 2002; 100:1410–1416.

20. Bennett JM, Catovsky D, Daniel MT, et al. Proposals for the classification of chronic (mature) B and T lymphoid leukaemias. French-American-British (FAB) Cooperative Group. J Clin Pathol 1989; 42:567–584.

21. DiRaimondo F, Albitar M, Huh Y, et al. The clinical and diagnostic relevance of CD23 expression in the chronic lymphoproliferative disease. Cancer 2002; 94:1721–1730.

22. Catovsky D, Foa R. The Lymphoid Leukaemias. London: Butterworths, 1990.

23. Stone RM. Prolymphocytic leukemia. Hematol Oncol Clin North Am 1990; 4:457.

24. Matutes E, Brito-Babapulle V, Swansbury J, et al. Clinical and laboratory features of 78 cases of T-prolymphocytic leukemia. Blood 1991; 78:3269–3274.

25. Ravandi F, O'Brien S. Chronic lymphoid leukemias other than chronic lymphocytic leukemia: diagnosis and treatment. Mayo Clin Proc 2005; 80:1660–1674.
26. Bartlett NL, Longo DL. T-small lymphocyte disorders. Semin Hematol 1999; 36:164–170.
27. Rai KR, Sawitsky A, Cronkite EP, et al. Clinical staging of chronic lymphocytic leukemia. Blood 1975; 46:219–234.
28. Rai KR. A critical analysis of staging in CLL. In: Gale RP, Rai KR, eds. Chronic Lymphocytic Leukemia: Recent Progress and Future direction. 1987 UCLA Symposia on Molecular and Cellular Biology, New Series, Vol. 59. New York: Alan R Liss, 1987:253.
29. Binet J-L, Auquier A, Dighiero G, et al. A new prognostic classification of chronic lymphocytic leukemia derived from a multivariate survival analysis. Cancer 1981; 48:198–206.
30. Muntañola A, Bosch F, Arguis P, et al. Abdominal computed tomography predicts progression in patients with Rai stage 0 chronic lymphocytic leukemia. J Clin Oncol 2007; 25(12):1576–1580.
31. Dohner H, Stilgenbauer S, Benner A, et al. Genomic aberrations and survival in chronic lymphocytic leukemia. N Engl J Med 2000; 343:1910–1916.
32. Montserrat E, Sanchez-Bisono J, Vinolas N, et al. Lymphocyte doubling time in chronic lymphocytic leukaemia: analysis of its prognostic significance. Br J Haematol 1986; 62:567–575.
33. Han T, Barcos M, Emrich L, et al. Bone marrow infiltration patterns and their prognostic significance in chronic lymphocytic leukemia: correlations with clinical, immunologic, phenotypic, and cytogenetic data. J Clin Oncol 1984; 2:562–570.
34. Kallander CF, Simonsson B, Hagberg H, et al. Serum deoxythymidine kinase gives prognostic information in chronic lymphocytic leukemia. Cancer 1984; 54:2450–2455.
35. Hallek M, Langenmayer I, Nerl C, et al. Elevated serum thymidine kinase levels identify a subgroup at high risk of disease progression in early, nonsmoldering chronic lymphocytic leukemia. Blood 1999; 93:1732–1737.
36. Keating MJ. Chronic lymphocytic leukemia in the next decade: where do we go from here? Semin Hematol 1998; 35:27–33.
37. Wierda WG, O'Brien S, Wang X, et al. Prognostic nomogram and index for overall survival in previously untreated patients with chronic lymphocytic leukemia. Blood 2007; 109(11):4679–4685.
38. Hamblin TJ, Davis Z, Gardiner A, et al. Unmutated Ig V(H) genes are associated with a more aggressive form of chronic lymphocytic leukemia. Blood 1999; 94:1848–1854.
39. Tobin G, Thunberg U, Johnson A, et al. Somatically mutated Ig V(H)3-21 genes characterize a new subset of chronic lymphocytic leukemia. Blood 2002; 99:2262–2264.
40. Tobin G, Thunberg U, Karlsson K, et al. Subsets with restricted immunoglobulin gene rearrangement features indicate a role for antigen selection in the development of chronic lymphocytic leukemia. Blood 2004; 104:2879–2885.
41. Crespo M, Bosch F, Villamor N, et al. ZAP-70 expression as a surrogate for immunoglobulin-variable-region mutations in chronic lymphocytic leukemia. N Engl J Med 2003; 348:1764–1775.
42. Krober A, Bloehdorn J, Hafner S, et al. Additional genetic high-risk features such as 11q deletion, 17p deletion, and V3-21 usage characterize discordance of ZAP-70 and VH mutation status in chronic lymphocytic leukemia. J Clin Oncol 2006; 24:969–975.
43. Orchard JA, Ibbotson RE, Davis Z, et al. ZAP-70 expression and prognosis in chronic lymphocytic leukaemia. Lancet 2004; 363:105–111.
44. Rassenti LZ, Huynh L, Toy TL, et al. ZAP-70 compared with immunoglobulin heavy-chain gene mutation status as a predictor of disease progression in chronic lymphocytic leukemia. N Engl J Med 2004; 351:893–901.
45. Le Garff-Tavernier M, Ticchioni M, Brissard M, et al. National standardization of ZAP-70 determination by flow cytometry: the French experience. Cytometry B Clin Cytom 2007; 2b:103–108.
46. Heintel D, Kienle D, Shehata M, et al. High expression of lipoprotein lipase in poor risk B-cell chronic lymphocytic leukemia. Leukemia 2005; 19:1216–1223.
47. van't Veer MB, Brooijmans AM, Langerak AW, et al. The predictive value of lipoprotein lipase for survival in chronic lymphocytic leukemia. Haematologica 2006; 91:56–63.

48. Oppezzo P, Vasconcelos Y, Settegrana C, et al. The LPL/ADAM29 expression ratio is a novel prognosis indicator in chronic lymphocytic leukemia. Blood 2005; 106(2):650–744.
49. Catovsky D, Richards S, Matutes E, et al. Assessment of fludarabine plus cyclophosphamide for patients with chronic lymphocytic leukaemia (the LRF CLL4 Trial): a randomised controlled trial. Lancet 2007; 370:230–239.
50. Döhner H, Stilgenbauer S, James MR, et al. 11q deletions identify a new subset of B-cell chronic lymphocytic leukaemia characterized by extensive nodal involvement and inferior prognosis. Blood 1997; 89:2516–2522.
51. Döhner H, Fischer K, Bentz M, et al. p53 gene deletion predicts for poor survival and non-response to therapy with purine analogs in chronic B-cell leukaemias. Blood 1995; 85:1580–1589.
52. Keating MJ, Flinn I, Jain V, et al. Therapeutic role of alemtuzumab (Campath-1H) in patients who have failed fludarabine: results of a large international study. Blood 2002; 99(10): 3554–3561.
53. Stilgenbauer S, Winkler D, Bühler A, et al. Subcutaneous alemtuzumab (MabCampath) in fludarabine-refractory CLL (CLL2H Trial of the GCLLSG). Blood 2007; 118:918A (abstr 3120).
54. Stilgenbauer S, Sander S, Bullinger L, et al. Clonal evolution in chronic lymphocytic leukemia: acquisition of high-risk genomic aberrations associated with unmutated VH, resistance to therapy, and short survival. Haematologica 2007; 92(9):1242–1245.
55. Lin K, Sherrington PD, Dennis M, et al. Relationship between p53 dysfunction, CD38 expression, and IgV(H) mutation in chronic lymphocytic leukemia. Blood 2002; 100:1404–1409.
56. Oscier DG, Gardiner AC, Mould SJ, et al. Multivariate analysis of prognostic factors in CLL: clinical stage, IGVH gene mutational status, and loss or mutation of the p53 gene are independent prognostic factors. Blood 2002; 100:1177–1184.

8

Frontline Therapy of Chronic Lymphocytic Leukemia

Barbara Eichhorst and Michael Hallek
Klinik I für Innere Medizin, Universität zu Köln, Köln, Germany

INTRODUCTION

The last decade has seen rapid progress in the management of chronic lymphocytic leukemia (CLL). Fludarabine and a monoclonal antibody, alemtuzumab, have been approved by the European and American regulatory agencies for treatment of CLL. Additional monoclonal antibodies (anti-CD20, anti-CD23, anti-MHC II, anti-CD40) as well as other drugs (flavopiridol, bendamustine, lenalidomide) are currently being tested in clinical trials. In addition, the increased experience with allogeneic progenitor cell transplantation provides an intensified treatment option to physically fit patients at very high risk of relapse. Similarly, rapid progress has been achieved with regard to new diagnostic tests to identify prognostic subgroups in CLL and to assess their response to therapy. However, the optimal use of these different therapeutic and diagnostic modalities remains to be determined. This chapter attempts to summarize the current state of the art in the initial management of CLL.

TREATMENT DECISION

Any decision to treat should be guided by clinical staging, the presence of symptoms and the disease activity (1). Criteria for initiating treatment may vary depending on whether or not the patient is treated in a clinical trial. In general practice, newly diagnosed patients with asymptomatic early-stage disease (Rai 0, Binet A) should be monitored without therapy until they have evidence of disease progression. Patients at intermediate (I and II) or high-risk (III and IV) according to the modified Rai classification or Binet stage B or C usually benefit from the initiation of treatment. Some of these patients can be monitored without therapy until they have evidence for progressive or symptomatic disease.

Active disease should be clearly documented for protocol therapy. At least one of the following criteria should be met:

1. Evidence of progressive marrow failure as manifested by the development of, or worsening of, anemia and/or thrombocytopenia.

2. Massive (i.e., >6 cm below the left costal margin) or progressive splenomegaly.
3. Massive nodes (i.e., >10 cm in longest diameter) or progressive lymphadenopathy.
4. Progressive lymphocytosis with an increase of >50% over a two-month period or lymphocyte doubling time (LDT) of less than six months. LDT can be obtained by linear regression extrapolation of WBC obtained at intervals of two weeks over an observation period of two to three months; patients with initial blood lymphocyte counts <30,000/µL may require a longer observation period to determine the LDT. Also, factors contributing to lymphocytosis or lymphadenopathy other than CLL (e.g., infections) should be excluded.
5. Autoimmune anemia and/or thrombocytopenia poorly responsive to corticosteroid therapy.
6. A minimum of any one of the following disease-related symptoms must be present:
   a. Unintentional weight loss ≥ 10% within the previous six months.
   b. Significant fatigue [i.e., Eastern Cooperative Oncology Group (ECOG) performance status 2 or worse; cannot work or unable to perform usual activities].
   c. Fevers of greater than 100.5°F or 38.0°C for ≥ two weeks without evidence of infection.
   d. Night sweats without evidence of infection.

Hypogammaglobulinemia or monoclonal or oligoclonal paraproteinemia does not constitute a basis for initiation of therapy in the absence of any of the above criteria for active disease.

Patients with CLL may present with a markedly elevated leukocyte count; however, the symptoms associated with leukocyte aggregates that develop in patients with acute leukemia rarely occur in patients with CLL. Therefore, the absolute lymphocyte count should not be used as the sole indication for treatment.

RESPONSE ASSESSMENT

Assessment of response should include a careful physical examination and evaluation of the blood and marrow. Response assessment should be performed according to the revised National cancer Institute (NCI)/International Workshop on CLL (IWCLL) guidelines (1).

Imaging studies, in particular CT scans, as outlined below, may not be necessary for patients in general practice. However, they are useful (and recommended) to assess the response in clinical trials. In a recent trial, the use of CT scans has changed the number of cases with complete remission (CR) or partial remission (PR) (2). Therefore, one CT scan should be performed before initiation of the study medication and a second CT scan after the end of treatment. No further CT scan is required for follow-up or to assess the time to progression.

As with other malignancies, eradication of the disease is a desired endpoint of CLL treatment, especially in younger patients. New detection technologies have found that many patients who achieve a complete response as defined by the National Cancer Institute-sponsored working group (NCI-WG) guidelines (3) typically have minimal residual disease (MRD). Critical in this assessment is a standardization of the techniques used to define MRD. The most sensitive techniques are four-color flow cytometry and real-time quantitative polymerase chain reaction (PCR). Fortunately, the techniques for assessing MRD have now become standardized (4). Nevertheless, the clinical relevance of MRD testing needs to be verified by prospective clinical trials and is not recommended for the general practice. Clinical trials that aim toward achieving long-lasting CRs should include a test for MRD, because eradication of leukemia may have a strong prognostic impact (5–8).

FRONTLINE THERAPY

Frontline Therapy of Early Stage

In early stages, treatment is necessary only if symptoms associated with the disease occur (e.g., B symptoms, decreased performance status, or symptoms or complications from hepatomegaly, splenomegaly, and lymphadenopathy).

Studies from both the French Cooperative Group on CLL (9), the Cancer and Leukemia Group B (CALGB) (10), the Spanish group Pethema (11), and the Medical Research Council (12) in patients with early-stage disease confirm that the use of alkylating agents in these patients does not prolong survival. In one study, treated patients with such early-stage CLL had an increased frequency of fatal epithelial cancers compared with untreated patients (9).

Moreover, several clinical trials evaluated the role of interferon α in early-stage CLL, but none of them was able to show a significant benefit from interferon treatment (13,14).

Therefore, the potential benefit, if any, of an early-intervention therapy with standard antileukemia drugs, alone or in combination with monoclonal antibodies, requires further study.

Frontline Therapy of Advanced Stage

Monotherapy with Alkylating Agents

The alkylating agent chlorambucil mainly acts by DNA cross-linking (15). In first-line treatment either as continuous (0.04–0.08 mg/kg/day for 4–8 weeks) or intermittent therapy (0.4–0.8 mg/kg every 4 weeks or 30 mg/m^2 every 2 weeks), it results in an overall response rate (ORR) of 30% to 70% (16–18). Chlorambucil should be given to the maximum response (median time 12 months), which may take up to 18 months (16). Higher remission rates (ORR 89%, CR 59%) had been observed when chlorambucil was administered at a fixed dose of 15 mg daily up to achievement of a CR or occurrence of grade 3 toxicity, for a maximum of six months (19). The combination regimen of chlorambucil with prednisone, although inducing higher response rates when compared with therapy based on either drug used alone, does not lead to improved survival compared with chlorambucil monotherapy (20). Because of the increased risk of infections by the steroid component, it is recommended to use chlorambucil as a single agent.

Besides chlorambucil, cyclophosphamide is another alkylating agent with activity in CLL. As a single agent, it is only infrequently used when chlorambucil is not tolerated and other agents are not indicated because of comorbidity (21).

Single-agent chlorambucil was equally potent when compared with combination therapy CVP (cyclophosphamide, vincristine, prednisone) or CHOP (cyclophosphamide, doxorubicin, vincristine, prednisone) (16,22). High-dose chlorambucil (15 mg/day up to 6 months) was even superior to the CHOP regimen including analysis of overall survival (68 vs. 47 months) (23). A meta-analysis by the CLL Trialists' Collaborative Group of clinical trials comparing chlorambucil with COP (Cyclophosphamide, vincristine and prednisolane), CHOP, or chlorambucil plus epirubicin revealed a similar five-year survival rate of 48% for both groups (24). Therefore, it can be summarized that chlorambucil is equally effective compared with more toxic alkylating agent–based combination therapy for patients with progressive or advanced CLL.

Monotherapy with Purine Analogs

Three purine analogs are currently used in CLL: fludarabine, pentostatin, and cladribine (2-CdA). Fludarabine remains by far the best-studied compound of the three in CLL.

Monotherapy with fludarabine   At the beginning of the nineties, fludarabine was introduced for treatment of CLL. Given intravenously, fludarabine is administered at 25 mg/m^2/day for five days. This regimen is repeated every 28 days. Fludarabine is now available in many countries (although not in the United States) as an oral formulation: It should be dosed at 40 mg/m^2/day p.o. for five days (25). Because of very promising results in the relapsed setting, fludarabine was then investigated as first-line therapy. Superior ORR and longer progression-free survival rates compared with other treatment regimens containing alkylating agents or corticosteroids were observed (26–28). In three phase III studies in treatment-naive CLL patients (Table 1), fludarabine induced more remissions and more CRs (7–40%) as well as a longer duration of remission than other chemotherapies, including CHOP, CAP (cyclophosphamide, doxorubicin, prednisone), or chlorambucil (29–31). Despite the superior efficacy of fludarabine, overall survival was not improved by this drug when used as a single agent (29–32). Two other phase III trials confirmed the above-mentioned data that fludarabine induces a higher rate of remission in comparison to chlorambucil, but interestingly no difference in progression-free survival was observed (Table 1) (33,34).

The main side effect of fludarabine, as well as of other purine analogs, is myelosuppression. Because of simultaneous depletion of T cells, opportunistic infections after fludarabine therapy have been reported (35–37). These infections are more frequent in the relapsed setting (38). The occurrence of autoimmune hemolytic anemias (AIHAs) is also related to T-cell imbalances (39,40). Interestingly, the incidence of AIHAs is decreased if fludarabine is combined with cyclophosphamide (33). Tumor lysis syndrome is another rare complication of fludarabine (41). So far, no significantly increased risk for secondary neoplasias after purine analog treatment has been reported (42), but some more preliminary data do indicate a tendency for more secondary neoplasias in older patients (34).

Monotherapy with cladribine   In CLL treatment, the purine analog cladribine is administered at 0.12 mg/kg/day intravenously for five consecutive days. Response rates of 77% and up to 34% CRs have been reported (43). Side effects are similar to fludarabine with the exception of an increased risk of lung cancer after cladribine therapy reported in one series (44).

The comparison of cladribine monotherapy to chlorambucil plus prednisone in one phase III trial has yielded a higher CR rate of 47% versus 12%, respectively (Table 1). However, this difference did not result in a longer survival after cladribine first-line treatment (chlorambucil plus prednisone vs. cladribine, 82% vs. 78% at 2 years), similar to the above-mentioned trials with fludarabine.

Other Monotherapies

Bendamustine, a hybrid of an alkylating nitrogen mustard group and a purine-like benzimidazole, was developed in the early 1960s for treatment of lymphoma and CLL. Data from a prospective phase III trial comparing bendamustine versus cyclophosphamide in 70 non-pretreated patients with B-CLL demonstrated marked activity of bendamustine

Table 1 Summary of Recent Major Randomized Trials for Advanced CLL in Treatment-Naive Patients

Study		N	CR (%)	PR (%)	Progression-free survival (median, months)	Survival (median, months)
Rai (30)	Fludarabine	170	20	43	25	66
	Chlorambucil	181	4	33	14	56
French Cooperative Group on CLL (29)	Fludarabine	52	23	48	NR	60% at 4 yr
	CAP	48	17	43	6.9	60% at 4 yr
Leporrier (31)	Fludarabine	341	40.1[a]	31	31.7	69
	CAP	240	15.2[a]	43	27.7	70
	CHOP	305	29.6[a]	41.9	29.5	67
Robak (98)	Cladribine + prednisone	126	47	40	21	78% at 2 yr
	Chlorambucil + prednisone	103	12	45	18	82% at 2 yr
Catovsky (33)	Chlorambucil	387	7	72	19	59% at 5 yr
	Fludarabine	194	15	80	28	52% at 5 yr
	Fludarabine, cyclophosphamide	196	38	94	43	54% at 5 yr
Eichhorst (2)	Fludarabine	182	4.9	78	20	Median not reached
	Fludarabine, cyclophosphamide	180	16.5	78	48	Median not reached
Flinn (53)	Fludarabine	137	4.6	59.5	19.2	79% at 2 yr
	Fludarabine, cyclophosphamide	141	23.4	50.9	31.6	80% at 2 yr
Robak (56)	Cladribine	166	21	56	23.5	51.2
	Cladribine, cyclophosphamide	162	29	54	22.4	Median not reached
	Cladribine, cyclophosphamide, mitoxantrone	151	36	44	23.6	Median not reached

[a]Included nPRs.

Please note that the response definitions varied considerably among the four trials. In the study by Leporrier et al. (31), a systematic evaluation of the bone marrow was not performed routinely to confirm a CR; thus, the CR rates are somewhat higher than in the other trials.

Abbreviations: CLL, chronic lymphocytic leukemia; CAP, cyclophosphamide, doxorubicin, prednisone; CHOP, cyclophosphamide, doxorubicin, vincristine, prednisone; CR, complete response; PR, partial response; NR, not reached.

in CLL with ORRs of 82% for the bendamustine arm versus 32% for the cyclophosphamide arm (45). Within another trial—including untreated and pretreated patients—bendamustine dose was adjusted for age: 60 mg/m^2 bendamustine for patients younger than 70 years and 50 mg/m^2 for those older than 70 years given on days 1 to 5 and repeated every 29 days (46). Six of 20 patients achieved a CR (30%), and 9 patients a PR (45%), yielding an ORR of 75%. In patients, receiving bendamustine as first-line treatment, the remission rate was 82% (9/11 patients). Median overall survival after treatment with bendamustine was 13.6 (1–46) months (all patients) and 16.6 (1–46) months for patients responding to therapy. Grade 3 or 4 leukocytopenia was observed in 51%, thrombocytopenia in 11%, and anemia in 6% of all evaluable courses. A European Intergroup phase III trial compared 100 mg/m^2 bendamustine (days 1 + 2 q4wk) to 0.8 mg/kg chlorambucil (days 1 and 15 q4wk) in first-line therapy of advanced CLL. A planned safety analysis revealed that both regimens were safe. The final results of this large trial were presented at the American Society of Hematology (ASH) meeting in 2007 showing a significantly higher ORR with bendamustine (68% vs. 39%) as well as a higher CR rate (30% vs. 2%) (47). Time to progression was better in the bendamustine arm with 21.7 months versus 9.3 months.

Several new substances—acting more specific by cell cycle inhibition, modulation of the immune system, or antiangiogenesis—are currently under investigation in the relapsed setting within phase II trials.

Combination Chemotherapies with Alkylating Agents

Combination therapies including an alkylating agent such as CVP, CAP, or CHOP did not show any advantage in comparison to the less toxic chlorambucil (16,22). These regimens can be effectively used in the relapsed setting in combination with monoclonal antibodies.

Combination Chemotherapy with Purine Analogs

Fludarabine has been evaluated in a variety of combination regimens. Fludarabine and another purine analog, cytarabine, appear to be less effective than fludarabine alone. The combination of fludarabine with chlorambucil or prednisone increases hematological toxicity as well as the incidence of opportunistic infections without improving the response rate compared with fludarabine alone (response rates 27–79%) (30,48).

The most thoroughly studied combination chemotherapy for CLL is fludarabine plus cyclophosphamide (FC). In preliminary, noncomparative trials, the ORRs did not appear to be better than with fludarabine alone, but the addition of cyclophosphamide appeared to improve the quality of the responses. This combination, with or without mitoxantrone, has achieved response rates of 64% to 100%, with CR rates of up to 50% (49–51). Variations on this regimen have shown that a slightly decreased cyclophosphamide dose improves the safety profile of the regimen without compromising efficacy and that results were similar with concurrent or sequential administration of the two therapies (52). The most frequently used dosing of this regimen is either fludarabine 30 mg/m^2/day plus cyclophosphamide 250 mg/m^2/day, both for three days intravenously (2,50) or fludarabine 20 mg/m^2/day for five days and cyclophosphamide 600 mg/m^2/day on day 1 intravenously (49,53). FC can also be administered as oral regimen with five days of fludarabine 24 mg/m^2/day and cyclophosphamide 150 mg/m^2/day day p.o.(33).

The addition of mitoxantrone to FC in 37 patients with relapsed/refractory CLL produced a high CR rate (50%), including 10 cases of MRD negativity, with a median duration of response of 19 months (5). All MRD-negative patients were alive at analysis; the median duration of response had not been reached in the CR patients compared with 25 months in non-CR patients. In frontline therapy, the FCM (fludarabine, cyclophosphamide, mitoxantrone) regimen has proved highly efficacious as well (54). The regimen administered to 69 patients younger than 65 years consisted of fludarabine 25 mg/m^2 and cyclophosphamide 200 mg/m^2, both administered for three days intravenously, as well as mitoxantrone 6mg/m^2 administered on day 1 for six courses. The CR rate in frontline therapy was 64%, including 26% MRD-negative CRs (54). The median response duration so far is 37 months with this regimen. Though these data are very promising, patients with 17p– deletion failed to respond.

In the relapsed setting, the combination of cladribine with cyclophosphamide (CC) has also demonstrated activity in advanced CLL, but the results appeared inferior to those of FC (55). This appeared to be different, when CC or CC plus mitoxantrone was administered frontline (56,57).

In a prospective trial of the German CLL Study Group comparing fludarabine with FC, results in 375 patients showed a superior response rate for the combination (2). FC chemotherapy resulted in a significantly higher CR rate (16%) and ORR (94%) compared with fludarabine alone (5% and 83%; $p = 0.004$ and 0.001, respectively). FC treatment also resulted in a longer progression-free survival (48 vs. 20 months, $p = 0.001$) and a longer event-free survival (49 vs. 33 months, $p = 0.001$). So far, no difference in the median overall survival was observed within a median observation period of 48 months (unpublished data). FC caused significantly more thrombocytopenia and neutropenia, but less anemia than fludarabine. FC did not increase the number of severe infections (38) (Table 1).

Two additional phase III trials have confirmed these findings. The American study (53) included 278 previously untreated patients with CLL randomly assigned to receive either fludarabine or FC. These cycles were repeated every 28 days for a maximum of six cycles. Treatment with fludarabine and cyclophosphamide was associated with a significantly higher CR rate (23.4% vs. 4.6%, $p < 0.001$) and a higher ORR (74.3% vs. 59.5%, $p = 0.013$) than treatment with fludarabine as a single agent. Progression-free survival was also superior in patients treated with fludarabine and cyclophosphamide (31.6 vs. 19.2 months, $p < 0.0001$). Fludarabine and cyclophosphamide caused additional hematologic toxicity, including more severe thrombocytopenia ($p = 0.046$), but it did not increase the number of severe infections ($p = .812$) (53).

The U.K. study compared chlorambucil versus fludarabine versus FC (33). Chlorambucil was administered in a higher dose of 10 mg/m^2 for seven days, fludarabine was dosed at 25 mg/m^2 for five days intravenously or 40 mg/m^2/day for five days orally. In the FC arm, 25 mg/m^2/day of fludarabine plus 250 mg/m^2/day of cyclophosphamide for three days were given intravenously or as oral formulation with five days of fludarabine 24 mg/m^2/day and cyclophosphamide 150 mg/m^2/day. In this trial, FC was confirmed to be better than fludarabine alone with regard to overall response, complete response, and progression-free survival. Interestingly, fludarabine was superior to chlorambucil for response rates only, but not for progression-free survival. FC was the best combination for all ages including patients older than 70 years and in prognostic subgroups defined by imnmunoglobulin heavy chain gene mutation status and cytogenetics, respectively (33). Patients treated with FC had more neutropenia and more days in hospital. Hemolytic anemia was less frequent with FC in comparison to fludarabine alone and chlorambucil.

A Polish study group compared 2-CdA alone to 2-CdA combined with cyclophosphamide (CC) or to cyclophosphamide and mitoxantrone (CMC) in 479 cases with untreated progressive CLL (56). Surprisingly, the CC combination therapy did not produce any benefit in terms of progression-free survival or response rates when compared with 2-CdA alone. Compared with 2-CdA, CMC induced a higher CR rate (36% vs. 21%, $p = 0.004$), and a trend for higher CR rate with CC was observed (29% vs. 21%, $p = 0.08$). Furthermore, the percentage of patients who were in CR and were MRD negative was higher in the CMC arm compared with 2-CdA (23% vs. 14%, $p = 0.042$). There were no differences in overall response, progression-free survival, and overall survival among treatment groups. Grade 3/4 neutropenia occurred more frequently in CC (32%) and CMC (38%) than in 2-CdA (20%) ($p = 0.01$ and $p = 0.004$, respectively). Infections were more frequent in CMC compared with 2-CdA (40% vs. 27%, $p = 0.02$). On the basis of these results, cladribine combination therapies do not seem to offer any advantage when used as a first-line treatment for CLL (Table 1).

Fludarabine may also be combined with anthracycline. In a phase II trial, 25 mg/m^2/day fludarabine was administered for five days along with 25 mg/m^2/day epirubicin on days 4 and 5. Similar efficacy (92% ORR and 40% CR) to the FC combination was observed (58). The median duration of response was 19 months. Side effects were mainly myelosuppression and infections. In rare cases, tumor lysis syndrome was reported (58). Results from a randomized trial are not yet published, but are expected to confirm the superiority of the fludarabine combination in comparison to fludarabine monotherapy (59). However, because the fludarabine and epirubicin combination shows no advantages in comparison to FC, but needs more careful monitoring of cardiac function because of the use of an anthracycline, the FC combination has become the standard frontline chemotherapy in CLL.

Rituximab-based Chemoimmunotherapy

Rituximab, an anti-CD20 monoclonal antibody, has provoked interest for the treatment of CLL. As a single agent, rituximab is less active than it is in follicular lymphoma (60), unless very high doses up to 2250 mg/m^2 (61) or more frequent administration such as three times (62) weekly are used. Somewhat surprisingly, combinations of rituximab with chemotherapy have proven to be very efficacious therapies for CLL. This may be because there is preclinical evidence for synergy between rituximab and fludarabine (63). The majority of rituximab combination studies in CLL have focused on combinations with fludarabine or fludarabine-based regimens (Table 2).

A multicenter phase II study of the German CLL Study Group evaluated the efficacy and safety of rituximab plus fludarabine in patients with previously treated or untreated CLL (64). All patients received standard dose fludarabine 25 mg/m^2/day for five days plus rituximab 375 mg/m^2/day given on days 57, 85, 113, and 153. Of 31 patients treated, 27 (87%) responded, with 10 patients (32%) achieving a complete response. ORR and CR rates in previously untreated patients were 85% and 20%, respectively.

Byrd and colleagues combined rituximab with fludarabine in either a sequential or concurrent regimen in a randomized study (CALGB 9712 protocol) (65). Patients ($N = 104$) with previously untreated CLL received six cycles of fludarabine, with (375 mg/m^2 rituximab on day 1 and 4 on cycle 1 of fludarabine, on day 1 only in cycles 2 to 6) or without rituximab, followed by four once-weekly doses of 375 mg/m^2 of rituximab. Overall and complete response rates were higher in the concurrent group (90% and 47% vs. 77% and 28%). No difference in the incidence of infections was observed. More recently, in a retrospective analysis, all patients of the CALGB 9712 protocol treated with fludarabine and rituximab were compared with 178 patients from the previous CALGB 9011 trial, who received only fludarabine (66). The basic characteristics of patients were comparable, except for an eight-year longer observation time in the CALGB 9011 protocol. The patients receiving fludarabine and rituximab had a better progression-free survival and overall survival than patients receiving fludarabine alone. Two-year progression-free survival probabilities were 67% versus 45% and 2-year overall survival probabilities were 93% versus 81%.

Similarly, a large phase II trial conducted at the M.D. Anderson Cancer Center on 224 patients with previously untreated CLL evaluated the combination of fludarabine/cyclophosphamide plus rituximab (FCR) (67). A dose of 25mg/m^2/day of fludarabine and 250 mg/m^2/day of cyclophosphamide were administered for five days. On day 1, 375 mg/m^2 of rituximab was administered in cycle 1 and 500 mg/m^2 in cycles 2 to 6, respectively. This regimen achieved a response rate of 95%, with 71% complete responses (67).

Table 2 Efficacy of Combination Regimens Using Purine Analogs Plus Concurrent Monoclonal Antibodies in CLL in Phase II Trials

Reference	No. of evaluable patients	Stage	Prior therapy	Treatment regimen	Clinical response		Survival/response-duration
					CR	CR + PR	
Fludarabine + rituximab							
Schulz (64)	31	100% Binet B or C	Yes: 20, no: 11	FLU 25 mg/m^2 d1-5 q4wk, rituxima b 375 mg/m^2 d1 q4wk	32%	87%	Median survival: 33 mo, median duration of response: 75 wk
Byrd (65) (Phase III, randomized)	104	Rai I/II: 59%, Rai III/IV: 41%	No	FLU 25 mg/m^2 d1-5 q4wk, rituxima b 375 mg q4wk, concurrent vs. sequential	47% concurrent, 28% sequential	90% concurrent, 77% sequential	After 23 months', median duration of response not yet reached in both arms
Fludarabine + cyclophosphamide + rituximab/pentostatin + cyclophosphamide + rituximab							
Wierda (99)	177	Rai IV 44%	Yes	FLU 25 mg/m^2 d1-3 q4wk, CYC 250 mg/m^2 d1-3 q4wk, rituximab [a]375/500 mg/m^2 d1 q4wk	25%	73%	Median survival: 42 mo, median time to progression: 28 mo
Keating (67)	224	Rai III + IV: 33%	No	FLU 25 mg/m^2 d1-3 q4wk, CYC 250 mg/m^2 d1-3 q4wk, rituximab [a]375/500 mg/m^2 d1 q4wk	70%	95%	69% failure free at 4 yr
Kay (68)	64	Rai III + IV: 53%	NO	PEN 2 mg/m^2 d1 q4wk, CYC 600 mg d1 q4wk, rituximab 375 mg/m^2 d1 q4wk	41%	91%	

[a]375 mg/m^2 rituximab were given at cycle 1; in the following cycles 500 mg/m^2 rituximab were administered.

Abbreviations: CLL, chronic lymphocytic leukemia; FLU, fludarabine; CYC, cyclophosphamide; PEN, pentostatin; CR, complete response; PR, partial response.

Median overall survival was not reached in patients treated with rituximab plus FC and was significantly longer than in patients treated with FC alone in an historical comparison (Table 2).

Recently, the purine analog pentostatin combined with cyclophosphamide and rituximab (PCR) was evaluated in previously untreated patients with CLL (68). Pentostatin was administered at 2 mg/m^2, cyclophosphamide at 600 mg/m^2, and rituximab at 375 mg/m^2. Fifty-eight of 64 evaluable patients had a response (91%), with 26 CRs (41%). The main toxicity was myelosuppression, especially severe neutropenia (41%) and thrombocytopenia (21%). With the routine addition of G-CSF (granulocyte colony stimulating factor), only 2% of all courses were complicated by severe infections (68). This regimen was similarly effective in younger and in elderly patients older than 70 years (69).

Taken together, these results suggest that rituximab plus fludarabine–based therapies represent a significant advance in therapy for CLL. However, the analysis by Byrd and colleagues is retrospective and could be confounded by differences in supportive care or different prognostic subsets included in the two trials. Therefore, these findings need to be confirmed by prospective trials. The results from the GCLLSG CLL8 trial comparing FC to FCR are expected in early 2008. In January 2008, the Data Safety Monitoring Board confirmed that the primary endpoint showing a longer progression-free survival after FCR in comparison to FC was reached.

Alemtuzumab-based Chemoimmunotherapy

Alemtuzumab is a recombinant, fully humanized, monoclonal antibody targeting the CD52 antigen. The antibody is given either intravenously or subcutaneously at 3×30 mg/wk for up to 8 to 12 weeks. For optimal response rates, 12 weeks of alemtuzumab administration or longer (70) should be used, if possible. One of the main side effects of alemtuzumab is the T-cell cytotoxicity, which is associated with an increased risk of infection especially cytomegalovirus (CMV) reactivation, which occurs in 10% to 66% of the patients (70,71). Moreover, by monitoring CMV antigenemia or CMV PCR as well as immediate treatment with ganciclovir or valganciclovir and discontinuation of alemtuzumab therapy, CMV infections can be prevented (71,72).

Monotherapy with alemtuzumab has produced response rates of 33% to 53%, with a median duration of response ranging from 8.7 to 15.4 months, in patients with advanced CLL who were previously treated with alkylating agents and had failed or relapsed after second-line fludarabine therapy (73–75).

First-line therapy with alemtuzumab reaches response rates up to 89% with 19% CRs (70) and 24 months of response duration (76). Recently, a large randomized trial compared alemtuzumab with chlorambucil in frontline therapy of 297 patients with CLL (77). Patients receiving alemtuzumab were additionally treated with the standard prophylaxis of famciclovir and cotrimoxazole. Response rates were significantly improved after alemtuzumab treatment (83% vs. 55%), including higher CR rates (24% vs. 2%). Progression-free survival was also significantly longer, showing 52% of the patients in the alemtuzumab arm had CMV viremia detected by PCR, 16% had a CMV infection. Though treatment-related neutropenia was more common with alemtuzumab, the incidence of anemia and thrombocytopenia was similar in both arms (77). This study demonstrates that alemtuzumab can be safely administered as first-line therapy of CLL.

In addition, alemtuzumab has proven efficacy even in patients with poor prognostic factors, including high-risk genetic markers such as deletions of chromosome 11 or 17 and p53 mutations (78,79).

Another regimen for CLL is the combination of the most effective single chemotherapeutic agent with the most effective monoclonal antibody—fludarabine plus alemtuzumab (Table 2). The synergistic activity of these two agents was initially suggested by the induction of responses, including one CR, in five of six patients who were refractory to each agent alone (80). The combination of fludarabine and alemtuzumab was investigated in a phase II trial enrolling patients with relapsed CLL (Table 2) (81). Using a four-weekly dosing protocol, this combination has proven feasible, safe, and very effective. Among the 36 patients, the ORR was 83% (30/36 patients), which included 11 CRs (30%) and 19 PRs (53%); in addition, one patient achieved stable disease. Sixteen of 31 (53%) evaluated patients achieved MRD negativity in the peripheral blood by three months' follow-up, and resolution of disease was observed in all disease sites, particularly in the blood, bone marrow, and spleen. The fludarabine and alemtuzumab combination therapy was well tolerated. Infusion reactions (fever, chills, and skin reactions) occurred primarily during the first infusion of alemtuzumab and were mild in the majority of patients. While 80% of patients were CMV IgG-positive before treatment, there were only two subclinical CMV reactivations. The primary grade 3/4 hematological events were transient, including leukocytopenia (44%) and thrombocyto-penia (30%). Stable $CD4^+$ T-cell counts ($>200/\mu L$) were seen after one year. A phase III prospective randomized study evaluating the effectiveness of fludarabine and alemtuzu-mab combination in comparison with fludarabine alone is currently under way.

The combination of both monoclonal antibodies (alemtuzumab and rituximab) has been studied in patients with lymphoid malignancies, including those with refractory/relapsed CLL, producing an ORR of 52% [8% CR, 4% nodular PR (nPR); 40% PR] (82). A larger trial with longer follow-up is needed to confirm these preliminary results and determine the long-term efficacy of this combination.

Because rituximab and alemtuzumab–based immunochemotherapeutic regimens are currently the most potent choices for treatment in CLL, several large study groups are now comparing these two regimens in frontline therapy of CLL.

CONSOLIDATION THERAPY

In contrast to other indolent lymphomas, there is currently no definitive role for consolidation or maintenance therapy in front line of CLL.

Consolidation with Interferon

Two clinical trials evaluated the role of interferon consolidation therapy after induction therapy with fludarabine. O'Brien and colleagues treated 31 patients with interferon α 3 $\times$ 10^6 U/wk with subcutaneous injections. Neither improvement of response rates nor prolongation of relapse-free survival in comparison to historical control was seen after interferon maintenance (83). Another trial evaluated the benefit of interferon α 2 $\times$ 10^6 U on days 1, 3, 5, 7, 9, 11, 13, and 15 after frontline therapy with fludarabine in a randomized setting of 133 patients (84). The addition of interferon had no influence on the ORR or the progression-free survival rate.

A third trial evaluated the role of interferon treatment in early stage CLL (14). Forty-four patients with high-risk CLL in Binet stage A—defined by elevated serum thymidine kinase or short LDT and nonnodular bone marrow infiltration—were randomized between interferon treatment or watch and wait. Though four patients in the interferon group achieved a partial response, no difference in progression-free survival or overall survival was assessed (14).

These study results indicate that there is no role for interferon maintenance or consolidation in CLL.

Consolidation with Monoclonal Antibodies

Several trials have evaluated consolidation with alemtuzumab; different dosing schemas have been used in these trials. Alemtuzumab consolidation therapy was administered after fludarabine-based chemotherapy. Alemtuzumab was shown to improve the quality of responses, provide molecular remissions in a substantial proportion of patients, and increased progression-free survival compared with patients who had no further treatment (8,85,86).

A phase III trial by the GCLLSG assessed in a randomized setting the efficacy of 3×30 mg alemtuzumab after induction therapy with fludarabine alone or FC (8). Of 21 evaluable patients, 11 were randomized to alemtuzumab before the study was stopped because of severe infections in 7 of 11 patients. These infections (1 life-threatening pulmonary aspergillosis IV, 4 CMV reactivations III requiring IV ganciclovir, 1 pulmonary tuberculosis III, 1 herpes zoster III) were successfully treated and not associated with the cumulative dose of alemtuzumab (8). After alemtuzumab treatment, five of six patients achieved a molecular remission in peripheral blood, while all patients in the observation arm remained MRD-positive ($p = 0.048$). A recent update of this trial after 48 months confirmed an improved progression-free survival with alemtuzumab consolidation therapy compared with the observation arm (median progression-free survival not reached vs. 20.6 months, $p = 0.004$) when calculated from the start of fludarabine-based treatment (87).

O'Brien and colleagues reported an ORR of 53% after alemtuzumab; responses were seen in 9 of 23 (39%) at a 10-mg dose and 17 of 26 (65%) at a 30-mg dose ($p = 0.066$) (86). Residual disease was cleared from the bone marrow in most patients, and 11 (38%) of the 29 patients with available data achieved a molecular remission. Median time-to-disease progression had not yet been reached for patients who achieved MRD negativity compared with 15 months for patients who still had residual disease after alemtuzumab consolidation treatment (86). While the GCLLSG trial was stopped early because of infectious adverse events, the study by O'Brien et al. had no such issue, perhaps due to a longer time interval between induction therapy and consolidation with alemtuzumab (6 months vs. 3 months in the GCLLSG study).

Montillo and colleagues found an improvement in ORR from 35% to 75% if three times 10 mg alemtuzumab was administered subcutaneously in 34 patients initially treated with a fludarabine-based regimen (85). Nine patients (56%) achieved even MRD negativity. The most common adverse events were injection-site reactions and fever. CMV reactivation occurred in 18 patients, all of whom were successfully treated with oral ganciclovir (85).

So far there are only two nonrandomized clinical trials assessing the role of rituximab consolidation therapy in CLL (88). Forty-four previously untreated patients with CLL and small lymphocytic lymphoma received rituximab 375 mg/m^2 weekly for four consecutive weeks. All patients with objective response or stable disease continued to receive identical four-week rituximab courses at six-month intervals, for a total of four courses. After a median follow-up of 20 months, the median progression-free survival time was 18.6 months, and the one- and two-year progression-free survival rates were 62% and 49%, respectively (88). No cumulative toxicity or opportunistic infections occurred. Within another small trial, 28 patients who were positive for MRD received four monthly cycles of rituximab (375 mg/m^2) followed by 12 monthly low doses of rituximab (150 mg/m^2) (89). In this nonrandomized setting, the 28 patients receiving consolidation therapy had a significantly longer response duration (87% vs. 32% at 5 years, $p = 0.001$) compared with a subset of 18 patients who did not receive consolidation therapy (89). These preliminary data have to be confirmed within large prospective randomized trials.

In summary these results show that consolidation improving the quality of remission and therapy with monoclonal antibodies in CLL may be a good treatment option for prolonging the duration of remissions, but the optimal dose of alemtuzumab and rituximab in this setting with an acceptable range of toxicity has yet to be established.

FRONTLINE THERAPY OF PATIENTS WITH del(17p) OR p53 MUTATION

Several clinical trials have shown that patients with the most unfavorable prognostic factor, the del(17p) or p53 mutation, do not respond well to fludarabine alone or FC combination (33,53,90) nor to fludarabine and rituximab (91). Complete responses in this patient group are very rare (33,91), and relapse usually occurs fast: In the largest clinical trial, the progression-free survival rate in this patient cohort after three years was 0% (33). The median overall survival after fludarabine containing regimens was shown to be dramatically diminished at only 15 months (92). These clinical data were recently confirmed by in vitro experiments showing significant resistance to apoptosis induced by fludarabine as well as a spontaneous resistance to apoptosis (93).

Alemtuzumab has efficacy in this very poor risk group of patients (78–80,94). A phase II trial of the GCLLSG showed an ORR of 50% in patients with del(17p) (94). In rare cases, CRs in patients who were refractory to all other agents were reported as well (79,80). However, the median reported response duration of eight months is still short and needs further improvement by combination with other agents (78). If these results are confirmed in larger, prospective trials, alemtuzumab might be a rational choice for first-line treatment of patients with these poor prognostic factors.

Young and physically fit patients in advanced stage and with del(17p) or p53 mutation should be offered the possibility of allogeneic progenitor cell transplantation from sibling or unrelated donor. Early results from clinical trials have shown that allogeneic stem cell transplantation may overcome the adverse prognosis of high-risk factors, such as unmutated IgVH status (95). According to the European Group for Blood and Bone Marrow Transplantation (EBMT) consensus, allogeneic transplantation is recommended for up-front therapy after induction in the very poor risk group of patients with del (17) or p53 mutation (96).

CONCLUSION

With the potential of potent chemoimmunotherapy regimens described above, choosing the right treatment for a patient with CLL has become a task that requires skill and experience. Table 3 proposes an algorithm for the selection of the best treatment option, which is based on three potentially relevant points to consider:

1. The physical condition (fitness and comorbidity) of the patient, which is independent of calendar age.
2. The prognostic risk of the leukemia as determined by the factors mentioned above.
3. The Rai or Binet stage of the disease.

Table 3 Summary of the Current Options for First- and Second-Line Treatment in CLL

Conclusion: CLL treatment 2007–2008

Binet stage	Fitness	First-line treatment
A, asymptomatic B	Irrelevant	None (except in clinical trials)
C, symptomatic B	Go go	FCR
	Slow go	CLB, F (dose reduced)
Relapse	Fitness	Second line
Late (> 1 yr)	Go go and slow go	Repeat first line
Early (< 1 yr) = refractory disease	Go go	Allo Tx
	Slow go	Alemtuzumab (17p–), Bendamustine, R-CHOP

Abbreviations: CLL, chronic lymphocytic leukemia; FCR, fludarabine, cyclophosphamide, rituximab; CLB, chlorambucil; F, fludarabine; R-CHOP, rituximab, cyclophosphamide, doxorubicin, vincristine, prednisone.

Patients at early stage (Binet A and B without symptoms) should not be treated outside clinical trials. Treatment may be indicated in clinical trials in patients at high risk of disease progression.

In patients with advanced disease (Binet C, or symptomatic stage A or B), treatment should be initiatied. In this situation, patients need to be evaluated for their physical condition (or comorbidity). Patients in good physical condition ("go go"), as defined by a normal creatinine clearance and a low score at the "cumulative illness rating scale" (CIRS) (97), should be offered more combination therapies such as FC or FR or FCR. Patients with a somewhat impaired physical condition ("slow go") may be offered either chlorambucil or a dose-reduced fludarabine monotherapy or FC regimen for symptom control.

Patients with symptomatic disease and with del(17p) or p53 mutations may be considered for an alemtuzumab-containing regimen as first-line treatment, because these patients respond poorly to fludarabine-based therapy. Up-front allogeneic stem cell transplantation should be considered in younger patients with these poor prognostic factors.

REFERENCES

1. Hallek M, Cheson BD, Catovsky D, et al. Guidelines for the diagnosis and treatment of chronic lymphocytic leukemia: a report from the International Workshop on Chronic Lymphocytic Leukemia (IWCLL) updating the National Cancer Institute-Working Group (NCI-WG) 1996 guidelines. Blood, 2008 [Epub ahead of print].
2. Eichhorst BF, Busch R, Hopfinger G, et al. Fludarabine plus cyclophosphamide versus fludarabine alone in first-line therapy of younger patients with chronic lymphocytic leukemia. Blood 2006; 107(3):885–891.
3. Cheson BD, Bennett JM, Grever M, et al. National Cancer Institute-sponsored Working Group guidelines for chronic lymphocytic leukemia: revised guidelines for diagnosis and treatment. Blood 1996; 87(12):4990–4997.
4. Rawstron AC, Villamor N, Ritgen M, et al. International standardized approach for flow cytometric residual disease monitoring in chronic lymphocytic leukaemia. Leukemia 2007; 21(5):956–964.
5. Bosch F, Ferrer A, Lopez-Guillermo A, et al. Fludarabine, cyclophosphamide and mitoxantrone in the treatment of resistant or relapsed chronic lymphocytic leukaemia. British Journal of Haematology 2002; 119(4):976–984.

6. Moreno C, Villamor N, Colomer D, et al. Clinical significance of minimal residual disease, as assessed by different techniques, after stem cell transplantation for chronic lymphocytic leukemia. Blood 2006; 107(11):4563–4569.

7. Moreton P, Kennedy B, Lucas G, et al. Eradication of minimal residual disease in B-cell chronic lymphocytic leukemia after alemtuzumab therapy is associated with prolonged survival. J Clin Oncol 2005; 23(13):2971–2979.

8. Wendtner CM, Ritgen M, Schweighofer CD, et al. Consolidation with alemtuzumab in patients with chronic lymphocytic leukemia (CLL) in first remission—experience on safety and efficacy within a randomized multicenter phase III trial of the German CLL Study Group (GCLLSG). Leukemia 2004; 18(6):1093–1101.

9. Dighiero G, Maloum K, Desablens B, et al. Chlorambucil in indolent chronic lymphocytic leukemia. French Cooperative Group on Chronic Lymphocytic Leukemia. N Engl J Med 1998; 338(21):1506–1514.

10. Shustik C, Mick R, Silver R, et al. Treatment of early chronic lymphocytic leukemia: intermittent chlorambucil versus observation. Hematol Oncol 1988;6(1):7–12.

11. Montserrat E, Fontanillas M. Estape J. Spanish PETHEMA Group. Chronic lymphocytic leukemia treatment: an interim report of PETHEMA trials. Leuk Lymphoma 1991; 5:89–92.

12. Catovsky D, Fooks J, Richards S. The UK Medical Research Council CLL trials 1 and 2. Nouv Rev Fr Hematol 1988; 30(5-6):423–427.

13. Boussiotis VA, Pangalis GA. Interferon alfa-2b therapy in untreated early stage, B-chronic lymphocytic leukaemia patients: one-year follow-up. Br J Haematol 1991; 79(suppl 1):30–33.

14. Langenmayer I, Nerl C, Knauf W, et al. Interferon-alpha 2b (IFN alpha) for early-phase chronic lymphocytic leukaemia with high risk for disease progression: results of a randomized multicentre study. Br J Haematol 1996; 94(2):362–369.

15. Begleiter A, Wang H, Verburg L, et al. In vitro cytotoxicity of 2-chlorodeoxyadenosine and chlorambucil in chronic lymphocytic leukemia. Leukemia 1996; 10(12):1959–1965.

16. Raphael B, Andersen JW, Silber R, et al. Comparison of chlorambucil and prednisone versus cyclophosphamide, vincristine, and prednisone as initial treatment for chronic lymphocytic leukemia: long-term follow-up of an Eastern Cooperative Oncology Group randomized clinical trial. J Clin Oncol 1991; 9(5):770–776.

17. Sawitsky A, Rai KR, Glidewell O, et al. Comparison of daily versus intermittent chlorambucil and prednisone therapy in the treatment of patients with chronic lymphocytic leukemia. Blood 1977; 50(6):1049–1059.

18. Montserrat E, Alcala A, Parody R, et al. Treatment of chronic lymphocytic leukemia in advanced stages. A randomized trial comparing chlorambucil plus prednisone versus cyclophosphamide, vincristine, and prednisone. Cancer 1985; 56(10):2369–2375.

19. Jaksic B, Brugiatelli M. High dose continuous chlorambucil vs intermittent chlorambucil plus prednisone for treatment of B-CLL—IGCI CLL-01 trial. Nouv Rev Fr Hematol 1988; 30(5-6): 437–442.

20. Han T, Ezdinli EZ, Shimaoka K, et al. Chlorambucil vs. combined chlorambucil-corticosteroid therapy in chronic lymphocytic leukemia. Cancer 1973; 31(3):502–508.

21. Montserrat E, Rozman C. Chronic lymphocytic leukaemia treatment. Blood Rev 1993; 7(3): 164–175.

22. Hansen MM, Andersen E, Christensen BE, et al. CHOP versus prednisolone + chlorambucil in chronic lymphocytic leukemia (CLL): preliminary results of a randomized multicenter study. Nouv Rev Fr Hematol 1988; 30(5-6):433–436.

23. Jaksic B, Brugiatelli M, Krc I, et al. High dose chlorambucil versus Binet's modified cyclophosphamide, doxorubicin, vincristine, and prednisone regimen in the treatment of patients with advanced B-cell chronic lymphocytic leukemia. Results of an international multicenter randomized trial. International Society for Chemo-Immunotherapy, Vienna. Cancer 1997; 79(11):2107–2114.

24. Chemotherapeutic options in chronic lymphocytic leukemia: a meta-analysis of the randomized trials. CLL Trialists' Collaborative Group. J Natl Cancer Inst 1999; 91(10):861–868.

25. Plosker GL, Figgitt DP. Oral fludarabine. Drugs 2003; 63(21):2317–2323.

26. Keating MJ, Kantarjian H, O'Brien S, et al. Fludarabine: a new agent with marked cytoreductive activity in untreated chronic lymphocytic leukemia. J Clin Oncol 1991; 9(1):44–49.

27. Keating MJ, O'Brien S, Kantarjian H, et al. Long-term follow-up of patients with chronic lymphocytic leukemia treated with fludarabine as a single agent. Blood 1993; 81(11):2878–2884.

28. Plunkett W, Gandhi V, Huang P, et al. Fludarabine: pharmacokinetics, mechanisms of action, and rationales for combination therapies. Semin Oncol 1993; 20(5 suppl 7):2–12.

29. French Cooperative Group on CLL, Johnson S, Smith AG, Löffler H, et al. Multicentre prospective randomised trial of fludarabine versus cyclophosphamide, doxorubicin, and prednisone (CAP) for treatment of advanced-stage chronic lymphocytic leukaemia. The French Cooperative Group on CLL. Lancet 1996; 347(9013): 1432–1438.

30. Rai KR, Peterson BL, Appelbaum FR, et al. Fludarabine compared with chlorambucil as primary therapy for chronic lymphocytic leukemia. N Engl J Med 2000; 343(24):1750–1757.

31. Leporrier M, Chevret S, Cazin B, et al. Randomized comparison of fludarabine, CAP, and ChOP in 938 previously untreated stage B and C chronic lymphocytic leukemia patients. Blood 2001; 98(8):2319–2325.

32. Steurer M, Pall G, Richards S, et al. Single-agent purine analogues for the treatment of chronic lymphocytic leukaemia: a systematic review and meta-analysis. Cancer Treat Rev 2006; 32(5): 377–389.

33. Catovsky D, Richards S, Matutes E, et al. Assessment of fludarabine plus cyclophosphamide for patients with chronic lymphocytic leukaemia (the LRF CLL4 Trial): a randomised controlled trial. Lancet 2007; 370(9583):230–239.

34. Eichhorst BF, Busch R, Stauch M, et al. No significant clinical benefit of first line therapy with fludarabine (F) in comparison to chlorambucil (Clb) in elderly patients (pts) with advanced chronic lymphocytic leukemia (CLL): results of a phase III study of the German CLL Study Group (GCLLSG). Blood 2007;110(11).

35. Anaissie E, Kontoyiannis DP, Kantarjian H, et al. Listeriosis in patients with chronic lymphocytic leukemia who were treated with fludarabine and prednisone. Ann Intern Med 1992; 117(6):466–469.

36. Anaissie EJ, Kontoyiannis D, O'Brien S, et al. Infections in patients with chronic lymphocytic leukemia treated with fludarabine. Ann Intern Med 1998; 129:559–566.

37. Morrison VA, Rai KR, Peterson BL, et al. Impact of therapy with chlorambucil, fludarabine, or fludarabine plus chlorambucil on infections in patients with chronic lymphocytic leukemia: Intergroup Study Cancer and Leukemia Group B 9011. J Clin Oncol 2001; 19(16):3611–3621.

38. Eichhorst BF, Busch R, Schweighofer C, et al. Due to low infection rates no routine anti-infective prophylaxis is required in younger patients with chronic lymphocytic leukaemia during fludarabine-based first line therapy. Br J Haematol 2007; 136(1):63–72.

39. Di Raimondo F, Giustolisi R, Cacciola E, et al. Autoimmune hemolytic anemia in chronic lymphocytic leukemia patients treated with fludarabine. Leuk Lymphoma 1993; 11(1-2):63–68.

40. Mauro FR, Foa R, Cerretti R, et al. Autoimmune hemolytic anemia in chronic lymphocytic leukemia: clinical, therapeutic, and prognostic features. Blood 2000; 95(9):2786–92.

41. Cheson BD, Frame JN, Vena D, et al. Tumor lysis syndrome: an uncommon complication of fludarabine therapy of chronic lymphocytic leukemia. J Clin Oncol 1998; 16(7):2313–2320.

42. Cheson BD, Vena DA, Barrett J, et al. Second malignancies as a consequence of nucleoside analog therapy for chronic lymphoid leukemias. J Clin Oncol 1999; 17(8):2454–2460.

43. Robak T, Blasinska-Morawiec M, Blonski JZ, et al. The effect of 2-h infusion of 2-chlorodeoxyadenosine (cladribine) with prednisone in previously untreated B-cell chronic lymphocytic leukaemia. Eur J Cancer 1997; 33(14):2347–2351.

44. Robak T, Blonski JZ, Gora-Tybor J, et al. Second malignancies and Richter's syndrome in patients with chronic lymphocytic leukaemia treated with cladribine. Eur J Cancer 2004; 40(3): 383–389.

45. Anger C, Fink R, und Fleischer J. Vergleichsuntersuchung zwischen Cytostasan (Bendamustin) und Cyclophosphamid bei der chronischen Lymphadenose, dem Plasmozytom, der Lymphogranulomatose und dem Bronchialkarzinom. Dtsch Gesundheitswesen 1975; 30:1280–1285.

46. Kath R, Blumenstengel K, Fricke HJ, et al. Bendamustine monotherapy in advanced and refractory chronic lymphocytic leukemia. J Cancer Res Clin Oncol 2001; 127(1):48–54.

47. Knauf WU, Lissichkov T, al. Aldaoud A. Bendamustine versus chlorambucil in treatment-naïve patients with B-cell chronic lymphocytic leukemia (B-CLL): results of an international phase III study. Blood 2007; 110(11).

48. O'Brien S, Kantarjian H, Beran M, et al. Results of fludarabine and prednisone therapy in 264 patients with chronic lymphocytic leukemia with multivariate analysis-derived prognostic model for response to treatment. Blood 1993; 82(6):1695–1700.

49. Flinn IW, Byrd JC, Morrison C, et al. Fludarabine and cyclophosphamide with filgrastim support in patients with previously untreated indolent lymphoid malignancies. Blood 2000; 96(1):71–75.

50. Hallek M, Schmitt B, Wilhelm M, et al. Fludarabine plus cyclophosphamide is an efficient treatment for advanced chronic lymphocytic leukaemia (CLL): results of a phase II study of the German CLL Study Group. Br J Haematol 2001; 114(2):342–348.

51. O'Brien SM, Kantarjian HM, Cortes J, et al. Results of the fludarabine and cyclophosphamide combination regimen in chronic lymphocytic leukemia. J Clin Oncol 2001; 19(5):1414–1420.

52. Hallek M, Eichhorst BF. Chemotherapy combination treatment regimens with fludarabine in chronic lymphocytic leukemia. Hematol J 2004; (5 suppl 1):S20–S30.

53. Flinn IW, Neuberg DS, Grever MR, et al. Phase III trial of fludarabine plus cyclophosphamide compared with fludarabine for patients with previously untreated chronic lymphocytic leukemia: US Intergroup Trial E2997. J Clin Oncol 2007; 25(7):793–798.

54. Bosch F, Ferrer A, Villamor N, et al. Fludarabine, cyclophosphamide, and mitoxantrone as initial therapy of chronic lymphocytic leukemia: high response rate and disease eradication. Clin Cancer Res 2008; 14(1):155–161.

55. Montillo M, Tedeschi A, O'Brien S, et al. Phase II study of cladribine and cyclophosphamide in patients with chronic lymphocytic leukemia and prolymphocytic leukemia. Cancer 2003; 97(1): 114–120.

56. Robak T, Blonski JZ, Gora-Tybor J, et al. Cladribine alone and in combination with cyclophosphamide or cyclophosphamide plus mitoxantrone in the treatment of progressive chronic lymphocytic leukemia: report of a prospective, multicenter, randomized trial of the Polish Adult Leukemia Group (PALG CLL2). Blood 2006; 108(2):473–479.

57. Robak T, Blonski JZ, Kasznicki M, et al. Cladribine combined with cyclophosphamide and mitoxantrone as front-line therapy in chronic lymphocytic leukemia. Leukemia 2001; 15(10): 1510–1516.

58. Rummel MJ, Kafer G, Pfreundschuh M, et al. Fludarabine and epirubicin in the treatment of chronic lymphocytic leukaemia: a German multicenter phase II study. Ann Oncol 1999; 10(2): 183–188.

59. Rummel MJ, Stilgenbauer S, Gamm H, et al. Fludarabine versus fludarabine plus epirubicin in the treatment of chronic lymphocytic leukemia (CLL)—preliminary results of a randomized phase III multicentre study. Blood 2002; 100(suppl. 1) (abstr. 1489).

60. Huhn D, von Schilling C, Wilhelm M, et al. Rituximab therapy of patients with B-cell chronic lymphocytic leukemia. Blood 2001; 98(5):1326–1331.

61. O'Brien SM, Kantarjian H, Thomas DA, et al. Rituximab dose-escalation trial in chronic lymphocytic leukemia. J Clin Oncol 2001; 19(8):2165–2170.

62. Byrd JC, Murphy T, Howard RS, et al. Rituximab using a thrice weekly dosing schedule in B-cell chronic lymphocytic leukemia and small lymphocytic lymphoma demonstrates clinical activity and acceptable toxicity. J Clin Oncol 2001; 19(8):2153–2164.

63. Di Gaetano N, Xiao Y, Erba E, et al. Synergism between fludarabine and rituximab revealed in a follicular lymphoma cell line resistant to the cytotoxic activity of either drug alone. Br J Haematol 2001; 114(4):800–809.

64. Schulz H, Klein SK, Rehwald U, et al. Phase 2 study of a combined immunochemotherapy using rituximab and fludarabine in patients with chronic lymphocytic leukemia. Blood 2002; 100(9):3115–3120.

65. Byrd JC, Peterson BL, Morrison VA, et al. Randomized phase 2 study of fludarabine with concurrent versus sequential treatment with rituximab in symptomatic, untreated patients with B-cell chronic lymphocytic leukemia: results from Cancer and Leukemia Group B 9712 (CALGB 9712). Blood 2003; 101(1):6–14.
66. Byrd JC, Rai K, Peterson BL, et al. Addition of rituximab to fludarabine may prolong progression-free survival and overall survival in patients with previously untreated chronic lymphocytic leukemia: an updated retrospective comparative analysis of CALGB 9712 and CALGB 9011. Blood 2005; 105(1):49–53.
67. Keating MJ, O'Brien S, Albitar M, et al. Early results of a chemoimmunotherapy regimen of fludarabine, cyclophosphamide, and rituximab as initial therapy for chronic lymphocytic leukemia. J Clin Oncol 2005; 23:4079–4088.
68. Kay NE, Geyer SM, Call TG, et al. Combination chemoimmunotherapy with pentostatin, cyclophosphamide, and rituximab shows significant clinical activity with low accompanying toxicity in previously untreated B chronic lymphocytic leukemia. Blood 2007; 109(2):405–411.
69. Shanafelt TD, Lin T, Geyer SM, et al. Pentostatin, cyclophosphamide, and rituximab regimen in older patients with chronic lymphocytic leukemia. Cancer 2007; 109(11):2291–2298.
70. Lundin J, Kimby E, Bjorkholm M, et al. Phase II trial of subcutaneous anti-CD52 monoclonal antibody alemtuzumab (Campath-1H) as first-line treatment for patients with B-cell chronic lymphocytic leukemia (B-CLL). Blood 2002; 100(3):768–773.
71. Laurenti L, Piccioni P, Cattani P, et al. Cytomegalovirus reactivation during alemtuzumab therapy for chronic lymphocytic leukemia: incidence and treatment with oral ganciclovir. Haematologica 2004; 89(10):1248–1252.
72. O'Brien SM, Keating MJ, Mocarski ES. Updated guidelines on the management of cytomegalovirus reactivation in patients with chronic lymphocytic leukemia treated with alemtuzumab. Clinical Lymphoma Myeloma 2006; 7(2):125–130.
73. Keating MJ, Flinn I, Jain V, et al. Therapeutic role of alemtuzumab (Campath-1H) in patients who have failed fludarabine: results of a large international study. Blood 2002; 99(10): 3554–3561.
74. Osterborg A, Mellstedt H, Keating M. Clinical effects of alemtuzumab (Campath-1H) in B-cell chronic lymphocytic leukemia. Med Oncol 2002; 19 suppl:S21–S26.
75. Rai KR, Freter CE, Mercier RJ, et al. Alemtuzumab in previously treated chronic lymphocytic leukemia patients who also had received fludarabine. J Clin Oncol 2002; 20(18):3891–3897.
76. Osterborg A, Fassas AS, Anagnostopoulos A, et al. Humanized CD52 monoclonal antibody Campath-1H as first-line treatment in chronic lymphocytic leukaemia. Br J Haematol 1996; 93(1):151–153.
77. Hillmen P, Skotnicki AB, Robak T, et al. Alemtuzumab compared with chlorambucil as first-line therapy for chronic lymphocytic leukemia. J Clin Oncol 2007; 25(35):5616–5623. [Epub 2007, Nov 5].
78. Lozanski G, Heerema NA, Flinn IW, et al. Alemtuzumab is an effective therapy for chronic lymphocytic leukemia with p53 mutations and deletions. Blood 2004; 103(9):3278–3281.
79. Stilgenbauer S, Dohner H. Campath-1H-induced complete remission of chronic lymphocytic leukemia despite p53 gene mutation and resistance to chemotherapy. N Engl J Med 2002; 347(6):452–453.
80. Kennedy B, Rawstron A, Carter C, et al. Campath-1H and fludarabine in combination are highly active in refractory chronic lymphocytic leukemia. Blood 2002; 99(6):2245–2247.
81. Elter T, Borchmann P, Schulz H, et al. Fludarabine in combination with alemtuzumab is effective and feasible in patients with relapsed or refractory B-cell chronic lymphocytic leukemia: results of a phase II trial. J Clin Oncol 2005; 23(28):7024–7031.
82. Faderl S, Thomas DA, O'Brien S, et al. Experience with alemtuzumab plus rituximab in patients with relapsed and refractory lymphoid malignancies. Blood 2003; 101(9):3413–3415.
83. O'Brien S, Kantarjian H, Beran M, et al. Interferon maintenance therapy for patients with chronic lymphocytic leukemia in remission after fludarabine therapy. Blood 1995; 86(4):1298–1300.
84. Mauro FR, Zinzani P, Zaja F, et al. Fludarabine + prednisone +/− alpha-interferon followed or not by alpha-interferon maintenance therapy for previously untreated patients with chronic

lymphocytic leukemia: long term results of a randomized study. Haematologica 2003; 88(12): 1348–1357.

85. Montillo M, Tedeschi A, Miqueleiz S, et al. Alemtuzumab as consolidation after a response to fludarabine is effective in purging residual disease in patients with chronic lymphocytic leukemia. J Clin Oncol 2006; 24(15):2337–2342.

86. O'Brien SM, Kantarjian HM, Thomas DA, et al. Alemtuzumab as treatment for residual disease after chemotherapy in patients with chronic lymphocytic leukemia. Cancer 2003; 98(12): 2657–2663.

87. Schweighofer C, Ritgen M, Eichhorst B, et al. Consolidation with alemtuzumab improves progression-free survival in patients with chronic lymphocytic leukemia (CLL) in first remission long-term follow-up of a randomized phase III trial of the German CLL Study Group (GCLLSG). Blood 2006; 108(11).

88. Hainsworth JD, Litchy S, Barton JH, et al. Single-agent rituximab as first-line and maintenance treatment for patients with chronic lymphocytic leukemia or small lymphocytic lymphoma: a phase II trial of the Minnie Pearl Cancer Research Network. J Clin Oncol 2003; 21(9):1746–1751.

89. Del Poeta G, Del Principe MI, Buccisano F, et al. Consolidation and maintenance immunotherapy with rituximab improve clinical outcome in patients with B-cell chronic lymphocytic leukemia. Cancer 2008; 112(1):119–128.

90. Eichhorst B, Hallek M. Revision of the guidelines for diagnosis and therapy of chronic lymphocytic leukemia (CLL). Best Pract Res Clin Haematol 2007; 20(3):469–477.

91. Byrd JC, Smith L, Hackbarth ML, et al. Interphase cytogenetic abnormalities in chronic lymphocytic leukemia may predict response to rituximab. Cancer Res 2003; 63(1):36–38.

92. Stilgenbauer S, Kröber A, Busch R, et al. 17p Deletion predicts for inferior overall survival after fludarabine-based first line therapy in chronic lymphocytic leukemia: first analysis of genetics in the CLL4 trial of the GCLLSG. Blood 2005; 106(11).

93. Turgut B, Vural O, Pala FS, et al. 17p Deletion is associated with resistance of B-cell chronic lymphocytic leukemia cells to in vitro fludarabine-induced apoptosis. Leuk Lymphoma 2007; 48(2):311–320.

94. Stilgenbauer S, Winkler D, Krober A, et al. Subcutaneous campath-1H (Alemtuzumab) in fludarabine-refractory CLL: interim analysis of the CLL2h study of the German CLL Study Group (GCLLSG). Blood 2004; 104(11).

95. Moreno C, Villamor N, Colomer D, et al. Allogeneic stem-cell transplantation may overcome the adverse prognosis of unmutated VH gene in patients with chronic lymphocytic leukemia. J Clin Oncol 2005; 23(15):3433–3438.

96. Dreger P, Corradini P, Kimby E, et al. Indications for allogeneic stem cell transplantation in chronic lymphocytic leukemia: the EBMT transplant consensus. Leukemia 2007; 21(7):12–17.

97. Extermann M, Overcash J, Lyman GH, et al. Comorbidity and functional status are independent in older cancer patients. J Clin Oncol 1998; 16(4):1582–1587.

98. Robak T, Blonski JZ, Kasznicki M, et al. Cladribine with prednisone versus chlorambucil with prednisone as first-line therapy in chronic lymphocytic leukemia: report of a prospective, randomized, multicenter trial. Blood 2000; 96(8):2723–2729.

99. Wierda W, O'Brien S, Wen S, et al. Chemoimmunotherapy with fludarabine, cyclophosphamide, and rituximab for relapsed and refractory chronic lymphocytic leukemia. J Clin Oncol 2005; 23(18):4070–4078.

9

Treatment of Patients with Relapsed or Refractory Chronic Lymphocytic Leukemia

Karen W.L. Yee
Department of Medical Oncology and Hematology, Princess Margaret Hospital, University Health Network, Toronto, Ontario, Canada

Michael J. Keating and Susan M. O'Brien
Department of Leukemia, University of Texas M.D. Anderson Cancer Center, Houston, Texas, U.S.A.

INTRODUCTION

Chronic lymphocytic leukemia (CLL) is the most common form of leukemia in adults in the Western world, accounting for nearly 25% of all leukemias with an estimated annual age-adjusted incidence of 3 per 100,000 persons in the United States (1,2). The median age at diagnosis is approximately 70 years, with 81% of the patients diagnosed at age $\geq$60 years (1). Under the World Health Organization (WHO) classification, CLL is a B-cell neoplasm, and the entity T-cell CLL has been reclassified as T-cell prolymphocytic leukemia (PLL) (3). Recent data from the Surveillance, Epidemiology, and End Results cancer statistics indicate that five-year survival of patients with CLL is 73% (4).

Significant changes in the understanding and management of CLL have occurred in the last two decades. With the advent of newer treatment modalities, such as purine analogs and monoclonal antibodies, substantial improvements have been made in achieving complete responses (CRs), with a proportion achieving molecular remissions and durable responses. Despite the advances in the treatment of patients with CLL, the majority of patients will relapse after primary therapy.

INDICATIONS FOR TREATMENT

Indications for salvage treatment are similar to those for first-line therapy (5,6). Criteria for therapy include B symptoms (i.e., fevers, sweats, or weight loss), progressive enlargement of lymph nodes or hepatosplenomegaly, obstructive adenopathy,

"

development of or worsening thrombocytopenia and anemia, immune hemolysis or thrombocytopenia not responsive to steroids, and rapid lymphocyte doubling time.

ASSESSMENT OF RESPONSE

The International Workshop on CLL (IWCLL)-National Cancer Institute (NCI)-sponsored working group (5) has refined the evaluation of response to therapy previously established by the NCI-sponsored working group (6), with more precision of lymph node diameters (Table 1). Assessment of minimal residual disease (MRD), by either multiparametric flow cytometry based on the immunophenotype of the CLL cell or polymerase chain reaction (PCR)-based strategies using either the qualitative consensus IgH PCR or the quantitative allele-specific oligonucleotide [to the complementarity-determining region 3 (CDR3)] PCR (7,8), should only be performed in a research setting. Techniques for assessing MRD require standardization, and prospective clinical studies are required to validate the role of MRD negativity as a surrogate marker for disease eradication and/or improved survival prior to its incorporation into routine clinical practice.

THERAPEUTIC OPTIONS FOR SALVAGE THERAPY

Choice of salvage therapy is guided by factors such as age, performance status, prior therapy, response and duration of response to such a therapy, and the goal of salvage therapy. At the current time, prognostic markers [such as del(17p), ZAP-70, mutational status of the immunoglobulin heavy-chain variable region genes, etc.] cannot be used to guide choice of salvage treatment (9). On the basis of retrospective data indicating that response to salvage therapy appears to be strongly associated with response to prior therapies and that most patients have been or will be treated with fludarabine or fludarabine-based regimens, relapsed patients have generally been classified into two groups on the basis of prior response or exposure to fludarabine: fludarabine naïve or fludarabine sensitive and fludarabine refractory. However, the choice of appropriate salvage therapy in relapsed patients is hampered by (*i*) the lack of randomized trials, including those involving stem cell transplant (SCT), in patients who have been previously exposed to purine analog–based regimens (10,11) and monoclonal antibodies, (*ii*) incomplete data in the currently reported phase II studies with respect to prior sensitivity or resistance to purine analog– and/or monoclonal antibody–based treatment regimens, and, (*iii*) usually, inclusion of both purine analog–sensitive and analog–resistant patients and/or alkylator-sensitive and alkylator-resistant patients in the same clinical trial.

Fludarabine (Purine Analog)-Naïve or Fludarabine (Purine Analog)-Sensitive Patients

Alkylating Agents

Although retreatment of patients who have received prior therapy with an alklyating agent with an alkylator-based regimen may induce responses in 21% to 62% of patients, the quality of responses is low (CR 0–31%), and the duration of responses is usually short (2–18 months) (10,12–15). In patients who relapsed after or were refractory to therapy with fludarabine, alkylator-based therapy can induce overall response (OR) rates of 7% to 44% with CR rates of 6% to 22% (10,16,17).

Table 1 Response Criteria

Criteria	Complete response (CR)	Partial response (PR)	Stable disease (SD)	Progressive disease (PD)
Symptoms	Absent	Absent or present	Absent or present	Absent or present
Lymphadenopathy[a]	None >1 cm	≥50% reduction	Change of −49% to +49%	≥50% increase
Hepato- and/or splenomegaly	Absent	≥50% reduction	Change of −49% to +49%	≥50% increase
Neutrophils ($\times 10^9$/L)	≥1.5	≥1.5% or ≥50% improvement from baseline	Any	Any
Lymphocytes ($\times 10^9$/L)	Normal	≥50% reduction from baseline	Change of −49% to +49%	≥50% increase
Platelets ($\times 10^9$/L)	>100	>100% or ≥50% improvement from baseline	Change of −49% to +49%	≥50% reduction from baseline
Hemoglobin (g/dL) (untransfused)	>11	>11% or ≥50% improvement from baseline	Increase of <11% or <50% improvement from baseline or decrease of <2	Decrease of >2% from baseline
Bone marrow aspirate and biopsy	Normocellular; <30% lymphocytes; no B-lymphoid nodules	Hypocellular or ≥30% lymphocytes or B-lymphoid nodules or not done	No change of marrow infiltrate	Increase of lymphocytes to >30% from normal

[a] sum of the products of multiple lymph nodes (as evaluated by CT scans, ultrasound, or physical examination).
Source: From Ref. 5.

Purine Analogs

Fludarabine   In previously treated CLL patients, where the majority of patients had failed therapy with an alkylator-based regimen, therapy with single agent fludarabine can yield OR rates of 12% to 58% with CR rates of 0% to 26% (18–23). Overall survival (OS) strongly correlated with quality of response achieved [i.e., CR vs. partial response (PR) vs. no response (NR)] (20,21). Long-term follow-up of 174 patients who received first-line therapy with single agent fludarabine indicated that 67% of patients who relapse will respond to salvage therapy with a fludarabine-based regimen, with 74% of patients responding to rechallenge with single agent fludarabine (16). However, no patient who initially failed to respond to fludarabine responded to retreatment with a fludarabine-containing regimen.

A single phase III study has compared fludarabine alone with CAP in previously treated and untreated CLL patients (Table 2) (10). Patients were stratified for prior or no prior therapy. However, the proportion of patients who received prior fludarabine was not specified. Subgroup analysis of the previously treated patients demonstrated a superior response rate in favor of fludarabine [OR 48% vs. 27%, $p = 0.036$; CR 13% vs. 6%, $p = $ NS (not significant)]. However, there was no significant difference in response duration or OS.

Several phase II studies have evaluated the efficacy of fludarabine in combination with alkylators [e.g., fludarabine and cyclophosphamide (FC)] (24–26), anthracyclines/ anthraquinones [e.g., fludarabine and doxorubicin or fludarabine and mitoxantrone (FM)] (27,28), both alkylators and anthracyclines/anthraquinones [e.g., fludarabine, cyclo-phosphamide, and mitoxantrone (FCM)] (29), or other nucleoside analogs (Table 3). Therapy with FC yielded OR rates of 60% to 94% (CR 10–29%) in previously treated patients, a proportion of patients who had received prior fludarabine (14–79%) (24–26). Treatment with fludarabine plus doxorubicin (28) or FM (27) appears to yield inferior results to those obtained with FC. However, the majority (72–83%) of these patients had received prior fludarabine in contrast to patients treated with FC. Treatment with FCM appears to yield higher quality response rates (CR 50%, with 33% having no detectable disease by flow cytometry and PCR analysis) in patients who have not received prior fludarabine, but may be associated with more myelosuppression (29). While fludarabine, ara-C (cytarabine), mitoxantrone, and dexamethasone (FAND) chemotherapy can induce CRs of 60% in previously treated patients (87%, who had received prior fludarabine, with at least 19% being fludarabine refractory), granulocyte-colony stimulating factor (G-CSF) was required to treat severe myelosuppression (30). It is unclear whether these results will be durable as 25% to 30% of the patients treated underwent SCT.

Preliminary results for a randomized trial comparing fludarabine alone with fludarabine and epirubicin (FE) in previously treated and untreated CLL patients have been presented (Table 2) (11). The proportion of patients who received prior fludarabine was not specified. Treatment with FE yielded superior response rates (OR 88% vs. 73%, respectively, $p = 0.026$; CR 29% vs. 9%, respectively, $p = 0.0029$). There was a trend to better progression-free survival (PFS) in favor of FE (26 months vs. 20 months, respectively, $p = 0.085$); however, this did not translate into an improved OS (76 months vs. 63 months, respectively, $p = 0.1$). Subgroup analysis of the previously treated patients has not been performed. Although response duration and/or OS after fludarabine-based salvage therapies appears to be strongly associated with response to prior therapies [i.e., prior alkylating agents only, prior alkylating agents and fludarabine (fludarabine sensitive but relapsed), and prior alkylating agents and fludarabine (alkylator and fludarabine refractory)] (24,29), the true magnitude of the efficacy of the various treatment regimens is hampered by incomplete data concerning patient refractoriness to prior alkylator and/or fludarabine therapies.

Table 2 Results of Randomized Trials Using Fludarabine Regimens in Previously Treated Patients

| | Patient characteristics | | | | | | Response | | |
Investigator, yr (reference)	Median age (yr)	N	Rai/Binet stage (%)	Prior F(%)	Median F/U	Chemotherapy regimen	Response rate (%)	Disease control (median)	Overall survival (median)
Johnson, 1996 (10)	62–63[a]	96[b]	A (1), B (54), C (45)[a]	NR	34 mo	F vs. CAP	OR 48 vs. 27[b,c]; CR 13 vs. 6[b]	Response duration 10.8 mo vs. 6 mo[b]	24.3 mo vs. 24.4 mo[b]
Rummel, 2005 (11)	62	150[d]	B (57), C (43)	NR	NR	F vs. FE	OR 73 vs. 88[d,e]; CR 29 vs. 9[d]	PFS 20 mo vs. 26 mo[d]; EFS 19 mo vs. 30 mo[f]	63 mo vs. 76 mo[d]

Note: Unless otherwise specified, p = NS.

[a]includes untreated ($n = 100$) and previously treated ($n = 96$) patients; [b]previously treated patients; [c]$p = 0.036$; [d]includes untreated and previously treated patients; [e]$p = 0.0026$; [f]$p = 0.0048$.

Abbreviations: CAP, cyclophosphamide, doxorubicin, and prednisone; CR, complete response; EFS, event-free survival; F, fludarabine; FE, fludarabine and epirubicin; F/U, follow-up; NR, not reported; PFS, progression-free survival; OR, overall response.

Table 3 Results of Phase II Trials Using Fludarabine-Containing Regimens in Previously Treated Patients

Investigator, yr (reference)	Patient characteristics						Response		
	Median age (range, yr)	N (evaluable)	Rai/Binet stage (%)	Prior F (%)	Median F/U	Chemotherapy regimen	Response rate (%)	Disease control (median)	Overall survival (median)
Fludarabine and cyclophosphamide									
Marotta, 2000 (84)	75 (61–87)	20	B (20), C (80)	0	NR	Low-dose FC	OR 85 CR 15; PR 70	NR	NR
Hallek, 2001 (25)	58.9[a] (41–72)	21[b] (18)	A (3), B (50), C (47)[+]	14[b]	14.4 mo	FC	OR 94.4[b] CR 11.1; PR 83.3[b]	NR	NR
O'Brien, 2001 (24)	58 (29–92)[c]	94[b]	0–II (53), III–IV (47)[c]	79	41 mo	FC	OR 69[b] CR 10; NPR 18; PR 41[b]	TTP 33 mo vs. 20 mo[d]	38 mo vs. 21 mo vs. 12 mo[e]
Schiavone, 2003 (85)	63[f] (42–75)	17[b]	II (31), III–IV (69)[f]	35[b]	24 mo	FC	OR 88[b] CR 29; PR 59[b]	TTP 18 mo[b]	20 mo[b]
Gonzalez, 2003 (26)	61.8[g] (38–82)	40[h]	A (4), B (52), C (44)[i]	NR	NR	FC	OR 60[h] CR 32.5; PR 27.5[h]	NR	NR
Fludarabine and an anthracycline/anthraquinone									
Robertson, 1995 (28)	61	30 (29)	0 (7), I–II (63), III–IV (30)	83	19 mo	FDox	OR 55 CR 3; NPR 17; PR 35	TTP not reached	Not reached

Rummel, 1999 (86)	54 (35–74)[j]	13[b]	B (38), C (62)[b]	NR	NR	FE	OR 62[b] CR 15; PR 46[b]	NR	28 mo[b]
Tsimberidou, 2004 (27)	59 (21–78)[k]	53[b]	III–IV (41)[k]	72[b]	8 yr	FM	OR 55[b] CR 8; NPR 9; PR 38[b]	TTP 16 mo vs. 17 mo vs. 5 mo[l]	31 mo vs. 36 mo vs. 9 mo[l]

Fludarabine and multi-agent therapy

Schmitt, 2002 (87)	62[m] (27)	63	B and C (100)	53[n]	NR	FCM vs. FCM + G-CSF	OR 77.8 CR 3.7; PR 74.1	RFS 18.2 mo	NR
Bosch, 2002 (29)	51 (30–71)	60	A (7), B (58), C (35)	8	NR	FCM	OR 78 CR 50; PR 28	DFS 19 mo	41 mo
Mauro, 2002 (30)	54 (22–60)	31	II (52), III–IV (48)[p]	87	34 mo	FAND	OR 70 CR 60; PR 16	TTP 28 mo	$OS_{67\ mo}$ 68%[q]

[a]includes untreated ($n = 15$) and previously treated ($n = 21$) patients; [b]previously treated patients only; [c]includes untreated ($n = 34$) and previously treated ($n = 94$) patients; [d]patients previously treated with alkylating agents only ($n = 20$) and with both fludarabine and alkylating agents ($n = 74$), respectively; [e]patients previously treated with alkylating agents only ($n = 20$), with both fludarabine and alkylating agents ($n = 46$), and fludarabine-refractory patients ($n = 28$), respectively; [f]includes untreated ($n = 15$) and previously treated ($n = 17$) patients; [g]includes NHL ($n = 6$), PLL ($n = 1$), and CLL ($n = 50$) of which 10 were previously untreated and 40 previously treated; [h]previously treated CLL patients only; [i]CLL patients only; [j]includes untreated ($n = 25$) and previously treated ($n = 13$) patients; [k]includes untreated ($n = 34$) and previously treated ($n = 53$) patients; [l]patients previously treated with alkylating agents only ($n = 15$) and with both fludarabine and alkylating agents ($n = 26$), and fludarabine-refractory patients ($n = 12$), respectively; [m]data from 32 patients only; [n]data from 19 patients only; [o]includes uncensored data from patients who subsequently received an autotransplant ($n = 12$) and allotransplant ($n = 4$); [p]data available for 23 patients only; [q]includes uncensored data from patients who subsequently received an autotransplant ($n = 9$) and allotransplant ($n = 1$).

Abbreviations: CR, complete response; F, fludarabine; FE, fludarabine and epirubicin; F/U, follow-up; NR, not reported; OR, overall response; DFS, disease-free survival; FAND, fludarabine, ara-C, mitoxantrone (Novantrone), and dexamethasone; FC, fludarabine and cyclophosphamide; FDox, fludarabine and doxorubicin; FCM, fludarabine, cyclophosphamide, and mitoxantrone (Novantrone); FM, fludarabine and mitoxantrone; NPR, nodular partial response; RFS, relapse-free survival; TTP, time to progression; OS, overall survival; OS_{67}, overall survival at 67 months; PR, partial response.

Cladribine (2-CdA)   Cladribine with or without steroids can induce OR rates of 31% to 68% with CRs of 0% to 31% in previously treated CLL patients (31–35). These results appear to be comparable to single agent fludarabine, although, the duration of responses appears to be shorter with cladribine (4–20 months vs. >18 months for fludarabine). However, 7% to 43% of these patients had received prior fludarabine (32–34). The European Organization for Research and Treatment of Cases (EORTC) has performed a randomized controlled trial comparing fludarabine with cladribine in previously treated CLL patients; no results have been reported to date.

A small number of CLL patients have received therapy with cladribine and cyclophosphamide (2-CdA/C) or cladribine, cyclophosphamide, and mitoxantrone (2-CdA/CM) (36–38). Treatment with 2-CdA/C yielded ORs of 45% to 62% (CR 8–15%) (36,38), which are similar to those obtained with FC therapy. However, these responses do not appear to be as durable (median, 11–12 months) as those obtained with FC, but a higher proportion of patients (85–95%) had received prior fludarabine therapy. Therapy with 2-CdA/CM appears to be inferior to both 2-CdA/C and FCM with an OR of only 37% (CR 5%) and median response duration of five months (37).

Pentostatin   Extremely poor results were seen when pentostatin monotherapy was used in previously treated CLL patients (OR 15–29%; CR 0–8%) (39–41). However, 59% of the patients in at least one study had been exposed to prior fludarabine (41). Twenty-one patients with CLL were treated with pentostatin plus cyclophosphamide (42). The majority had advanced disease, and 87% had received prior fludarabine. OR was 81% (CR 19%), with median response duration of only seven months. Similar to what has been observed with fludarabine-based regimens, response to salvage therapy with cladribine- or pentostatin-based regimens appears to be affected by prior fludarabine exposure.

Rituximab

Rituximab induction therapy   Single agent rituximab administered at the standard dose and schedule yielded unimpressive responses in previously treated CLL/small lymphocytic leukemia (SLL) patients (OR 0–35%; CR 0%) (43–46). Alternative doses (up to 2250 mg/m^2/week) and schedules of administration (thrice a week) have improved response rates of single agent rituximab induction therapy (OR 36% and 52%; CR 0% and 4%) with median time to disease progression (TTP) of 8 to 11 months (47,48).

The German CLL Study Group (GCLLSG) has evaluated fludarabine and rituximab (FR) in previously untreated ($n = 20$) and treated ($n = 11$) CLL patients (Table 4) (49). Of the 11 previously treated patients, OR was 90% [CR 27%; complete response unconfirmed (CRu) 18%]. Median duration of response for this subset of patients was not stated. No survival data were reported. Inferior results were obtained when rituximab was combined with either pentostatin or cladribine (50,51).

Fludarabine, cyclophosphamide, and rituximab (FCR) therapy has been evaluated in 143 previously treated CLL patients (Table 4) (52). An OR of 73% [CR 25%; nodular partial response (NPR) 16%; PR 32%] was obtained. Twenty-five of 35 (71%) patients in CR had <1% CD5$^+$/CD19$^+$ cells in the marrow by flow cytometry, and 12 of 37 (32%) patients in CR achieved a molecular remission. With a follow-up of 28 months, the estimated median survival was 42 months (Fig. 1). These results have been compared with historical controls treated with FC and fludarabine with or without prednisone (F+/−P) (53). OR and CR for FC and F+/−P were 67% and 12%, and 59% and 13%, respectively. Estimated median survival was 31 and 19 months, respectively. Multivariate analysis showed that the FCR group had a significantly higher CR rate and longer survival compared with FC and F+/−P ($p = 0.0001$ and $p < 0.0001$, respectively) (Fig. 2).

Table 4 Results of Trials Using Rituximab-Containing Regimens

	Patient characteristics						Response		
Investigator, yr (reference)	Median age (range, yr)	N (evaluable)	Rai/Binet stage (%)	Prior F (%)	Median F/U	Regimen	Response rate (%)	Disease control (median)	Overall survival (median)
Rituximab induction									
Robak, 2007 (50)	57 (40–80)	18	II (22) III–IV (78)	NR[a]	16 mo	2-CdA/R	OR 67 CR 6; PR 61	NR	NR
Robak, 2007 (50)	59 (45–76)	28	II (29) III–IV (71)	NR[b]	16 mo	2-CdA/CR	OR 78 CR 7; PR 71	NR	NR
Drapkin, 2002 (51)	61 (41–85)[d]	38[c]	II (21), III–IV (52)[d]	NR	NR	DCF/R	OR 33.4[c]	Response duration 9.8 mo[d]	NR
Lamanna, 2006 (54)	62 (30–80)[f]	32[e]	NR	78[e]	NR	DCF/CR	OR 75[e] CR 25; NPR 3; PR 47[e]	Response duration 25 mo[e]	44 mo[e]
Schulz, 2002 (49)	59 (30–70)[g]	11[c]	B (68), C (32)[g]	0	13.5 mo	FR	OR 90[c] CR 27; CRu 18; PR 45[c]	Response duration 18.8 mo[g]	NR
Wierda, 2005 (52)	59 (36–81)	177	I–II (47) III–IV (50)	82	28 mo	FCR	OR 73 CR 25; NPR 16; PR 32	TTP 28 mo	42 mo

[a]patients previously treated with cladribine ($n = 11$); [b]patients previously treated with cladribine ($n = 18$); [c]previously treated patients only; [d]includes untreated ($n = 24$) and previously treated ($n = 38$) patients; [e]CLL patients only; [f]includes patients with CLL ($n = 38$) and other low-grade B-cell neoplasms ($n = 14$); [g]includes untreated ($n = 20$) and previously treated ($n = 11$) patients.

Abbreviations: CR, complete response; F, fludarabine; F/U, follow-up; NR, not reported; OR, overall response; NPR, nodular partial response; TTP, time to progression; PR, partial response; 2-CdA/R, cladribine and rituximab; 2-CdA/CR, cladribine, cyclophosphamide, and rituximab; DCF/R, pentostatin and rituximab; DCF/CR, pentostatin, cyclophosphamide, and rituximab; FCR, fludarabine, cyclophosphamide, and rituximab; FR, fludarabine and rituximab.

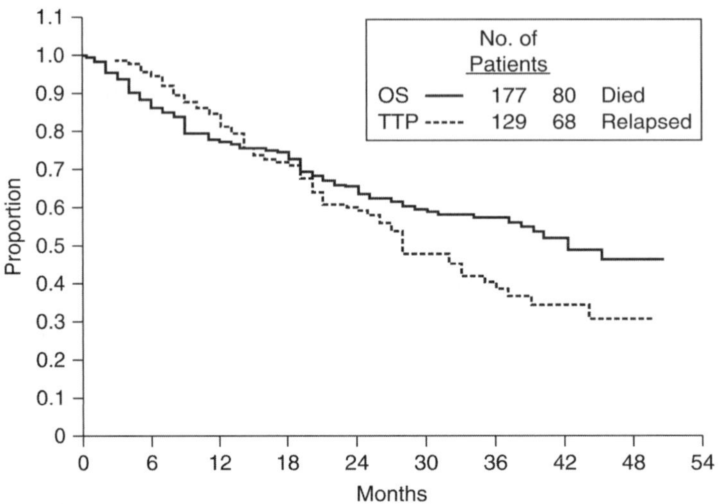

Figure 1 Kaplan-Meier estimates of time to progression for responding patients and overall survival for all patients treated with fludarabine, cyclophosphamide, and rituximab (FCR) with a median follow-up of 28 months for all patients. *Source*: From Ref. 52.

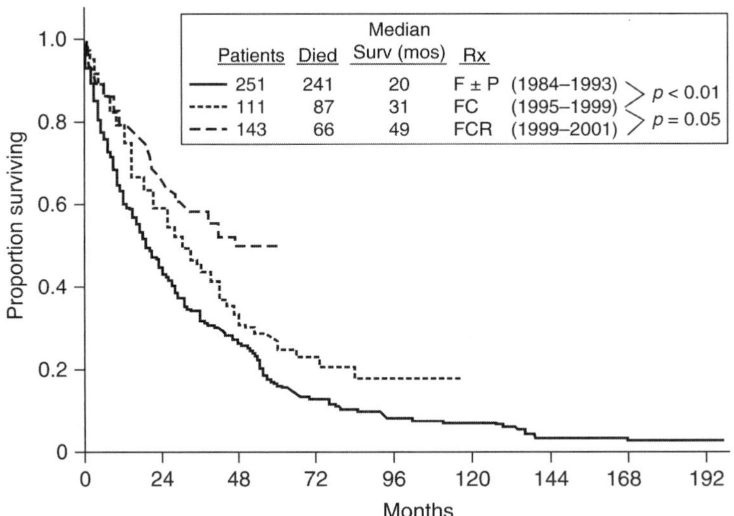

Figure 2 Kaplan-Meier survival curves for patients treated with F+/−P, FC, and FCR at a single institution. The estimated median overall survival was 19 months, 31 months, and 42+ months for the F+/−P, FC, and FCR groups respectively ($p \leq 0.05$). *Abbreviations*: F+/−P, fludarabine with or without prednisone; FC, fludarabine and cyclophosphamide; FCR, fludarabine, cyclophosphamide, and rituximab. *Source*: From Ref. 53.

Median survival for the nonresponders was similar for all three groups, suggesting that improved supportive care over time did not have a major impact on survival. A phase III trial comparing FCR with FC in previously treated patients with CLL is currently under way. The OR rates obtained with FCR appear comparable to those obtained with FR therapy, albeit in a significantly smaller cohort of previously treated patients (49).

However, in this study, MRD was not evaluated, and follow-up is too short to draw conclusions about survival (49). A formal comparison of FR with FCR therapy is warranted.

Therapy with pentostatin, cyclophosphamide, and rituximab (DCF/CR) can yield OR rates of 75% (CR 25%), with all eight patients who achieved a CR being negative for MRD by immunophenotyping (Table 4) (54). Median response duration and time to treatment failure (TTF) were 25 and 40 months, respectively. Median survival was 44 months. Although response frequencies were similar between the DCF/CR regimen and pentostatin and cyclophosphamide regimen, response duration and OS with DCF/CR appeared superior to results historically obtained with pentostatin and cyclophosphamide (42,54). Results with DCF/CR appear to be comparable to that obtained with FCR therapy, although a relatively small number of patients were treated with DCF/CR compared with those treated with FCR therapy (52,54). In contrast, inferior results appear to be obtained with cladribine, cyclophosphamide, and rituximab (OR 78% with a CR rate of only 7%) (Table 4) (50).

Alemtuzumab

Alemtuzumab induction therapy   Alemtuzumab has been approved for the treatment of patients with refractory CLL (Table 5) (55–60). The majority of these patients had advanced-stage disease and had received prior fludarabine (55–100%) and ≤3 prior therapies. Standard-dose alemtuzumab was administered intravenously in all except one study (55) until a maximum response was achieved or a maximum of 12 weeks (56–58,60). The OR rates were 31% to 70% with CRs of 0% to 30%. Patients were less likely to respond if they had high-risk disease (57,59), enlarged lymph nodes, especially >5 cm in diameter (56,57,59), WHO performance status of 2 (57), and >5 prior therapeutic regimens (60). The higher quality of the responses (CR 30% and 36%; with no detectable bone marrow disease by immunophenotyping in 20% of patients) achieved in two trials may be due to differences in patient characteristics and the duration of therapy with alemtuzumab (55,61). Median OS was reported only in three studies and ranged from 16 to 27.5 months (57,59,61). Median OS and treatment-free survival may be significantly longer for patients with MRD-negative CR compared with those achieving a MRD-positive CR or PR or with nonresponders (61,62). However, a significant proportion of patients (47%) with MRD-negative remission will convert to MRD positivity over time (61). Major toxicities were infusion related, infections [including cytomegalovirus (CMV) reactivation], neutropenia, and thrombocytopenia.

On the basis of promising preliminary results with fludarabine and alemtuzumab in patients with fludarabine-refractory CLL (see below) (63), the efficacy and safety of this combination was further evaluated in 36 patients with relapsed or refractory CLL fludarabine (Table 6) (64). Twenty-two patients had received prior fludarabine, and four had received prior alemtuzumab. Twenty-five percent were fludarabine refractory. Fifteen of 36 patients did not receive the target number of cycles for a variety of reasons (prolonged aplasia, poor response/disease progression, lack of compliance, infections, and Richter's transformation). Most toxicities were infusion related (predominantly with initial alemtuzumab doses) and myelosuppression. Patients with massive adenopathy were prone to signs of cytokine release syndrome during the first two cycles of therapy. CMV reactivation occurred in only two patients. The OR rate was 83% (CR 30%; PR 53%). Responses were observed in 18 (82%) of 22 patients who had received prior fludarabine (CR 27%; PR 55%), including 6 (67%) of the 9 patients with fludarabine-refractory CLL. Three (75%) of four patients who had received prior alemtuzumab achieved a PR. With a median follow-up time of 15 months, the median OS for all patients was 35.6 months with a median TTP of 12.97 months.

Table 5 Results of Trials in Fludarabine-Refractory Patients with Single Agent Alemtuzumab

Investigator, yr (reference)	Patient characteristics						Response		
	Median age (range, yr)	N (evaluable)	Rai/Binet stage (%)	F refractory (%)	Median F/U	Chemotherapy regimen	Response rate (%)	Disease control (median)	Overall survival (median)
Moreton, 2005 (61)	58 (32–75)	91	0–I (14), II (25), III–IV (60)	50[a]	NR	Cam to maximum response then FCam ($n = 8$) or SCT ($n = 23$)	OR 54; CR 35; PR 19 [OR 50[b]; CR 27; PR23[b]]	TFS not reached vs. 20 mo vs. 13 mo vs. 6 mo[c]	Not reached vs. 41 mo vs. 30 mo vs. 15 mo[c]
Keating, 2002 (57)	66 (31–86)	93	0 (1), I–II (23), III–IV (76)	99	29 mo	Cam	OR 33; CR 2; NPR 5; PR 26	Response duration 8.7 mo	16 mo
Rai, 2002 (59)	NR	24[d]	0 (4), I–II (25), III–IV (71)[c]	71[d]	NR	Cam	OR 30[b]; CR 0; PR 30[b]	Response duration 15.4 mo[d]	27.5 mo[d]
Ferrajoli, 2003 (56)	61 (35–75)[e]	42[f]	I–II (24), III–IV (76)	55[f]	NR	Cam	OR 31[f]; CR 5; NPR 2; PR 24[f]	NR	NR
Lozanski, 2004 (79)	61 (47–74)	36	I–II (25), III–IV (75)	81	NR	Cam	OR 31; CR 6; PR 25	Response duration 10 mo	NR

[a]purine analogs not specified; [b]fludarabine-refractory patients only; [c]MRD-negative CR vs. MRD-positive CR vs. PR vs. nonresponder; [d]includes CLL ($n = 23$) and PLL ($n = 1$) patients; [e]includes CLL ($n = 42$), PLL ($n = 21$), CTCL ($n = 6$), and others ($n = 9$); [f]CLL patients only.

Abbreviations: CR, complete response; F, fludarabine; F/U, follow-up; NR, not reported; OR, overall response; NPR, nodular partial response; PR, partial response; Cam, alemtuzumab; CTCL, cutaneous T-cell lymphoma; FCam, fludarabine and alemtuzumab; MRD, minimal residual disease; PLL, prolymphocytic leukemia; CLL, chronic lymphocytic leukemia; TFS, treatment-free survival.

Table 6   Results of Trials Using Alemtuzumab-Containing Regimens

	Patient characteristics						Response		
Investigator, yr (reference)	Median age (range, yr)	N (evaluable)	Rai/Binet stage (%)	Prior F (%)	Median F/U	Regimen	Response rate (%)	Disease control (median)	Overall survival (median)
Alemtuzumab induction									
Nabhan, 2004 (66)	69.5 (53–73)	12	II (25)	NR[a]	NR	RCam	OR 8	Response duration 2.5 mo	NR
Faderl, 2003 (67)	62 (44–79)[b]	48[b]	IV (75) III–IV (79)	54+ [b]	6.5 mo	RCam	PR 8 OR 63[c] CR 6; NPR 7; PR 50[c]	TTP 6 mo[b]	11 mo[b]
Faderl, 2005 (68)	57	28[d]	III–IV (50)[d]	30+	NR	RCam[e]	OR 55[d] CR 30; NPR 5; PR 20[d]	NR	NR
Kennedy, 2002 (63)	(39–78)[d] 52 (40–71)	(20) 6	B (50), C (50)	83	12 mo	FCam	OR 83	NR	NR
Elter, 2005 (64)	61 (38–80)	36	B (22), C (78)	61	15 mo	FCam	CR 16; PR 67 OR 83 CR 30; PR 53	TTP 13 mo	35.6 mo
Wierda, 2006 (65)	58 (39–79)	79 (74)	NR	67+	12 mo	CFAR	OR 65 CR 24; NPR 3; PR 38	TTP 26 mo	19 mo
Alemtuzumab consolidation									
O'Brien, 2003 (69,70)	60 (44–79)	58 (49)	NR	41+	24 mo	Response to chemotherapy (i.e., ≥PR) + Cam consolidation	OR 53; CR 47; NPR/CR 46	TTP not reached	NR

[a]purine analogs not specified; [b]includes CLL ($n = 32$), CLL/PLL ($n = 9$), PLL ($n = 1$), MCL ($n = 4$), and RS ($n = 2$) patients; [c]CLL patients only; [d]includes CLL ($n = 26$), CLL/SLL ($n = 1$), and marginal zone lymphoma ($n = 1$) patients; [e]continuous infusion followed by subcutaneous injection of alemtuzumab.

Abbreviations: CR, complete response; F, fludarabine; F/U, follow-up; NR, not reported; OR, overall response; NPR, nodular partial response; PR, partial response; Cam, alemtuzumab; PLL, prolymphocytic leukemia; CLL, chronic lymphocytic leukemia; CFAR, cyclophosphamide, fludarabine, alemtuzumab, and rituximab; FCam, fludarabine and alemtuzumab; MCL, mantle cell lymphoma; TTP, time to progression; SLL, small lymphocytic leukemia; RCam, rituximab and alemtuzumab; RS, Richter's syndrome.

In an attempt to improve upon results obtained with FCR in previously treated patients, alemtuzumab was added to the FCR regimen [cyclophosphamide, fludarabine, alemtuzumab, and rituximab (CFAR)] (Table 6) (65). Seventy-nine patients with relapsed/refractory CLL had been enrolled onto the study. Thirty-two (40%) patients were fludarabine refractory. Of 74 evaluable patients, the OR rate was 65% (CR 24%; NPR 3%; PR 38%). Of the 43 patients previously treated with FCR, 19% achieved a CR and 37% a PR; similarly, for the 10 patients previously treated with FC, 10% achieved a CR and 60% a PR. Among the fludarabine-refractory patients, the OR rate was 51% (CR 13%; PR 38%). Responses were also observed in patients with unfavorable cytogenetics [i.e., del(17p), del(11q), complex, and del(6q)] (CR14%; PR 50%), with 44% of patients with del(17p) responding. Eradication of MRD as evaluated by two-color flow cytometry occurred in 100% of patients in CR. Median follow-up time was 12 months. Estimated median TTP for all responders and OS for all patients were 26 and 19 months, respectively. Toxicities included grade 3 or 4 neutropenia and thrombocytopenia. CMV reactivation occurred in 12 patients.

Three studies have evaluated the efficacy and safety of alemtuzumab combined with rituximab in patients with relapsed or refractory CLL (OR 0–67%; CR 0–44%) (Table 6) (66–68). No responses were seen in the Nabhan et al. study; possibly because 6 of 12 patients received lower doses of alemtuzumab and only one course of therapy was administered (66). Responses may be higher in patients who are not fludarabine/purine analog refractory (67,68) and have less advanced disease (68). No study reported response duration or OS. In general, a higher frequency and severity of adverse events were seen with alemtuzumab than with rituximab. CMV reactivation occurred in up to 27% of patients.

Alemtuzumab consolidation therapy   Administration of alemtuzumab consolidation therapy to patients with CLL who have achieved a PR, NPR, or CR after chemotherapy can improve response rates (Table 6) (69,70). The OR rate was 53% with a response of 39% at the 10-mg tiw dose compared with 65% at the 30-mg tiw dose ($p = 0.066$). Forty-seven percent of patients in NPR achieved CR, and 46% in PR achieved NPR or CR. Residual bone marrow disease cleared in most patients with 11 of 29 patients (38%) achieving a molecular remission. Median TTP has not been reached in responders after a median follow-up of 24 months. Subgroup analysis indicated a longer TTP in patients with no detectable MRD (not reached vs. 15 months, respectively) after a median follow-up of 18 months. Toxicities included Grade 1 to 2 infusion-related events (common) and infections (mainly CMV reactivation). There was one death from pneumonia, and three patients developed Epstein-Barr virus (EBV)-positive large cell lymphoma (all resolved: two spontaneously and one after treatment with cidofovir and immunoglobulin).

Fludarabine-Refractory Patients

Up to 37% of previously untreated and 76% of previously treated CLL patients will not respond to single agent fludarabine (defined as either failure to achieve PR or CR to at least one fludarabine-containing regimen, or disease progression while on fludarabine treatment) (10,16–23,71,72), and an additional 7% to 14% of patients who were initially sensitive to fludarabine (i.e., CR or PR) will relapse within six months of therapy (10,17,22,23). Treatment of fludarabine-refractory patients has met with limited success. Furthermore, a significant proportion (40–89%) of these patients will develop serious infections (73,74). Historically, OR rates of 22% (CR 1%) with a median survival of 10 to 13 months have been obtained after first salvage therapy with a variety of agents, including single agent purine analogs, purine analogs combined with alkylators or other chemotherapeutic agents, and anthracycline-based regimens (Table 7) (73,74). This contrasts with results obtained in patients with fludarabine-sensitive disease, where ORs of 50% to 80% (CR 12–30%) and median survivals of 21 to 36 months can be achieved (24,27,52).

The mechanisms implicated in resistance to purine analogs include (*i*) a low intracellular deoxycytidine kinase (dCK) to 5′-nucleotidase (5′NT) ratio, leading to decreased phosphorylation of the purine analogs, (*ii*) mutations, deletions, and/or epigenetic silencing via promoter methylation of the tumor suppressor protein p53, which is required for apoptosis, and (*iii*) overexpression of the anti-apoptotic *bcl-2* family members, which can impair p53 activity (75).

Purine Analogs

Cladribine (2-CdA)   Although structurally similar, cladribine and fludarabine differ in their mechanism of inducing apoptosis and therefore, may not lead to the development of cross-resistance (50,51). Unfortunately, this has not translated into clinical benefit for fludarabine-refractory patients (52–54) (Table 7). In a very select group of fludarabine-refractory patients (i.e., intermediate stage, good baseline hematological parameters, ≤3 prior types of therapy, ≤6 cycles of fludarabine), a modest response may be seen (OR 32%; CR 0%) with an OS of 26 months with single agent cladribine (76). However, few patients will fulfill these characteristics, as demonstrated by an accrual time of four years for 28 patients.

Pentostatin   In a small series of patients, the combination of pentostatin and cyclophosphamide appears to improve OR rates (77%) with few CRs (8%) (Table 7) (42). However, the durability of these responses and effect on OS are unknown.

Rituximab

Rituximab induction therapy   Modest responses of short duration have been achieved with single agent rituximab (47,48). Higher response rates (OR 59%) can be obtained with FCR therapy; but, CRs are infrequent (5%), and the durability of responses are unknown (52). Responses have also been observed with combination DCF/CR therapy (54) and with rituximab plus CHOP (cyclophosphamide, hydroxydoxorubicin (doxorubicin hydrochloride), oncovin (vincristine) and prednisone) chemotherapy (77).

Alemtuzumab

Alemtuzumab induction therapy   Alemtuzumab is currently the only approved drug for the treatment of patients with fludarabine-refractory CLL (Table 5) (57–60). Single agent alemtuzumab can induce OR rates of 31% to 46% (CR 0–29%) in this group of patients (56,57,59,61,78,79), with a proportion of complete responders having no detectable marrow disease by immunophenotyping (61). Higher responses were seen in patients with ≤3 prior types of therapy (61) and no significant adenopathy (none or <2 cm in diameter) (57,61). Response duration ranged from 8.7 to 15.4 months (57,59,79) with reported median OS for all patients being 16 to 27.5 months (57,59).

The combination of alemtuzumab and fludarabine (FCam) may yield higher responses, even in patients refractory to single agent alemtuzumab and single agent fludarabine (Table 8) (63). Of the six patients treated with FCam, the OR was 83% (CR 16%; PR 67%), with two of five patients having no detectable marrow disease on immunophenotyping. Two patients underwent stem cell harvesting followed by autologous

Table 7 Results of Trials in Fludarabine-Refractory Patients with Purine Analogs

Investigator, yr (reference)	Patient characteristics						Response		
	Median age (range, yr)	N (evaluable)	Rai/Binet stage (%)	F refractory (%)	Median F/U	Chemotherapy regimen	Response rate (%)	Disease control (median)	Overall survival (median)
Fludarabine-containing regimens									
Tsimberidou, 2004 (27)	59 (21–78)[b]	12[a]	III–IV (41)[b]	100[a]	8 yr	FM	OR 25[a] CR 0; NPR 0; PR 25[a]	TTP 5 mo[a]	9 mo[a]
O'Brien, 2001 (24)	58 (29–92)[c]	28[a]	0–II (53), III–IV (47)[c]	100[a]	41 mo	FC	OR 39[a] CR 3; NPR 13; PR 26[a]	NR	12 mo[a]
Wierda, 2005 (52)	59 (36–81)[d]	33[a]	I–II (47) III–IV (50)	100[a]	28 mo	FCR	OR 58[a] CR 6; NPR 9; PR 42[a]	TTP 28 mo[d]	42 mo[d]
Non-fludarabine purine analog–containing regimens									
O'Brien, 1994 (88)	63 (43–80)	28	III–IV (82)	100	NR	2-CdA	OR 7 CR 0; PR 7	Response duration 4 mo and 14 mo for PRs	mo
Byrd, 2003 (76)	62 (30–87)	28	I–II (46),	100	NR	2-CdA	OR 32; CR 0; PR 32	Response duration 12 mo; PFS 9 mo	26 mo
Weiss, 2003 (42)	64 (32–79)[e]	13[a]	III–IV (54) I–II (29), III–IV (71)[e]	100[a]	NR	DCF/C	OR 77[a]; CR 8; NPR+ PR 69[a]	NR	NR

[a]fludarabine-refractory patients only; [b]includes untreated ($n = 34$) and previously treated ($n = 53$) patients of which 15 were refractory to alkylating agents, 26 were fludarabine sensitive but relapsed, and 12 fludarabine refractory; [c]includes untreated ($n = 34$) and previously treated ($n = 94$) patients of which 28 were fludarabine refractory; [d]includes fludarabine refractory ($n = 37$) and fludarabine sensitive ($n = 108$) patients and others ($n = 32$); [e]includes CLL ($n = 42$), PLL ($n = 21$), CTCL ($n = 6$), and others ($n = 9$).

Abbreviations: CR, complete response; F, fludarabine; F/U, follow-up; NR, not reported; OR, overall response; NPR, nodular partial response; PR, partial response; TTP, time to progression; 2-CdA, cladribine; DCF/C, pentostatin and cyclophosphamide; PFS, progression-free survival; FC, fludarabine and cyclophosphamide; FM, fludarabine and mitoxantrone; FCR, fludarabine, cyclophosphamide, and rituximab.

Table 8   Results of Trials in Fludarabine-Refractory Patients with Chemo- or Immunotherapy

| | Patient characteristics | | | | | | Response | | |
Investigator, yr (reference)	Median age (range, yr)	N (evaluable)	Rai/Binet stage (%)	F refractory (%)	Median F/U	Chemotherapy regimen	Response rate (%)	Disease control (median)	Overall survival (median)
Kennedy, 2002 (63)	52 (40–71)	6	B (50), C (50)	83	NR	FCam	OR 83	NR	NR
Elter, 2005 (64)	61 (38–80)	36	B (22), C (78)	25	15 mo	FCam	CR 16; PR67 OR 67[a]	TTP 13 mo	35.6 mo
Sayala, 2006 (80)	64 (41–79)	53 (49)	NR	100	NR	Cam then FCam[b] if PD or nonresponder	OR 49 CR16; PR 33	NR	25 mo vs. 13 mo[c]
Nabhan, 2004 (66)	69.5 (53–73)	12	II (25) IV (75)	NR[d]	NR	RCam	OR 8 PR 8	Response duration 2.5 mo	NR
Faderl, 2003 (67)	62 (44–79)[e]	48[e]	III–IV (79)[e]	54[e]	6.5 mo[e]	RCam	OR 63[f] CR 6; NPR 7; PR 50[f]	NR	NR
Faderl, 2005 (68)	57 (39–78)[g]	28[g] (20)	III–IV (50)[g]	30+	NR	RCam[h]	OR 55[g] CR 30; NPR 5; PR 20[g]	NR	NR
Wierda, 2006 (65)	58 (39–79)	79 (74)	NR	40	12	CFAR	OR 51[a] CR 13; PR 38[a]	TTP 26 mo	19 mo

[a]fludarabine-refractory patients only; [b]oral fludarabine and subcutaneous alemtuzemab; [c]responders vs. nonrepsonders; [d]all had failed purine analogs (fludarabine in 11 and cladribine in 1); [e]includes CLL ($n = 32$), CLL/PLL ($n = 9$), PLL ($n = 1$), MCL ($n = 4$), and RS ($n = 2$) patients; [f]CLL patients only; [g]includes CLL ($n = 26$), CLL/SLL ($n = 1$), and marginal zone lymphoma ($n = 1$) patients; [h]continuous infusion followed by subcutaneous injection of alemtuzumab.

Abbreviations: CR, complete response; F, fludarabine; F/U, follow-up; NR, not reported; OR, overall response; NPR, nodular partial response; PR, partial response; Cam, alemtuzumab; CFAR, cyclophosphamide, fludarabine, alemtuzumab, and rituximab; FCam, fludarabine and alemtuzumab; RCam, rituximab and alemtuzumab; TTP, time to progression; PD, progressive disease.

stem cell transplantation. Toxicity was acceptable with one patient requiring hospitalization for pneumonia during neutropenia, and two patients required G-CSF for neutropenia. There were no cases of CMV reactivation. Nine other patients with fludarabine-refractory CLL have been treated with FCam, six of whom achieved a response (64). A phase II study conducted by the United Kingdom National Cancer Research Institute (NCRI) involving 50 patients with fludarabine-refractory CLL confirmed that OR rates of 45% (CR 16%; PR 29%) can be achieved with single agent alemtuzumab; however, only 2 of 11 (18%) patients who were refractory to both fludarabine and single agent alemtuzumab achieved a PR with oral fludarabine and subcutaneous alemtuzumab combination therapy (Table 8) (80). At this time, it is unclear whether the addition of rituximab to alemtuzumab will yield better results (Table 8) (66,67).

The combination of CFAR has activity in patients with fludarabine-refractory CLL (OR 51%; CR 13%; PR 38%) (Table 8) (65). Responses were observed in patients who had previously been treated with FCR and FC combination chemotherapy.

Patients who are both fludarabine and alemtuzumab refractory (defined as failure to achieve a response following at least eight weeks of single agent alemtuzumab or an alemtuzumab-based regimen or disease progression within three months of completing therapy) have a poor outcome. Salvage therapy with a variety of agents can induce OR rates of only 20% (CR 0%) with a median survival of eight months (81). Major infections occurred in 60% of patients during first salvage therapy.

Bcl-2 Family–Targeted Therapies

Oblimersen sodium   One of the mechanisms implicated in resistance to purine analogs is overexpression of the anti-apoptotic *bcl-2* family members, which can impair p53 activity (75). Therefore, in an attempt to reduce *bcl-2* levels and render cells more susceptible to apoptosis-inducing agents, a randomized phase III trial evaluating FC with or without oblimersen sodium in 241 patients with relapsed or refractory CLL has been conducted (82). Oblimersen sodium is a first-generation phosphorothioate antisense oligodeoxynucleotide of 18 nucleotides in length that is directed against the first six codons of the open reading frame of the *bcl-2* mRNA.

Patients were stratified on the basis of number of prior treatment regimens, fludarabine refractoriness, and response duration to last therapy. All patients received FC chemotherapy for three days. Patients randomized to receive oblimersen received 3 mg/kg/day for seven days by intravenous infusion, beginning four days prior to and during FC therapy ($n = 120$). The cycle was repeated every 28 days until achievement of CR or a maximum of six cycles. Approximately half of the patients in both groups had failed ≥ 3 prior treatment regimens; all patients had received prior fludarabine. All patients have completed at least two years of follow-up. More nausea, fever, fatigue, and intravenous catheter complications occurred in the oblimersen sodium and FC arm. Grade 4 thrombocytopenia, neutropenic fever, and hypotension were more common in the oblimersen and FC arm. Anemia and leukopenia were more common in the FC arm, with more patients receiving filgrastim and erythropoietin; whereas more patients in the oblimersen and FC arm received platelet transfusions and had a greater incidence of bleeding events (19% vs. 8%). The incidence of opportunistic infections and second malignancies was similar in the two groups. Serious adverse events resulted in discontinuation of therapy in 36% and 35% of patients in oblimersen sodium and FC and FC-only arms, respectively.

The overall response rate (ORR) (i.e., CR, NPR, and PR) was similar for both groups ($p = $ NS). However, a higher proportion of patients who were treated with

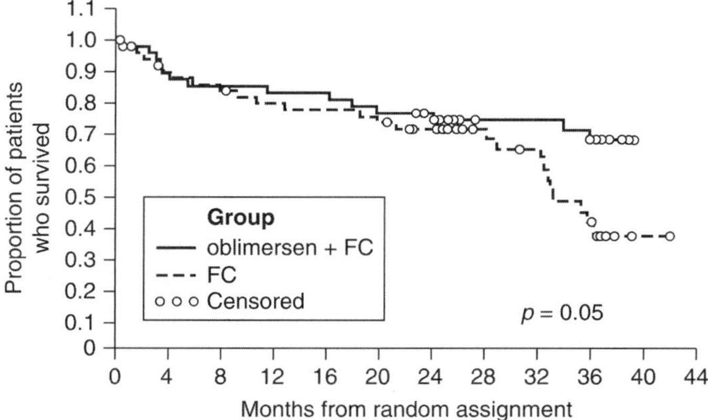

Figure 3   Kaplan-Meier survival curves for fludarabine-sensitive patients by treatment group. Median overall survival not reached for the oblimersen sodium and FC arm versus 33.2 months for the FC-only arm (hazard ratio = 0.53, p = 0.05). *Abbreviation*: FC, fludarabine and cyclophosphamide. *Source*: From Ref. 82 (*See Color Insert*).

oblimersen sodium and FC achieved a major response (i.e., CR or NPR) [17% (CR 9%; NPR 8%) vs. 7% (CR 3%; NPR 4%), respectively; $p = 0.025$]. For responders (i.e., CR or NPR), the median response duration was significantly shorter in the FC-only arm compared with the oblimersen sodium and FC arm (20 months vs. not reached, respectively; $p = 0.002$). Five of the 20 major responders (25%) in the oblimersen sodium and FC arm have relapsed compared with 6 of 8 (75%) in the FC arm. The median TTP was similar for both arms. However, the TTP correlated with response; in patients achieving a CR or NPR, TTP was ≥ 2 years in 70% of patients in the oblimersen sodium and FC arm compared with 50% in the FC-only arm ($p < 0.001$). The estimated median OS was similar for both arms (33.8 months for oblimersen sodium and FC arm vs. 32.9 months for FC arm; $p = $ NS). As observed for TTP, in patients achieving a CR or NPR, survival was ≥ 3 years in 70% of patients in the oblimersen sodium and FC arm compared with 38% in the FC-only arm ($p < 0.001$). Furthermore, among fludarabine-sensitive patients, the addition of oblimersen sodium to FC chemotherapy resulted in a significant survival benefit ($p = 0.05$) (Fig. 3).

These response rates are lower than what has been reported with FC chemotherapy (ORR 80–100%; CR 21–60%) (83); this may be attributable to a combination of factors including use of CT scans to document CR, independent review of bone marrow pathology, and a high proportion of fludarabine-refractory patients. On the basis of the above results, discussions are under way with the food and drug administration (FDA) concerning approval for a new drug application of oblimersen sodium in patients with relapsed or refractory CLL.

SUMMARY

Despite the advances made in the understanding and treatment of CLL, the majority of patients will relapse after initial therapy. There is a paucity of data to guide choice of appropriate salvage therapy in patients with relapsed or refractory CLL. This is in part due to (i) the lack of randomized trials in patients who have been previously exposed to purine analog–based regimens (10,11), (ii) incomplete data in the currently reported phase II studies with respect to prior sensitivity or resistance to purine analog– and/or monoclonal antibody–based treatment regimens, and, (iii) usually, inclusion of both purine analog–sensitive and analog-resistant patients and/or alkylator-sensitive and alkylator-resistant patients in the same clinical trial.

Furthermore, prior to the development of the revised IWCLL-NCI-sponsored working group guidelines, there was no widely accepted definition for relapsed and refractory CLLs. This lack of a standardized definition for relapse or refractory disease has impeded comparability between studies and the evaluation of the clinical significance of new therapeutic agents. In the revised guidelines, relapse is defined as disease progression after 12 or more months in a patient who had previously achieved a CR or PR (5), whereas refractory disease is defined as failure to respond to a purine analog–based treatment regimen or stem cell transplantation, or disease progression within 12 months of such a therapy (5).

Although allogeneic myeloablative and nonmyeloablative stem cell transplantation have not been discussed in this section, they may be reasonable and feasible options in the setting of patients with relapsed and/or refractory CLL. However, responses and remission durations are not satisfactory with the currently available salvage therapies. Novel agents need to be evaluated, and newer treatment strategies need to be developed to circumvent or overcome resistance, optimize responses, and potentially cure CLL. In the absence of data to guide salvage therapy in these patients, enrollment onto a clinical trial should be considered.

REFERENCES

1. Diehl LF, Karnell LH, Menck HR. The American College of Surgeons Commission on Cancer and the American Cancer Society. The National Cancer Data Base report on age, gender, treatment, and outcomes of patients with chronic lymphocytic leukemia. Cancer 1999; 86:2684–2692.
2. Group USCSW. United States Cancer Statistics: 2000 Incidence. Atlanta: Department of Health and Human Services, Centers for Disease Control and Prevention and National Cancer Institute, 2003.
3. Jaffe ES, Harris N, Stein H, et al. Pathology and Genetics of Tumours of Haematopoietic and Lymphoid Tissues. Lyon, France: IARC Press, 2001.
4. Jemal A, Clegg LX, Ward E, et al. Annual report to the nation on the status of cancer, 1975-2001, with a special feature regarding survival. Cancer 2004; 101:3–27.
5. Eichhorst B, Hallek M. Revision of the guidelines for diagnosis and therapy of chronic lymphocytic leukemia (CLL). Best Pract Res Clin Haematol 2007; 20:469–477.
6. Cheson BD, Bennett JM, Grever M, et al. National Cancer Institute-sponsored Working Group guidelines for chronic lymphocytic leukemia: revised guidelines for diagnosis and treatment. Blood 1996; 87:4990–4997.
7. Bottcher S, Ritgen M, Pott C, et al. Comparative analysis of minimal residual disease detection using four-color flow cytometry, consensus IgH-PCR, and quantitative IgH PCR in CLL after allogeneic and autologous stem cell transplantation. Leukemia 2004; 18:1637–1645.
8. Moreno C, Villamor N, Colomer D, et al. Clinical significance of minimal residual disease, as assessed by different techniques, after stem cell transplantation for chronic lymphocytic leukemia. Blood 2006; 107:4563–4569.
9. Kay NE, O'Brien SM, Pettitt AR, et al. The role of prognostic factors in assessing 'high-risk' subgroups of patients with chronic lymphocytic leukemia. Leukemia 2007; 21:1885–1891.
10. Johnson S, Smith AG, Loffler H, et al. Multicentre prospective randomised trial of fludarabine versus cyclophosphamide, doxorubicin, and prednisone (CAP) for treatment of advanced-stage chronic lymphocytic leukaemia. The French Cooperative Group on CLL. Lancet 1996; 347:1432–1438.

11. Rummel MJ, Stilgenbauer S, Gamm H, et al. Fludarabine versus fludarabine plus epirubicin in the treatment of chronic lymphocytic leukemia - final results of a German randomized phase III study. Blood 2005; 106: 600a.

12. Sawitsky A, Rai KR, Glidewell O, et al. Comparison of daily versus intermittent chlorambucil and prednisone therapy in the treatment of patients with chronic lymphocytic leukemia. Blood 1977; 50:1049–1059.

13. Montserrat E, Alcala A, Alonso C, et al. A randomized trial comparing chlorambucil plus prednisone vs cyclophosphamide, melphalan, and prednisone in the treatment of chronic lymphocytic leukemia stages B and C. Nouv Rev Fr Hematol 1988; 30:429–432.

14. Itala M, Remes K. The COP regimen is not a feasible treatment for advanced, refractory chronic lymphocytic leukemia. Leuk Lymphoma 1996; 23:137–141.

15. Liepman M, Votaw ML. The treatment of chronic lymphocytic leukemia with COP chemotherapy. Cancer 1978; 41:1664–1669.

16. Keating MJ, O'Brien S, Lerner S, et al. Long-term follow-up of patients with chronic lymphocytic leukemia (CLL) receiving fludarabine regimens as initial therapy. Blood 1998; 92:1165–1171.

17. Rai KR, Peterson BL, Appelbaum FR, et al. Fludarabine compared with chlorambucil as primary therapy for chronic lymphocytic leukemia. N Engl J Med 2000; 343:1750–1757.

18. Grever MR, Kopecky KJ, Coltman CA, et al. Fludarabine monophosphate: a potentially useful agent in chronic lymphocytic leukemia. Nouv Rev Fr Hematol 1988; 30:457–459.

19. Puccio CA, Mittelman A, Lichtman SM, et al. A loading dose/continuous infusion schedule of fludarabine phosphate in chronic lymphocytic leukemia. J Clin Oncol 1991; 9:1562–1569.

20. Keating MJ, O'Brien S, Kantarjian H, et al. Long-term follow-up of patients with chronic lymphocytic leukemia treated with fludarabine as a single agent. Blood 1993; 81:2878–2884.

21. Kemena A, O'Brien S, Kantarjian H, et al. Phase II clinical trial of fludarabine in chronic lymphocytic leukemia on a weekly low-dose schedule. Leuk Lymphoma 1993; 10:187–193.

22. Sorensen JM, Vena DA, Fallavollita A, et al. Treatment of refractory chronic lymphocytic leukemia with fludarabine phosphate via the group C protocol mechanism of the National Cancer Institute: five-year follow-up report. J Clin Oncol 1997; 15:458–465.

23. Zinzani PL, Bendandi M, Magagnoli M, et al. Long-term follow-up after fludarabine treatment in pretreated patients with chronic lymphocytic leukemia. Haematologica 2000; 85:1135–1139.

24. O'Brien SM, Kantarjian HM, Cortes J, et al. Results of the fludarabine and cyclophosphamide combination regimen in chronic lymphocytic leukemia. J Clin Oncol 2001; 19:1414–1420.

25. Hallek M, Schmitt B, Wilhelm M, et al. Fludarabine plus cyclophosphamide is an efficient treatment for advanced chronic lymphocytic leukaemia (CLL): results of a phase II study of the German CLL Study Group. Br J Haematol 2001; 114:342–348.

26. Gonzalez H, Maloum K, Tezenas du Montcel S, et al. Fludarabine + cyclophosphamide in chronic lymphoproliferative disorders. Blood 2003; 102: 357b.

27. Tsimberidou AM, Keating MJ, Giles FJ, et al. Fludarabine and mitoxantrone for patients with chronic lymphocytic leukemia. Cancer 2004; 100:2583–2591.

28. Robertson LE, O'Brien S, Kantarjian H, et al. Fludarabine plus doxorubicin in previously treated chronic lymphocytic leukemia. Leukemia 1995; 9:943–945.

29. Bosch F, Ferrer A, Lopez-Guillermo A, et al. Fludarabine, cyclophosphamide and mitoxantrone in the treatment of resistant or relapsed chronic lymphocytic leukaemia. Br J Haematol 2002; 119:976–984.

30. Mauro FR, Foa R, Meloni G, et al. Fludarabine, ara-C, novantrone and dexamethasone (FAND) in previously treated chronic lymphocytic leukemia patients. Haematologica 2002; 87:926–933.

31. Robak T, Blonski JZ, Kasznicki M, et al. Cladribine with or without prednisone in the treatment of previously treated and untreated B-cell chronic lymphocytic leukaemia—updated results of the multicentre study of 378 patients. Br J Haematol 2000; 108:357–368.

32. Tallman MS, Hakimian D, Zanzig C, et al. Cladribine in the treatment of relapsed or refractory chronic lymphocytic leukemia. J Clin Oncol 1995; 13:983–988.

33. Juliusson G, Liliemark J. Long-term survival following cladribine (2-chlorodeoxyadenosine) therapy in previously treated patients with chronic lymphocytic leukemia. Ann Oncol 1996; 7:373–379.

34. Rondelli D, Lauria F, Zinzani PL, et al. 2-Chlorodeoxyadenosine in the treatment of relapsed/ refractory chronic lymphoproliferative disorders. Eur J Haematol 1997; 58:46–50.

35. Betticher DC, Ratschiller D, Hsu Schmitz SF, et al. Reduced dose of subcutaneous cladribine induces identical response rates but decreased toxicity in pretreated chronic lymphocytic leukaemia. Swiss Group for Clinical Cancer Research (SAKK). Ann Oncol 1998; 9:721–726.

36. Van Den Neste E, Louviaux I, Michaux JL, et al. Phase I/II study of 2-chloro-2′-deoxyadenosine with cyclophosphamide in patients with pretreated B cell chronic lymphocytic leukemia and indolent non-Hodgkin's lymphoma. Leukemia 2000; 14:1136–1142.

37. Robak T, Gora-Tybor J, Lech-Maranda E, et al. Cladribine in combination with mitoxantrone and cyclophosphamide(CMC) in the treatment of heavily pre-treated patients with advanced indolent lymphoid malignancies. Eur J Haematol 2001; 66:188–194.

38. Montillo M, Tedeschi A, O'Brien S, et al. Phase II study of cladribine and cyclophosphamide in patients with chronic lymphocytic leukemia and prolymphocytic leukemia. Cancer 2003; 97:114–120.

39. Dillman RO, Mick R, McIntyre OR. Pentostatin in chronic lymphocytic leukemia: a phase II trial of Cancer and Leukemia group B. J Clin Oncol 1989; 7:433–438.

40. Ho AD, Thaler J, Stryckmans P, et al. Pentostatin in refractory chronic lymphocytic leukemia: a phase II trial of the European Organization for Research and Treatment of Cancer. J Natl Cancer Inst 1990; 82:1416–1420.

41. Johnson SA, Catovsky D, Child JA, et al. Phase I/II evaluation of pentostatin (2′-deoxycoformycin) in a five day schedule for the treatment of relapsed/refractory B-cell chronic lymphocytic leukaemia. Invest New Drugs 1998; 16:155–160.

42. Weiss MA, Maslak PG, Jurcic JG, et al. Pentostatin and cyclophosphamide: an effective new regimen in previously treated patients with chronic lymphocytic leukemia. J Clin Oncol 2003; 21:1278–1284.

43. McLaughlin P, Grillo-Lopez AJ, Link BK, et al. Rituximab chimeric anti-CD20 monoclonal antibody therapy for relapsed indolent lymphoma: half of patients respond to a four-dose treatment program. J Clin Oncol 1998; 16:2825–2833.

44. Foran JM, Rohatiner AZ, Cunningham D, et al. European phase II study of rituximab (chimeric anti-CD20 monoclonal antibody) for patients with newly diagnosed mantle-cell lymphoma and previously treated mantle-cell lymphoma, immunocytoma, and small B-cell lymphocytic lymphoma. J Clin Oncol 2000; 18:317–324.

45. Huhn D, von Schilling C, Wilhelm M, et al. Rituximab therapy of patients with B-cell chronic lymphocytic leukemia. Blood 2001; 98:1326–1331.

46. Itala M, Geisler CH, Kimby E, et al. Standard-dose anti-CD20 antibody rituximab has efficacy in chronic lymphocytic leukaemia: results from a Nordic multicentre study. Eur J Haematol 2002; 69:129–134.

47. Byrd JC, Murphy T, Howard RS, et al. Rituximab using a thrice weekly dosing schedule in B-cell chronic lymphocytic leukemia and small lymphocytic lymphoma demonstrates clinical activity and acceptable toxicity. J Clin Oncol 2001; 19:2153–2164.

48. O'Brien SM, Kantarjian H, Thomas DA, et al. Rituximab dose-escalation trial in chronic lymphocytic leukemia. J Clin Oncol 2001; 19:2165–2170.

49. Schulz H, Klein SK, Rehwald U, et al. Phase 2 study of a combined immunochemotherapy using rituximab and fludarabine in patients with chronic lymphocytic leukemia. Blood 2002; 100:3115–3120.

50. Robak T, Smolewski P, Cebula B, et al. Rituximab plus cladribine with or without cyclophosphamide in patients with relapsed or refractory chronic lymphocytic leukemia. Eur J Haematol 2007; 79:107–113.

51. Drapkin R, Di Bella NJ, Cuasay LC, et al. Phase II multicenter trial of pentostatin and rituximab in patients with previously treated or untreated chronic lymphocytic leukemia. Blood 2002; 100:803a.

52. Wierda W, O'Brien S, Wen S, et al. Chemoimmunotherapy with fludarabine, cyclophosphamide, and rituximab for relapsed and refractory chronic lymphocytic leukemia. J Clin Oncol 2005; 23:4070–4078.

53. Wierda W, O'Brien S, Faderl S, et al. A retrospective comparison of three sequential groups of patients with Recurrent/Refractory chronic lymphocytic leukemia treated with fludarabine-based regimens. Cancer 2006; 106:337–345.

54. Lamanna N, Kalaycio M, Maslak P, et al. Pentostatin, cyclophosphamide, and rituximab is an active, well-tolerated regimen for patients with previously treated chronic lymphocytic leukemia. J Clin Oncol 2006; 24:1575–1581.

55. Ciolli S, Gigli F, Mannelli F, et al. High response rates and reduced first-dose reactions with subcutaneous alemtuzumab in patients with relapsed and refractory CLL. Blood 2003; 102:357b.

56. Ferrajoli A, O'Brien SM, Cortes JE, et al. Phase II study of alemtuzumab in chronic lymphoproliferative disorders. Cancer 2003; 98:773–778.

57. Keating MJ, Flinn I, Jain V, et al. Therapeutic role of alemtuzumab (Campath-1H) in patients who have failed fludarabine: results of a large international study. Blood 2002; 99:3554–3561.

58. Rai KR, Coutre S, Rizzieri D, et al. Efficacy and safety of alemtuzumab (Campath-1H) in refractory B-CLL patients treated on a compassionate basis. Blood 2001; 98:365a.

59. Rai KR, Freter CE, Mercier RJ, et al. Alemtuzumab in previously treated chronic lymphocytic leukemia patients who also had received fludarabine. J Clin Oncol 2002; 20:3891–3897.

60. Rai KR, Keating MJ, Coutre S, et al. Patients with refractory B-CLL and T-PLL treated with alemtuzumab (Campath^{O}) on a compassionate basis. A report on efficacy and safety of CAM 511 trial. Blood 2002; 100:802a.

61. Moreton P, Kennedy B, Lucas G, et al. Eradication of minimal residual disease in B-cell chronic lymphocytic leukemia after alemtuzumab therapy is associated with prolonged survival. J Clin Oncol 2005; 23:2971–2979.

62. Anderson JR, Neuberg DS. Analysis of outcome by response flawed. J Clin Oncol 2005; 23: 8122–8123 (author reply 8123–8124).

63. Kennedy B, Rawstron A, Carter C, et al. Campath-1H and fludarabine in combination are highly active in refractory chronic lymphocytic leukemia. Blood 2002; 99:2245–2247.

64. Elter T, Borchmann P, Schulz H, et al. Fludarabine in combination with alemtuzumab is effective and feasible in patients with relapsed or refractory B-cell chronic lymphocytic leukemia: results of a phase II trial. J Clin Oncol 2005; 23:7024–7031.

65. Wierda WG, O'Brien S, Faderl S, et al. Combined cyclophosphamide, fludarabine, alemtuzumab, and rituximab (CFAR), an active regimen for heavily treated patients with CLL. Blood 2006; 108:14a.

66. Nabhan C, Patton D, Gordon LI, et al. A pilot trial of rituximab and alemtuzumab combination therapy in patients with relapsed and/or refractory chronic lymphocytic leukemia (CLL). Leuk Lymphoma 2004; 45:2269–2273.

67. Faderl S, Thomas DA, O'Brien S, et al. Experience with alemtuzumab plus rituximab in patients with relapsed and refractory lymphoid malignancies. Blood 2003; 101:3413–3415.

68. Faderl S, Ferrajoli A, Wierda W, et al. Continuous infusion/subcutaneous alemtuzumab (Campath-1H) plus rituximab is active for patients with relapsed/refractory chronic lymphocytic leukemia (CLL). Blood 2005; 106:831a.

69. O'Brien SM, Kantarjian HM, Thomas DA, et al. Alemtuzumab as treatment for residual disease after chemotherapy in patients with chronic lymphocytic leukemia. Cancer 2003; 98:2657–2663.

70. O'Brien SM, Gribben JG, Thomas DA, et al. Alemtuzumab for minimal residual disease in CLL. Blood 2003; 102:109a.

71. Leporrier M, Chevret S, Cazin B, et al. Randomized comparison of fludarabine, CAP, and ChOP in 938 previously untreated stage B and C chronic lymphocytic leukemia patients. Blood 2001; 98:2319–2325.

72. Eichhorst BF, Busch R, Stauch M, et al. Fludarabine (F) induces higher response rates in first line therapy of older patients (pts) with advanced chronic lymphocytic leukemia (CLL) than chlorambucil: interim analysis of a phase III study of the German CLL Study Group (GCLLSG). Blood 2003; 102:109a.

73. Keating MJ, O'Brien S, Kontoyiannis D, et al. Results of first salvage therapy for patients refractory to a fludarabine regimen in chronic lymphocytic leukemia. Leuk Lymphoma 2002; 43:1755–1762.

74. Perkins JG, Flynn JM, Howard RS, et al. Frequency and type of serious infections in fludarabine-refractory B-cell chronic lymphocytic leukemia and small lymphocytic lymphoma: implications for clinical trials in this patient population. Cancer 2002; 94:2033–2039.
75. Pettitt AR. Mechanism of action of purine analogues in chronic lymphocytic leukaemia. Br J Haematol 2003; 121:692–702.
76. Byrd JC, Peterson B, Piro L, et al. A phase II study of cladribine treatment for fludarabine refractory B cell chronic lymphocytic leukemia: results from CALGB Study 9211. Leukemia 2003; 17:323–327.
77. Eichhorst BF, Busch R, Duehrsen U, et al. CHOP plus rituximab (CHOP-R) in fludarabine (F) refractory chronic lymphocytic leukemia (CLL) or CLL with autoimmune hemolytic anemia (AIHA) or Richter's transformation (RT): first interim analysis of a phase II trial of the German CLL Study Group (GCLLSG). Blood 2005; 106:601a.
78. Stilgenbauer S, Winkler D, Krober A, et al. Subcutaneous Campath-1H (alemtuzumab) in fludarabine-refractory CLL: interim analysis of the CLL2h study of the German CLL Study Group (GCLLSG). Blood 2004; 104:140a.
79. Lozanski G, Heerema NA, Flinn IW, et al. Alemtuzumab is an effective therapy for chronic lymphocytic leukemia with p53 mutations and deletions. Blood 2004; 103:3278–3281.
80. Sayala HA, Moreton P, Jones RA, et al. Final report of the UKCLL02 trial: a phase II study of subcutaneous alemtuzumab plus fludarabine in patients with fludarabine refractory CLL (on behalf of the NCRI CLL Trials Sub-Group). Blood 2006; 108:14a–15a.
81. Tam CS, O'Brien S, Lerner S, et al. The natural history of fludarabine-refractory chronic lymphocytic leukemia patients who fail alemtuzumab or have bulky lymphadenopathy. Leuk Lymphoma 2007; 48:1931–1939.
82. O'Brien S, Moore JO, Boyd TE, et al. Randomized phase III trial of fludarabine plus cyclophosphamide with or without oblimersen sodium (Bcl-2 antisense) in patients with relapsed or refractory chronic lymphocytic leukemia. J Clin Oncol 2007; 25:1114–1120.
83. Yee KW, O'Brien SM, Giles FJ. An update on the management of chronic lymphocytic leukaemia. Expert Opin Pharmacother 2004; 5:1535–1554.
84. Marotta G, Bigazzi C, Lenoci M, et al. Low-dose fludarabine and cyclophosphamide in elderly patients with B-cell chronic lymphocytic leukemia refractory to conventional therapy. Haematologica 2000; 85:1268–1270.
85. Schiavone EM, De Simone M, Palmieri S, et al. Fludarabine plus cyclophosphamide for the treatment of advanced chronic lymphocytic leukemia. Eur J Haematol 2003; 71:23–28.
86. Rummel MJ, Kafer G, Pfreundschuh M, et al. Fludarabine and epirubicin in the treatment of chronic lymphocytic leukaemia: a German multicenter phase II study. Ann Oncol 1999; 10:183–188.
87. Schmitt B, Franke A, Burkhard O, et al. Fludarabine, mitoxantrone and cyclophosphamide combination therapy in relapsed chronic lymphocytic leukemia (CLL) with or without G-CSF: results of the first interim ana[n]lysis of a phase III study of the German CLL Study Group (GCLLSG). Blood 2002; 100:364b.
88. O'Brien S, Kantarjian H, Estey E, et al. Lack of effect of 2-chlorodeoxyadenosine therapy in patients with chronic lymphocytic leukemia refractory to fludarabine therapy. N Engl J Med 1994; 330:319–322.

10

New Therapies in Chronic Lymphocytic Leukemia

John C. Byrd, Farrukh Awan, Thomas S. Lin, and Michael R. Grever
Division of Hematology and Oncology, Department of Internal Medicine and Division of Medicinal Chemistry and Pharmacognosy, College of Pharmacy, The Ohio State University, Columbus, Ohio, U.S.A.

INTRODUCTION

As outlined in previous chapters in this book, significant progress has been made in the predictive biomarkers for early disease progression and poor response to initial therapy in chronic lymphocytic leukemia (CLL). The applicability of many of these biomarkers to CLL relapsing from initial therapy is less well defined. More important to the outcome of patients relapsing after initial therapy is the duration of the initial remission and, potentially, the initial treatment utilized. Patients relapsing within six months of completing initial therapy have an extremely poor prognosis as compared with those with extended remissions following fludarabine-based therapy (1,2). Similarly, patients relapsing after combination chemoimmunotherapy have less therapeutic options available to them and, in general, have a lower response to subsequent therapy. In one study, complex karyotype also predicted poor outcome of therapy, but to date, there have been no large definitive studies demonstrating that del(17p13.1) or del(11q22.3) contributes to poor outcome in the relapse setting (3). This is likely reflective of the poor outcome of the majority of patients relapsing after initial treatment of symptomatic CLL.

The approach to reinitiating therapy for CLL patients who relapsed after initial therapy is similar to that practiced prior to the first treatment. There is no evidence that early treatment at first evidence of relapse improves outcome as compared with delaying therapy until symptoms develop. Patients therefore need not receive therapy at the first sign of relapse. Rather, patients should have an indication for treatment, as discussed above. Patients should have repeat interphase cytogenetic analysis of the peripheral blood or bone marrow aspirate, as they may acquire additional cytogenetic abnormalities as their CLL becomes more advanced, most notably del(17p13.1). The incidence of del(17p13.1) or p53 mutations increases from 5% of patients at initial diagnosis (4) to nearly half of heavily treated patients with advanced CLL, and acquisition of this abnormality has profound implications for treatment, as will be discussed below (5). IgV$_H$ mutational analysis does not need to be performed if such information has been obtained previously, as a patient's IgV_H mutational status does not change with time. A bone marrow should be performed if cytopenias are present, to confirm that CLL is the cause and to exclude other potential causes of cytopenias such as transformed lymphoma, prolonged marrow toxicity from prior therapy, or development of treatment-related myelodysplasia (MDS). Patients should be treated according to the indications put forth by the 2008 National Cancer Institute (NCI) Treatment Guidelines for CLL (6). In general, for patients under the age of 70 who have experienced a good remission with initial therapy (>12 months), an FCR regimen, preferably in combination with an investigational agent, is chosen (3). For patients relapsing who are 70 years or greater, re-treatment with the same therapy or an alternative antibody or investigational agent can be considered. Fludarabine, cyclophosphamide, and rituximab (FCR) is not routinely administered to this patient population because of concerns of increasing toxicity. This review will focus predominately on therapeutic agents that are in late phase II/III clinical trials for CLL. A brief discussion of select agents in late preclinical or early phase I clinical development will follow.

INVESTIGATIONAL AGENTS CURRENTLY IN PHASE II TO III TESTING FOR RELAPSED CLL

Ofatumumab (HuMax CD20) is a fully humanized, high-affinity monoclonal antibody, which targets a different epitope on the CD20 molecule than rituximab (7). Ofatumumab has higher affinity for binding to CD20 and activates complement dependent cytoxicity more effectively than rituximab in primary CLL cells, suggesting that it may have more antitumor activity (7,8). Results from a phase I/II clinical trial have been reported and included 27 patients treated at the phase II dose 500 mg IV as the initial dose and then three weekly doses of 2 g (9). This study demonstrated an overall response rate (ORR) of 44% (14 of 33 enrolled patients) with 1 nPR and 13 partial response (PR); the ORR at the phase II dose was 50%. Nine of the 33 patients (27%) maintained their response to week 19, and 2 (7%) to week 27. The median progression-free survival (PFS) for the entire group was 106 days, but the median time to next treatment was 1 year. Thirty-two of the 33 patients received all four weekly infusions. The most common toxicities were infusion related, including fever, chills, fatigue, and rash. These side effects tended to decrease in number and intensity on subsequent infusions. Infectious toxicity occurred in 51% of patients; three infections were grade 3 (varicella zoster, nasopharyngitis, and pneumonia), and one grade 5 case of fatal infectious interstitial pneumonitis occurred. To date, no data are available on the impact of high-risk genomic features on response to ofatumumab. On the basis of the promising data from this phase I/II clinical trial, a phase III registration study of ofatumumab in patients with fludarabine- and alemtuzumab-resistant CLL is ongoing. Other studies are examining ofatumumab in combination with fludarabine or fludarabine/cyclophosphamide.

Lumiliximab (IDEC-152)

CD23, a 45-kDa low-affinity IgE receptor, is another potential target of monoclonal antibody therapy, as the antigen is expressed on almost all CLL cells (10,11). In vitro studies of a chimeric macaque–human anti-CD23 monoclonal antibody lumiliximab (IDEC-152) demonstrated that cross-linked lumiliximab was able to induce apoptosis in primary CLL cells, and that this apoptosis was enhanced by fludarabine and rituximab (12). Given these encouraging preclinical data, a phase I clinical trial was pursued. In the phase I study, 46 patients with relapsed CLL received lumiliximab 125 to 500 mg/m^2 IV weekly or thrice weekly for four weeks (13). Lumiliximab was well tolerated with minimal infusion toxicity and mild to absent cytopenias; only 15% of patients developed grade 3 or 4 toxicity. No depression in T cells or natural killer (NK) cells was observed during therapy. Lumiliximab produced no complete or partial responses by NCI criteria, although a decrease in peripheral lymphocytosis was observed in 91% of patients, and 28% experienced more than a 50% reduction in their lymphocyte count. Changes in lymphocyte count occurred predominately in patients with lower total leukocyte counts. Reduction of nodal disease was seen in 52% of patients, although predominately in smaller nodes. On the basis of preclinical data demonstrating synergy of lumiliximab with either fludarabine or rituximab (12) and the favorable, nonoverlapping toxicity profile of this agent (13), a decision was made to pursue a phase I/II study of lumiliximab with FCR in patients with relapsed CLL (14). Thirty-one patients received fludarabine 25 mg/m^2 and cyclophosphamide 250 mg/m^2 on days 2 to 4 of cycle 1 and on days 1 to 3 of cycles 2 to 6, rituximab 50 and 325 mg/m^2 on days 1 and 3 of cycle 1 and 500 mg/m^2 on day 1 of cycle 2 to 6, and lumiliximab 50 and 325 or 450 mg/m^2 on days 2 and 4 of cycle 1 and 375 or 500 mg/m^2 on day 1 of cycle 2 to 6, every 28 days for up to six cycles. Grade 3 or 4 toxicity, primarily hematologic, was observed in 65% of patients. These toxicities were similar to those observed with FCR alone, with exception of rash potentially referable to lumiliximab; this rash was generally reversible and of little clinical consequence. In this phase I/II study, The ORR was 71%, with 52% of patients attaining CR. Progression-free survival with FCR and lumiliximab was also favorable as compared with single-institution phase II studies. Examining the impact of high-risk genomic features demonstrated that patients with del(11q22.3) but not del(17p13.1) had high response rates and durable remissions to this therapy. On the basis of these promising results, a randomized phase III study comparing FCR alone with the combination of FCR and lumiliximab is under way in patients with relapsed CLL.

Lenalidomide

Lenalidomide, or 3-(4-amino-1,3-dihydro-1-oxo-2H-isoindol-2-yl)-2,6-piperidinedione (Revlimid), is a synthetic analog of thalidomide that was developed to eliminate many of its unfavorable properties including neurotoxicity while preserving favorable findings including antiangiogenesis, T-cell co-stimulation, and inhibition of monocyte production of tumor necrosis factor-α (TNF-α) (15,16). Unlike many cancer therapeutics that are developed using structural activity relationship (SAR) analysis based on tumor kill, lenalidomide and other immune modulatory derivatives of thalidomide were chosen based on their ability to downregulate TNF-α produced by monocytes in response to bacterial lipopolysaccharide exposure (16). Other mechanisms include interfering with tumor cell: stromal cell interaction (17), enhancing SPARC expression (18), and activating T cells (19) and NK cells (20–22) to enhance their antitumor surveillance. Two second-generation molecules (CC-4047, actimid and CC-5013, lenalidomide) were brought forward. Actimid is a member of the selective cytokine inhibitory drugs (SelCID) and inhibits phosphodiesterase 4. In contrast, lenalidomide is a member of the immunomo-dulatory drugs (IMiDs); these agents are mechanistically similar to thalidomide but have significantly greater potency. While the exact mechanism of action of lenalidomide is uncertain, it appears to downregulate TNF-α (19) more potently than thalidomide. On the basis of data available at the time of lenalidomide's clinical development that thalidomide was an active agent in both relapsed multiple myeloma (MM) and myelodysplastic syndrome, clinical trials were undertaken; they showed significant activity of lenalidomide in both del(5q) MDS and MM (23–26). In phase I/II studies in these diseases, dose-dependent myelosuppression was observed. In patients with MM, lenalidomide was administered at 50 mg/day without grade 3 or 4 myelosuppression after 28 days of therapy (23). However, with additional therapy beyond one month, myelosuppression was noted in the large majority of patients. In these patients, dose reductions to 25 mg/day resulted in a well-tolerated therapy. Patients with MDS receiving 25 mg of lenalidomide daily also experienced myelosuppression with delayed onset; 77% required dose reduction because of myelosuppression after a median 4.6 weeks of therapy (range, 3–9 weeks) (23). Dose reductions were also required at lower doses but were not necessary until after 6 to 8.5 weeks of treatment. For the indications of MM and MDS (with 5q- in particular), significant clinical activity was seen. These data suggest that the maximally tolerated dose of lenalidomide might vary by the disease treated. In neither MM nor MDS has the toxicity of tumor flare or signs and symptoms of cytokine release been observed.

Three recent phase II studies have demonstrated that lenalidomide has clinical activity in CLL (27–29). The first of these by Chanan-Khan (27) was a phase II study, which included 45 previously treated patients with CLL and utilized 25 mg of lenalidomide orally daily on days 1 through 21 of a 28-day cycle. This regimen was associated with a 47% overall response rate and a 9% complete response rate. The most commonly reported toxicities were fatigue, thrombocytopenia, and neutropenia. Tumor flare reactions occurred in 58% of patients (grade 1–2 in 50%; grade 3–4 in 8%) typically involving painful enlargement of lymph nodes and/or spleen with associated low-grade fever and rash. Tumor flare in this study was managed with either nonsteroidal anti-inflammatory agents or prednisone. Two patients developed atypical tumor lysis syndrome associated with renal insufficiency. There was one death, which was attributed to worsening congestive heart failure. While correlative studies performed in this trial have not been formally reported, two preliminary abstract reports by this group have demonstrated response to CLL therapy correlated with baseline pretreatment NK cell number similar to what was observed in patients with MM (30–32). The second study by Ferrajoli et al. (28) included 35 patients, with 22 evaluable for response and toxicity. Patients received lenalidomide 10 mg/day for 28 days with dose escalation to a maximum of 25 mg/day as tolerated. The average dose that patients were ultimately able to receive was 10 mg. The overall response rate was 32%, with one complete response. Tumor flare was observed in 27% of patients. No patients were reported to have tumor lysis syndrome. Limited correlative studies demonstrated evidence of cytokine release (TNF-α and IL-6 mediated) (29). Combined data from these trials in relapsed CLL were presented at the 2007 ASH meeting, where the impact of lenalidomide on high-risk genomic and fludarabine-refractory CLL was examined. The combined experience demonstrated that lenalidomide had efficacy in the subset of patients with del(17p13.1) and del(11q22.3) (33) or fludarabine-refractory disease, similar to what was seen in patients without these poor prognostic features (33,34).

The Ohio State University (OSU) group pursued a phase I study with inclusion of detailed correlative studies (35). This study demonstrated that the 25 mg/day schedule was not tolerated by all three patients in this cohort with developing a dose limiting toxicity during the first cycle of therapy. These toxicities included life-threatening tumor flare in two patients and neutropenic fever with sepsis in another patient. Correlative studies done in conjunction with this trial demonstrated that B-cell activation occurred in the CLL cells with upregulation of CD40, CD80, and CD86, and that the degree of this upregulation correlated with the severity of tumor flare. A large multi-institutional randomized study that administered lenalidomide 25 mg/day as done by Chanan-Khan et al. (27) or continuous dosing at 10 mg/day as reported by Ferrajoli et al. (28) was initiated at multiple U.S. and European sites. The results were similar to the experience at OSU (36). This trial had early suspension of accrual due to unexpected deaths due to rapid disease progression, tumor flare, and possible atypical tumor lysis syndrome. These events suggest that the 25 mg/day schedule cannot be safely administered to patients with CLL and active disease and that lower doses of lenalidomide should be pursued.

Concurrent with the lenalidomide studies in relapsed CLL, a trial in previously untreated patients with CLL is being conducted by the NCI Canada CLL group (29). Twelve patients were reported who received a 10-mg starting dose of lenalidomide with weekly 5-mg dose escalations to the target dose of 25 mg/day × 21 days every 28-day cycle. Prophylactic allopurinol and aspirin were mandated. Steroids were allowed for management of tumor flare symptoms, but routine prophylaxis was not used. The first two patients were enrolled at the starting dose of 10 mg/day. The first patient reached the target dose of 25 mg with a lymphocyte reduction but at six weeks developed acute tumor lysis with renal failure and was removed from study. The second patient developed grade 4 neutropenia on day 21 of cycle 1, leading to a septic death. The study was halted, and the protocol was revised with reduced starting and target doses (2.5 and 10 mg, days 1–21), slower dose escalations (2.5 mg cycle 1, 5 mg cycle 2, 10 mg cycle 3, and thereafter), and extension of allopurinol prophylaxis to a minimum of three cycles. Eight evaluable patients had been accrued at the time of a preliminary report. Five of eight patients developed grade 3 to 4 neutropenia, leading to dose reductions in three patients and hospitalization for febrile neutropenia in one patient. One patient had grade 4 thrombocytopenia, whereas nonhematologic toxicity included grade 1 to 2 fatigue ($n = 5$), tumor flare ($n = 4$), non-desquamating rash ($n = 3$), and infections ($n = 3$). Tumor flare was often noted with each dose escalation but was responsive to prednisone. All eight patients achieved a partial response by the end of cycle 2 using 5-mg doses. Thus, the toxicities of lenalidomide use in CLL including tumor lysis, tumor flare, and myelosuppression may be more common in previously untreated CLL. This suggests that a lower dose will be required for safe administration for this population.

The development of lenalidomide at this time has been somewhat hampered by inability to identify the safe starting dose and dose escalation schedule to avoid the occurrence of tumor flare in CLL. It is clear that lenalidomide is an active agent in CLL, and that completion of studies to identify a safe dose in CLL is essential in its development. In addition, mechanistic studies to elucidate how lenalidomide works in CLL and to provide a better understanding of the etiology of tumor flare will be critically important.

Flavopiridol

Flavopiridol is a synthetic flavone with a novel structure, compared with polyhydroxylated flavones such as quercetin and genistein. Flavopiridol, as currently used in clinical trials, is obtained from a synthetic process, but its chemical structure is identical to a product obtained from *Dysoxylum binectariferum,* an indigenous plant found in India. Initially flavopiridol was presented to the National Cancer Institute as a tyrosine kinase antagonist, with in vitro activity against the epidermal growth factor receptor tyrosine kinase with an IC_{50} of approximately 20 µM. Subsequent studies revealed that flavopiridol was not, in fact, a cytotoxic agent to stationary MDA-MB-468 breast carcinoma cell lines, but reversibly inhibited growth via inhibition of cyclin-dependent kinase (CDK)1 and CDK2 (37–39). Flavopiridol induced cell cycle inhibition by altering phosphorylation of tyrosine residues on these cell cycle kinases (40). Additionally, flavopiridol directly antagonized CDK1 and CDK2 activity as a result of competitive inhibition with ATP. On the basis of these initial observations, investigators hypothesized that flavopiridol would be effective in rapidly dividing tumor systems where a minimum volume of tumor exists. In addition, since flavopiridol initially appeared to allow collection of cells in G1 or G2 as a consequence of CDK1 and CDK2 inhibition, it is possible that this agent could also be used to synchronize cells in vivo and thereby make them more sensitive to cell cycle–independent agents. Subsequent work has demonstrated that flavopiridol also inhibits other kinases including CDK 9 (41,42). CDK 9, along with the regulatory subunit cyclin T, is part of the positive transcription elongation factor b (P-TEFb), which phosphorylates the carboxyl-terminal domain (CTD) of RNA polymerase II (RNAPII). Inhibition of this complex by flavopiridol leads to secondary inactivation of RNAPII, ultimately resulting in global inhibition of gene transcription (43).

A variety of different schedules of administration have been explored with flavopiridol including 72-hour continuous infusion (44,45), 24-hour continuous infusion (46), and 1-hour bolus (47). The one-hour bolus schedule recommended a phase II dose of 50 mg/m^2 administered on days 1, 2, and 3 (47). Toxicities have included short-duration neutropenia, diarrhea, cytokine release syndrome (48), and fatigue. No significant clinical activity was observed in phase II testing (49–51). Modest activity was seen in mantle cell NHL (52); a 14% partial response rate was noted with the 1-hour 50 mg/m^2 QD × 3 days schedule. Attempts at combining flavopiridol were also unsuccessful because of either enhanced toxicity or lack of defined benefit as compared with what would be expected without the addition of flavopiridol. Development of flavopiridol in 2002 ceased temporarily on the basis of these results.

Studies of flavopiridol in CLL have been pursued by several groups and have demonstrated that this agent induces apoptosis in both cell lines and primary leukemic cells favoring a caspase 3–dependent mechanism (53–55). Additionally, induction of apoptosis by flavopiridol was shown to be p53 independent (53,56). Flavopiridol also induced profound decreases in the Mcl-1 and XIAP expression in CLL cells in vitro (55,57,58), and this loss of Mcl-1 has been related by different groups to alteration in ERK activity (59)or inhibition of CDK9, which contributes to the cellular transcriptional machinery. In addition, Hussain et al. showed that depolarization of the mitochondrial membrane occurs as early as six hours following in vitro exposure of leukemic cells to flavopiridol (55,57,58).

Unfortunately, phase II studies administering flavopiridol by 24- to 72-hour CIVI failed to show any clinical activity (60,61). A 1-hour infusion of flavopiridol for three consecutive days of 21-day cycles resulted in a 11% partial response in previously treated patients with CLL (60).

The lack of clinical activity in the earlier studies using flavopiridol was in part due to increased binding of the agent to human serum proteins leading to an underestimation of the dose required to induce apoptosis in CLL cells. Thus, neither CIVI nor bolus dosing of flavopiridol achieved pharmacologically effective drug concentrations. Pharmacokinetic (PK) modeling indicated that a dosing schedule of 30-min IVB followed by 4-hour CIVI would achieve a target $C_{4.5hr}$ of 1.5 µM and induce apoptosis of CLL cells in vivo. On the basis of this PK model, a phase I study of flavopiridol in relapsed CLL was conducted at OSU (62). DLT was observed at dose level 2 (40 mg/m^2 30-min IVB + 40 mg/m^2 4-hour CIVI), with two of three patients developing grade 4 to 5 TLS. Decreasing the dose to 30 mg/m^2 30-min IVB + 30 mg/m^2 4-hour CIVI, increased safety precautions, aggressive monitoring of serum potassium, and prompt intervention for hyperkalemia allowed safe administration of the drug. Subsequent cohorts in the phase I study demonstrated that the four-hour CIVI could be safely escalated to 50 mg/m^2 after the initial treatment if tumor lysis did not occur on the first course of therapy. This increase in the four-hour CIVI dose from 30 to 50 mg/m^2 increased $C_{4.5hr}$ from 0.96 µM to 1.55 µM, with a concomitant increase in antitumor activity, as measured in median rise in LDH. TLS requiring hemodialysis with the first treatment dose was observed in only 3% of patients with WBC < 200 × 10^9/L, but this procedure was required in 63% of patients with WBC $\geq 200 \times 10^9$/L. Patients with marked peripheral lymphocytosis should undergo cytoreduction before receiving flavopiridol. Nineteen of the first 42 patients in the phase I study responded (45%), including 5 of 12 patients (42%) with del(17p), 13 of 18 patients (72%) with del(11q), and 16 of 31 patients (51%) with bulky lymph nodes >5 cm in size. Median PFS was 11 months.

Preliminary results of a phase II trial in CLL presented in late 2007 demonstrated similar activity with 15 of the first 31 (48%) patients responding; two individuals attained a complete response by NCI criteria (63). Flavopiridol is active in del(17p13.1) disease (64) and is associated with a low frequency of opportunistic infections compared with other agents such as alemtuzumab (65). Currently, flavopiridol is in a pivotal phase II trial targeting treatment of patients with fludarabine-refractory CLL. Combination studies of flavopiridol with other active agents including cyclophosphamide/rituximab and lenalidomide are ongoing.

Oblimersen (G3139)

Oblimersen sodium (Genasense) is an 18-mer phosphothiorate oligonucleotide antisense molecule that binds to Bcl-2 transcript. A phase I to II trial in patients with relapsed CLL used a five-day continuous infusion at doses of 3 to 7 mg/kg/day (66). The initial dose of 7 mg was previously established to be safe in patients with solid tumors. However, a cytokine release syndrome including fever, chills, and hypotension was seen in all the three patients with this dose and led to dose reduction. A lower dose was pursued in this trial with the addition of corticosteroids which was safe and feasible to administer. Two (8%) of 26 assessable patients achieved a partial remission. Other evidence of antitumor activity included $\geq$50% reduction in: splenomegaly in 7 of 17 patients (41%), adenopathy in 7 of 22 patients (32%), and lymphocytosis in 11 of 22 patients (50%). A large randomized phase III study of oblimersen combined with fludarabine and cyclophosphamide (FC) was compared with FC alone in patients with relapsed CLL (67). This trial demonstrated a higher nodular PR and CR rate in those receiving the three-drug combination. CR/nPR was also more durable in patients receiving oblimersen; with a minimum follow-up of two years, 5 (25%) of 20 patients in the oblimersen group relapsed compared with 6 (75%) of 8 patients who received chemotherapy alone. Median duration of CR/nPR was 20 months in the chemotherapy-only group and was not reached in the oblimersen group; it was estimated to exceed 31 months.

Whereas fludarabine-refractory patients had no significant increase in CR rate with oblimersen, patients still sensitive to fludarabine had a fourfold increase in CR rate with the addition of this agent to FC. Further analysis of this study demonstrated no overall improvement in progression-free survival or overall survival for the entire group of patients enrolled on the study. At the present time, these retrospective analyses are not deemed sufficient to merit approval by the United States Food and Drug Administration (FDA) for marketing of this product in the United States.

SELECT LATE PRECLINICAL OR EARLY PHASE I AGENTS RELEVANT TO CLL

A variety of novel therapies have come forward for the treatment of CLL over the past five years that have an immunologic mechanism of action or, alternatively, target specific genes in CLL that prevent apoptosis or enhance proliferation. A comprehensive summary of these is included in Table 1. A few interesting agents in clinical trials for CLL are highlighted below. Figure 1 depicts the chemical diversity of several of these exciting small molecules with promising preclinical or clinical activity in CLL.

(*text continues on page 176*)

Table 1 List of Agents Currently in Early-Stage Clinical Trials for the Treatment of CLL

Name	Comments
Antibodies	
BU-12	Radioactive yttrium (Y-90)-labeled anti-CD19
MDX-1342	Anti-CD19
Low-dose rituximab	Anti-CD20
Ofatumumab (HuMax)	Anti-CD20
R7159	Anti-CD20
IMMU-106 (veltuzumab, hA20)	Anti-CD20
PRO131921	Anti-CD20
Tositumomab	Radioactive iodine (I-131)-labeled anti-CD20
Epratuzumab	Radioactive yttrium (Y-90)-labeled anti-CD22
Lumiliximab	Anti-CD23
CAT-8015 immunotoxin	Anti-CD22 linked to pseudomonas exotoxin A
LMB-2 immunotoxin	Anti-CD25 (IL-2R) linked to pseudomonas Exotoxin A
HCD122 (CHIR-12.12)	Anti-CD40
Milatuzumab (hLL1)	Anti-CD74
ALXN6000	Anti-CD200
Apolizumab (Hu-1D10)	Anti-1D10 (HLA-DR β)
A27.15	Anti-transferrin receptor
E2.3	Anti-transferrin receptor
Bevacizumab	Anti-VEGF
Kinase inhibitors	
Dasatinib (BMS-354825)	Tyrosine and LYN kinase inhibitor
Imatinib	Tyrosine kinase inhibitor
Enzastaurin (LY317615)	Serine-threonine kinase inhibitor
Sorafenib (BAY 43-9006)	Raf, platelet-derived growth factor (PDGF), VEGF kinase, and c-kit inhibitor
Sunitinib	Vascular endothelial growth factor (VEGF), PDGF kinase, and FLT3 and c-kit inhibitor
Cediranib	VEGF tyrosine kinase inhibitor
7-hydroxystaurosporine (UCN-01)	Serine-threonine, AKT, protein kinase C (PKC), and CDK inhibitor
Bryostatin	Inhibits PKC
Alvocidib (flavopiridol)	Cyclin-dependent kinase (CDK) and adenosine triphosphate inhibitor
SNS-032	CDK 2, 7, and 9 inhibitor
Bcl-2-targeted agents	
SPC2996	Antisense oligonucleotide against Bcl-2 mRNA
Obatoclax (GX15-070)	Small-molecule pan-Bcl-2 family inhibitor
ABT-263	Bcl-2 family inhibitor
GX15-070MS	Inhibits BH3 domain–mediated interaction of Bcl-2 with proapoptotic members of Bcl-2 proteins
AT-101	Binds BH3 domain of endogenous antagonists of Bcl-2
Dolastatin 10	Inhibits microtubule assembly, may also inhibit bcl-2
Nucleoside analogs	
Clofarabine	Purine nucleoside analog
Nelarabine (506U78)	Purine nucleoside analog
Acadesine	Purine nucleoside analog
Triciribine (TCN-PM, VD-0002)	Purine nucleoside analog, inhibits the Akt pathway.
GS-9219	Pro-form of purine nucleoside analog
Gemcitabine	Pyrimidine nucleoside analog
CP-4055	Pyrimidine nucleoside analog

Table 1   List of Agents Currently in Early-Stage Clinical Trials for the Treatment of CLL (*Continued*)

Name	Comments
Topoisomerase inhibitors	
Topotecan	Inhibits topoisomerase I
Epirubicin	Inhibits topoisomerase II
Pixantrone (BBR 2778)	Inhibits topoisomerase II
XK469R	Inhibits topoisomerase IIB
AQ4N	Inhibits topoisomerase II, concentrates in hypoxic tumor cells
Mitoxantrone	Inhibits topoisomerase II, intercalates into and cross-links DNA
Elsamitrucin	Inhibits topoisomerase I and II
Immunomodulatory agents	
Lenalidomide	Stimulates B and T cells, reduces VEGF and bFGF levels, and inhibits angiogenesis
CpG 7909	Toll-like receptor 9 (TLR9) agonist. Activates dendritic, B, and cytotoxic T cells
Thalidomide	
Demethylating agents	
5-Azacytidine	
Decitabine	
Proteasome inhibitors	
Bortezomib	
NPI 0052	
Mammalian target of rapamycin (mTOR)	
Inhibitors	
Temsirolimus (CCI-779)	
Everolimus	
RAD001	
Alkylating agents	
Bendamustine	
Heat shock protein (Hsp)-90 inhibitors	
BIIB021 (CNF2024)	
KW-2478	
SNX-5422	
CNF1010 (17-AAG)	
Histone deacetylase (HDAC) inhibitors	
Valproic acid	
MG-0103	
Suberoylanilide hydroxamic acid (SAHA, vorinostat)	
PCI-24781	
Pyroxamide	
Romidepsin (depsipeptide, FK228)	
DNA and RNA repair and synthesis inhibitors	
Triapine	Inhibits ribonucleotide reductase and DNA synthesis

(*Continued*)

Table 1 List of Agents Currently in Early-Stage Clinical Trials for the Treatment of CLL (*Continued*)

Name	Comments
Cloretazine (VNP40101M)	Chloroethylates guanine residues and induces interstrand DNA cross-links
Oxaliplatin	Forms DNA adducts and inhibits DNA and RNA
Quarfloxin (CX-3543)	Selectively inhibits ribosomal RNA (rRNA)
SJG-136 (NSC 694501)	DNA cross-linking agent
GRN163L	Telomerase inhibitor
APO866	Inhibits the synthesis of NAD, protein modification, and mRNA synthesis
Selective apoptotic antineoplastic drugs (SAANDs) and SAAND-like agents	
OSI-461	Sulindac derivative. May impair microtubule function and protein kinase G activation
CP-461	Specifically inhibit cGMP phosphodiesterase (PDE) but not cycloxygenase (COX)-1 or COX-2
SDX-101 (R-etodolac)	Non-COX-2-inhibiting R-enantiomer of the NSAID drug etodolac
Cytokines and other targeted agents	
Ontak (denileukin diftitox)	Interleukin-2 (IL-2) protein sequences fused to diphtheria toxin that act through IL-2R (CD25)
Aldesleukin (IL-2)	Recombinant IL-2 receptor agonist
Interleukin-12	Recombinant interleukin-12
Etanercept	Recombinant tumor necrosis factor receptor conjugated to Fc region of IgG
TRU-016	Small modular immuno-pharmaceutical (SMIP) against CD-37
EL625	Antisense oligonucleotide against p53 mRNA
ABT-888	Poly(ADP-ribose) polymerase inhibitor
Forodesine	Purine nucleoside phosphorylase (PNP) inhibitor
Talabostat	Inhibits dipeptidyl peptidases
Fenretinide	Activates retinoic acid receptors
Tipifarnib	Inhibits the enzyme farnesyl protein transferase
Miscellaneous	
GCS-100	Antagonistic polysaccharide to Bcl-2, Hsp-27, and NF-KB
β-glucan	Polysaccharide that induces complement-mediated leukocyte activation and tumor death
Epigallocatechin gallate (EGCG) or polyphenon E	May inhibit PDGF, ligand-receptor cross-linking, and growth factor receptor activation
Plerixafor (AMD3100)	CXCR4 inhibitor and stem cell mobilizer
R7112	HDM2 or MDM2 inhibitor
Motexafin gadolinium	Increases reactive oxygen species (ROS) production in the tumor cells and lowers the tumor cell apoptotic threshold to ionizing radiation and chemotherapy
Arsenic trioxide	Induces apoptosis, promotes cell differentiation, and suppresses cell proliferation
Noscapine	Disrupts microtubule assembly
Ixabepilone	Binds to tubulin and promotes polymerization and microtubule stabilization

Table 1 List of Agents Currently in Early-Stage Clinical Trials for the Treatment of CLL (*Continued*)

Name	Comments
Theophylline	Inhibits PDE and prostaglandin (PG) production, regulates calcium flux and intracellular calcium distribution, and antagonizes adenosine
Sodium salicylate	Irreversibly acetylates COX-1 and COX-2 and inhibits PG synthesis. May also activate MAPK
Perifosine	Modulates membrane permeability, lipid composition, and metabolism. Inhibits the anti-apoptotic mitogen-activated protein kinase (MAPK) pathway
EMD 121974 (cilengitide)	Inhibits α- and β-integrins
Tetradecanoylphorbol acetate (TPA)	Induces maturation and differentiation of leukemic cells and may induce gene expression and PKC activity

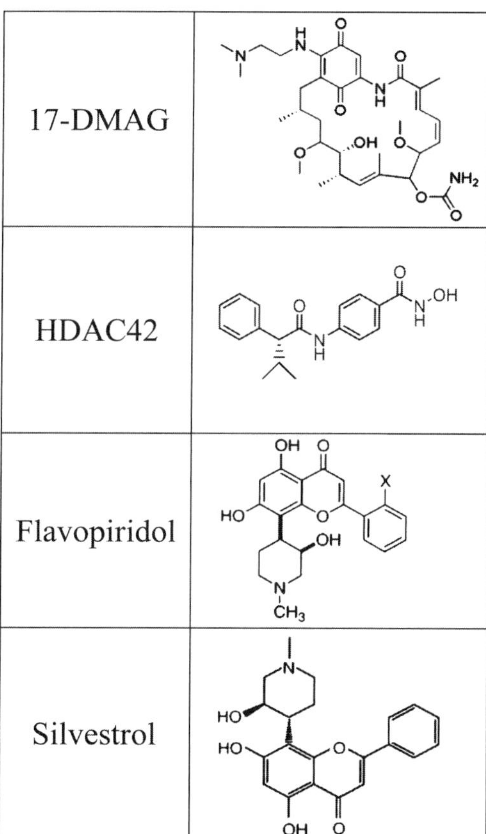

Figure 1 Novel agents with diverse chemical structure for the treatment of CLL.

BIOLOGIC AGENTS OF PARTICULAR INTEREST

Interleukin 21

IL-21 is a γ receptor family member cytokine that has the unique property of mediating direct apoptosis toward both normal B cells and transformed B cells including those from patients with CLL (68–72). Apoptosis mediated by IL-21 against CLL cells occurs via induction of the BH3-only domain protein BIM (73). This induction of BIM by IL-21 is similar to that observed during B-cell activation (72). Additionally, our group has shown that IL-21 also enhances direct apoptosis mediated by both rituximab and fludarabine (73). IL-21 has similar effects on natural killer cells as compared to IL-2, mediating enhanced antibody-dependent cellular cytotoxicity (ADCC) against CLL cells coated with rituximab and other therapeutic antibodies (73).

Preliminary reports of a phase I study combining IL-21 and rituximab demonstrated a favorable safety profile and clinical activity in both CLL and NHL (74). A phase II study of this novel combination regimen in elderly CLL is being considered at this time.

FcγR Engineered Anti-CD20 Antibodies

The introduction of rituximab in the treatment of CLL has perhaps represented the biggest advance made during the past decade. While the mechanism of action of rituximab is uncertain, it is likely that ADCC, CDC lysis, and direct apoptosis contribute. Studies previously performed in follicular lymphoma have demonstrated that response to rituximab is influenced by the presence or absence of specific FcγRIIIa and FcγRIIa single nucleic polymorphisms (SNP) that modify the affinity to IgG1 antibodies (75–77). Follicular lymphoma, Waldenstrom's macroglobulinemia, and large-cell lymphoma patients with low affinity SNPs have a lower response rate to rituximab (75–77). This has prompted several groups to modify the backbone of CD20 antibodies to enhance FcγRIIIa binding with the hope of improving therapeutic efficacy. PRO131921 is one such therapeutic antibody that targets CD20 with an engineered Fc binding domain. This agent is in early clinical trials for CLL. While studies in CLL demonstrated no definite association of response to rituximab with specific FcγRIIIa or FcγRIIa SNPs (78), these tumor cells are sensitive to NK cell–mediated rituximab ADCC (73), thereby justifying clinical trials with PRO131921 in CLL.

Tru16

This molecule represents a new class of drugs called small modular immune pharmaceutics (SMIP), which contain variable regions derived from specific antibodies and engineered constant regions encoding human IgG$_1$ domains (hinge, CH$_2$, and CH$_3$) (79). Two such SMIPS are under clinical development, one targeting CD20 (Tru15) and another targeting CD37 (Tru16). CD37 is a tetraspan superfamily member and a heavily glycosylated glycoprotein with a molecular weight of 40 to 52 kDa (80). Despite the fact that little is known about the function of this cell surface antigen, CD37 is an attractive target for treatment against CLL and other types of B-cell malignancies because, similar to CD20, it is specifically expressed on B cells, and has minimal or no expression on other types of blood cells, including T cells, neutrophils, monocytes, and NK cells (81–83). The expression level of CD37 on malignant B cells has made it appropriate for development of CD37-targeted immunotherapy, since CLL, NHL, and hairy cell leukemia cells all have

CD37 positivity (84,85). This is particularly attractive for CLL, because the CD37 expression levels on CLL cells are relatively high, in contrast to the dim and variable expression of CD20 on CLL cells (86,87). Preclinical work with CD37SMIP (79) has demonstrated that it mediates caspase-independent apoptosis against primary CLL cells and a variety of B-cell lymphoma cell lines. Additionally, CD37SMIP mediates superior ADCC against CLL cells as compared with rituximab and alemtuzumab, two alternative therapies currently approved for this disease. In vivo activity in xenograft models of disseminated leukemia has been demonstrated with Tru16 that is dependent on NK cell function (79). These promising data with relative specificity to B-cell diseases have led to initiation of a phase I trial in CLL.

Milatuzumab (hLL1)

Milatuzumab (hLL1) is a humanized monoclonal antibody directed at CD74, the innominate chain of HLA-DR. CD74 is the receptor for MIF-1α, and when it is ligated in CLL cells, CD74 is translocated to the nucleus where it enhances NF-κB activation and transcription of anti-apoptotic genes such as bcl-xl (88). Preclinical studies of milatuzumab have demonstrated that this antibody mediates potent apoptosis against B-cell lymphoma cell lines (89,90). Additionally, milatuzumab mediates potent in vivo activity in lymphoma xenograft models (89). On the basis of these results, early phase I/II clinical trials of milatuzumab in CLL and NHL are being initiated.

TARGETED SMALL MOLECULES

HSP90 Inibitors

A variety of small molecules (17AAG, DMAG, CNF2024) that inhibit HSP90 are in clinical development. These agents target the ATP binding site of HSP90, a ubiquitously expressed protein involved in chaperoning a variety of peptides relevant to CLL survival including AKT, PDK1, ZAP70, and IKK. Preclinical data from several groups have demonstrated that HSP90 inhibitors are effective at inducing apoptosis in a subset of patients with CLL and also enhance the efficacy of commonly utilized therapies including fludarabine, chlorambucil, and rituximab (91–94). Of particular interest was the finding by one group that CLL cell death induced by HSP90 inhibitors occurred only in ZAP-70-expressing cells (95). Over time it has become apparent from several other published papers that this association may extend to all patients with CLL. Efforts are currently under way to test the efficacy of HSP90-inhibiting agents in CLL.

SRC Inhibitors

A recent paper demonstrated that lyn kinase, a member of the src kinase family, is constitutively activated in CLL (96). Dasatinib is a src inhibitor that showed significant efficacy in chronic myelogenous leukemia (CML), leading to its recent approval in the United States and Europe in patients with CML failing imatinib. Subsequent preclinical work by several groups has demonstrated that dasatinib has both in vitro activity against CLL cells and also enhances the sensitivity to fludarabine (97,98). A preliminary report of a clinical trial of dasatinib in CLL demonstrated some clinical activity with acceptable toxicity (99). While dasatinib will likely not be viable as a single-agent therapy in CLL, its application in combination might be significant given its ability to sensitize tumor cells to fludarabine-mediated apoptosis.

Histone Deacetylase Inhibitors

Histone deacetylase (HDAC) enzymes represent a wide range of peptides that deacetylate nuclear and cytoplasmic proteins thereby modifying their function. Class I HDAC enzymes predominately reside in the nucleus and remove acetyl groups from histone and other nuclear proteins. With respect to histone proteins, deacetylation by HDAC enzymes promotes silencing of genes. HDACs often form repressor complexes on specific genes, preventing their transcription. The addition of HDAC inhibitors in this setting would be predicted to increase gene transcription. Class II HDAC inhibitors generally acetylate proteins in the cytoplasm such as p53, HSP90, and tubulin and modulate function. For instance, LBH589, a broad class I/II inhibitor has been demonstrated to inhibit HSP90 binding to specific client proteins (100). These agents have promising preclinical activity in CLL by virtue of their ability to activate novel apoptotic pathways not utilized by other therapies in this disease (101–109). To date, only one trial with a class I specific HDAC inhibitor depsipeptide has been performed in CLL with some evidence of clinical activity (110). Patients were generally unable to receive this therapy for more than one to two cycles because of profound fatigue and other constitutional symptoms. To date, no broad-class HDAC inhibitors have been explored in CLL. OSU-HDAC42, a class I and class II HDAC inhibitor, has promising preclinical activity in CLL, and trials in this disease will likely be pursued in the early development of this molecule (111).

BH-3 Mimetics

While the antisense molecule oblimersen targets bcl-2 alone, several small molecules antagonizing multiple bcl-2 protein family members (bcl-2, bcl-xl, bcl-w, A1, and mcl-1) have entered clinical trials for the treatment of CLL. AT-101 is an orally active agent that inhibits the anti-apoptotic activity of Bcl-2, Bcl-XL, and Mcl-1 (112). Gastrointestinal toxicity is the most notable adverse event. Obatoclax is a novel small molecule that also inhibits Bcl-2, Bcl-XL, and Mcl-1 (113). It induces apoptosis of human B-CLL cells treated ex vivo and is additive with both fludarabine and chlorambucil. In a phase I trial in patients with heavily pretreated CLL (median 4 prior regimens, 22 of 26 patients fludarabine refractory), obatoclax was administered as a short infusion every three weeks. The predominant side effect was euphoria/somnolence during the infusion that rapidly dissipated thereafter. The recommended phase II dose was 28 mg/m^2 over three hours every three weeks. Reductions in lymphocyte counts were observed in 18 of 26 patients, and 1 PR was noted. In addition, significant improvements in cytopenias were seen with some patients becoming transfusion independent while on treatment with obatoclax. A potent inhibitor of bcl-2 and Bcl-xl, ABT263 has also recently entered phase I clinical trials in CLL and NHL where responses have been noted, particularly in patients with bulky lymph node enlargement (114).

SILVESTROL

Silvestrol, a novel plant-derived natural product, is undergoing preclinical evaluation at the NCI. This agent was selected for preclinical drug development on the basis of B-cell selectivity and its potent in vitro activity against leukemic cells obtained from patients with CLL. Furthermore, the agent is effective against cells with del17p, suggesting that p53-defective cells would retain sensitivity. In leukemic cell lines overexpressing Bcl-2, effective cytotoxicity was still observed. Lucas et al. have shown that silvestrol mediates an early reduction in Mcl-1 protein, and that this is mediated through inhibition of translation and not transcription (personal communication, M.R. Grever). Reduction in Mcl-1 in leukemic cells from patients with CLL can induce mitochondrial instability and apoptosis. Preclinical work has confirmed that this agent has in vivo efficacy against B cells in murine models of leukemia. Therefore, the preclinical development of this exciting new agent will be followed with interest as it moves progressively toward phase I studies in human.

In selecting new therapeutic strategies for CLL, all avenues deserve exploration. Rational targeted therapies with selectivity and effectiveness may take the form of a small synthetic agent or a monoclonal antibody. Intriguing new leads may also arise from biologic observations from natural products research. Many sources of interesting new agents have provided a wide spectrum of promising agents for strategic en route investigation to find a better therapy for this disease.

ACKNOWLEDGMENTS

This work was supported by the National Cancer Institute P01 CA95426, The Leukemia and Lymphoma Society, and The D. Warren Brown Foundation.

REFERENCES

1. Perkins JG, Flynn JM, Howard RS, et al. Frequency and type of serious infections in fludarabine-refractory B-cell chronic lymphocytic leukemia and small lymphocytic lymphoma: implications for clinical trials in this patient population. Cancer 2002; 94:2033–2039.
2. Keating MJ, O'Brien S, Kontoyiannis D, et al. Results of first salvage therapy for patients refractory to a fludarabine regimen in chronic lymphocytic leukemia. Leuk Lymphoma 2002; 43:1755–1762.
3. Wierda W, O'Brien S, Wen S, et al. Chemoimmunotherapy with fludarabine, cyclophosphamide, and rituximab for relapsed and refractory chronic lymphocytic leukemia. J Clin Oncol 2005; 23:4070–4078.
4. Dohner H, Stilgenbauer S, Benner A, et al. Genomic aberrations and survival in chronic lymphocytic leukemia. N Engl J Med 2000; 343:1910–1916.
5. Lozanski G, Heerema NA, Flinn IW, et al. Alemtuzumab is an effective therapy for chronic lymphocytic leukemia with p53 mutations and deletions. Blood 2004; 103:3278–3281.
6. Hallek M, Cheson BD, Catovsky D, et al. Guidelines for the diagnosis and treatment of chronic lymphocytic leukemia: a report from the International Workshop on Chronic Lymphocytic Leukemia (IWCLL) updating the National Cancer Institute-Working Group (NCI-WG) 1996 guidelines. Blood 2008; 111:5446–5456.
7. Teeling JL, Mackus WJ, Wiegman LJ, et al. The biological activity of human CD20 monoclonal antibodies is linked to unique epitopes on CD20. J Immunol 2006; 177:362–371.
8. Teeling JL, French RR, Cragg MS, et al. Characterization of new human CD20 monoclonal antibodies with potent cytolytic activity against non-Hodgkin lymphomas. Blood 2004; 104:1793–1800.
9. Coiffier B, Lepretre S, Pedersen LM, et al. Safety and efficacy of ofatumumab, a fully human monoclonal anti-CD20 antibody, in patients with relapsed or refractory B-cell chronic lymphocytic leukemia: a phase 1-2 study. Blood 2008; 111:1094–1100.
10. Sarfati M. CD23 and chronic lymphocytic leukemia. Blood Cells 1993; 19:591–596; discussion 597–599.
11. Sarfati M, Bron D, Lagneaux L, et al. Elevation of IgE-binding factors in serum of patients with B cell-derived chronic lymphocytic leukemia. Blood 1988; 71:94–98.
12. Pathan NI, Chu P, Hariharan K, et al. Mediation of apoptosis by and antitumor activity of lumiliximab in chronic lymphocytic leukemia cells and CD23+ lymphoma cell lines. Blood 2008; 111:1594–1602.

13. Byrd JC, O'Brien S, Flinn IW, et al. Phase 1 study of lumiliximab with detailed pharmacokinetic and pharmacodynamic measurements in patients with relapsed or refractory chronic lymphocytic leukemia. Clin Cancer Res 2007; 13:4448–4455.

14. Byrd JC, Castro J, O'Brien S, et al. Comparison of results from a phase 1/2 study of lumiliximab (anti-CD23) in combination with FCR for patients with relapsed CLL with published FCR results. Blood 2006; 108:32 (abstr).

15. Bartlett JB, Dredge K, Dalgleish AG. The evolution of thalidomide and its IMiD derivatives as anticancer agents. Nat Rev Cancer 2004; 4:314–322.

16. Melchert M, List A. The thalidomide saga. Int J Biochem Cell Biol 2007; 39:1489–1499.

17. James DF, Betty MR, Mosadeghi R, et al. Lenalidomide abrogates the protective influence of nurse-like cells on primary chronic lymphocytic leukemia cells in vitro. Blood 2007; 110: 3116 (abstr).

18. Pellagatti A, Jadersten M, Forsblom AM, et al. Lenalidomide inhibits the malignant clone and up-regulates the SPARC gene mapping to the commonly deleted region in 5q- syndrome patients. Proc Natl Acad Sci U S A 2007; 104:11406–11411.

19. Marriott JB, Clarke IA, Dredge K, et al. Thalidomide and its analogues have distinct and opposing effects on TNF-alpha and TNFR2 during co-stimulation of both CD4(+) and CD8(+) T cells. Clin Exp Immunol 2002; 130:75–84.

20. Tai YT, Li XF, Catley L, et al. Immunomodulatory drug lenalidomide (CC-5013, IMiD3) augments anti-CD40 SGN-40-induced cytotoxicity in human multiple myeloma: clinical implications. Cancer Res 2005; 65:11712–11720.

21. Reddy N, Hernandez-Ilizaliturri FJ, Deeb G, et al. Immunomodulatory drugs stimulate natural killer-cell function, alter cytokine production by dendritic cells, and inhibit angiogenesis enhancing the anti-tumour activity of rituximab in vivo. Br J Haematol 2008; 140:36–45.

22. Hernandez-Ilizaliturri FJ, Reddy N, Holkova B, et al. Immunomodulatory drug CC-5013 or CC-4047 and rituximab enhance antitumor activity in a severe combined immunodeficient mouse lymphoma model. Clin Cancer Res 2005; 11:5984–5992.

23. List A, Kurtin S, Roe DJ, et al. Efficacy of lenalidomide in myelodysplastic syndromes. N Engl J Med 2005; 352:549–557.

24. List A, Dewald G, Bennett J, et al. Lenalidomide in the myelodysplastic syndrome with chromosome 5q deletion. N Engl J Med 2006; 355:1456–1465.

25. Richardson PG, Blood E, Mitsiades CS, et al. A randomized phase 2 study of lenalidomide therapy for patients with relapsed or relapsed and refractory multiple myeloma. Blood 2006; 108:3458–3464.

26. Richardson PG, Schlossman RL, Weller E, et al. Immunomodulatory drug CC-5013 overcomes drug resistance and is well tolerated in patients with relapsed multiple myeloma. Blood 2002; 100:3063–3067.

27. Chanan-Khan A, Miller KC, Musial L, et al. Clinical efficacy of lenalidomide in patients with relapsed or refractory chronic lymphocytic leukemia: results of a phase II study. J Clin Oncol 2006; 24:5343–5349.

28. Ferrajoli A, Lee BN, Schlette EJ, et al. Lenalidomide induces complete and partial remissions in patients with relapsed and refractory chronic lymphocytic leukemia. Blood 2008 [Epub ahead of print].

29. Chen CI, Paul H, Mariela P, et al. A phase II study of lenalidomide in previously untreated, symptomatic chronic lymphocytic leukemia (CLL). Blood 2007; 110:2042.

30. Chanan-Khan AA, Cheson BD. Lenalidomide for the treatment of B-cell malignancies. J Clin Oncol 2008; 26:1544–1552.

31. Padmanabhan S, Ersing N, Wallace PK, et al. First Clinical evidence of in vivo natural killer (NK) cell modulation in chronic lymphocytic leukemia (CLL) patients (pts) treated with lenalidomide (L). Blood 2006; 108: 2109 (abstr).

32. Chanan-Khan AA, Padmanabhan S, Miller KC, et al. In vivo evaluation of immunomodulating effects of lenalidomide (L) on tumor cell microenvironment as a possible underlying mechanism of the antitumor effects observed in patients (pts) with chronic lymphocytic leukemia (CLL). Blood 2005; 106: 2975 (abstr).

33. Ferrajoli A, Keating MJ, Wierda WG, et al. Lenalidomide is active in patients with relapsed/ refractory chronic lymphocytic leukemia (CLL) carrying unfavorable chromosomal abnormalities. Blood 2007; 110:754 (abstr).

34. Chanan-Khan AA, Czuczman MS, Padmanabhan S, et al. Clinical efficacy of lenalidomide in fludarabine-refractory chronic lymphocytic leukemia patients. Blood 2007; 110: 3108 (abstr).

35. Andritsos LA, Johnson AJ, Lozanski G, et al. Higher doses of lenalidomide are associated with unacceptable toxicity including life-threatening tumor flare in patients with chronic lymphocytic leukemia. J Clin Oncol 2008; 26(15):2519–2525.

36. Moutouh-de Parseval LA, Weiss L, DeLap RJ, et al. Tumor lysis syndrome/tumor flare reaction in lenalidomide-treated chronic lymphocytic leukemia. J Clin Oncol 2007; 25:5047.

37. Carlson BA, Dubay MM, Sausville EA, et al. Flavopiridol induces G1 arrest with inhibition of cyclin-dependent kinase (CDK) 2 and CDK4 in human breast carcinoma cells. Cancer Res 1996; 56:2973–2978.

38. Losiewicz MD, Carlson BA, Kaur G, et al. Potent inhibition of CDC2 kinase activity by the flavonoid L86-8275. Biochem Biophys Res Commun 1994; 201:589–595.

39. Kaur G, Stetler-Stevenson M, Sebers S, et al. Growth inhibition with reversible cell cycle arrest of carcinoma cells by flavone L86-8275. J Natl Cancer Inst 1992; 84:1736–1740.

40. Worland PJ, Kaur G, Stetler-Stevenson M, et al. Alteration of the phosphorylation state of p34cdc2 kinase by the flavone L86-8275 in breast carcinoma cells. Correlation with decreased H1 kinase activity. Biochem Pharmacol 1993; 46:1831–1840.

41. Chao SH, Fujinaga K, Marion JE, et al. Flavopiridol inhibits P-TEFb and blocks HIV-1 replication. J Biol Chem 2000; 275:28345–28348.

42. Chao SH, Price DH. Flavopiridol inactivates P-TEFb and blocks most RNA polymerase II transcription in vivo. J Biol Chem 2001; 276:31793–31799.

43. Lam LT, Pickeral OK, Peng AC, et al. Genomic-scale measurement of mRNA turnover and the mechanisms of action of the anti-cancer drug flavopiridol. Genome Biol 2001; 2: RESEARCH0041.

44. Senderowicz AM, Headlee D, Stinson SF, et al. Phase I trial of continuous infusion flavopiridol, a novel cyclin-dependent kinase inhibitor, in patients with refractory neoplasms. J Clin Oncol 1998; 16:2986–2999.

45. Thomas JP, Tutsch KD, Cleary JF, et al. Phase I clinical and pharmacokinetic trial of the cyclin-dependent kinase inhibitor flavopiridol. Cancer Chemother Pharmacol 2002; 50:465–472.

46. Schwartz GK, O'Reilly E, Ilson D, et al. Phase I study of the cyclin-dependent kinase inhibitor flavopiridol in combination with paclitaxel in patients with advanced solid tumors. J Clin Oncol 2002; 20:2157–2170.

47. Tan AR, Headlee D, Messmann R, et al. Phase I clinical and pharmacokinetic study of flavopiridol administered as a daily 1-hour infusion in patients with advanced neoplasms. J Clin Oncol 2002; 20:4074–4082.

48. Messmann RA, Ullmann CD, Lahusen T, et al. Flavopiridol-related proinflammatory syndrome is associated with induction of interleukin-6. Clin Cancer Res 2003; 9:562–570.

49. Schwartz GK, Ilson D, Saltz L, et al. Phase II study of the cyclin-dependent kinase inhibitor flavopiridol administered to patients with advanced gastric carcinoma. J Clin Oncol 2001; 19:1985–1992.

50. Stadler WM, Vogelzang NJ, Amato R, et al. Flavopiridol, a novel cyclin-dependent kinase inhibitor, in metastatic renal cancer: a University of Chicago Phase II Consortium study. J Clin Oncol 2000; 18:371–375.

51. Shapiro GI, Supko JG, Patterson A, et al. A phase II trial of the cyclin-dependent kinase inhibitor flavopiridol in patients with previously untreated stage IV non-small cell lung cancer. Clin Cancer Res 2001; 7:1590–1599.

52. Kouroukis CT, Belch A, Crump M, et al. Flavopiridol in untreated or relapsed mantle-cell lymphoma: results of a phase II study of the National Cancer Institute of Canada Clinical Trials Group. J Clin Oncol 2003; 21:1740–1745.

53. Byrd JC, Shinn C, Waselenko JK, et al. Flavopiridol induces apoptosis in chronic lymphocytic leukemia cells via activation of caspase-3 without evidence of bcl-2 modulation or dependence on functional p53. Blood 1998; 92:3804–3816.

54. Konig A, Schwartz GK, Mohammad RM, et al. The novel cyclin-dependent kinase inhibitor flavopiridol downregulates Bcl-2 and induces growth arrest and apoptosis in chronic B-cell leukemia lines. Blood 1997; 90:4307–4312.

55. Kitada S, Zapata JM, Andreeff M, et al. Protein kinase inhibitors flavopiridol and 7-hydroxy-staurosporine down-regulate antiapoptosis proteins in B-cell chronic lymphocytic leukemia. Blood 2000; 96:393–397.

56. Parker BW, Kaur G, Nieves-Neira W, et al. Early induction of apoptosis in hematopoietic cell lines after exposure to flavopiridol. Blood 1998; 91:458–465.

57. Chen R, Keating MJ, Gandhi V, et al. Transcription inhibition by flavopiridol: mechanism of chronic lymphocytic leukemia cell death. Blood 2005; 106:2513–2519.

58. Hussain SR, Lucas DM, Johnson AJ, et al. Flavopiridol causes early mitochondrial damage in chronic lymphocytic leukemia cells with impaired oxygen consumption and mobilization of intracellular calcium. Blood 2008; 111:3190–3199.

59. Pepper C, Thomas A, Fegan C, et al. Flavopiridol induces apoptosis in B-cell chronic lymphocytic leukaemia cells through a p38 and ERK MAP kinase-dependent mechanism. Leuk Lymphoma 2003; 44:337–342.

60. Byrd JC, Peterson BL, Gabrilove J, et al. Treatment of relapsed chronic lymphocytic leukemia by 72-hour continuous infusion or 1-hour bolus infusion of flavopiridol: results from Cancer and Leukemia Group B study 19805. Clin Cancer Res 2005; 11:4176–4181.

61. Flinn IW, Byrd JC, Bartlett N, et al. Flavopiridol administered as a 24-hour continuous infusion in chronic lymphocytic leukemia lacks clinical activity. Leuk Res 2005; 29:1253–1257.

62. Byrd JC, Lin TS, Dalton JT, et al. Flavopiridol administered using a pharmacologically derived schedule is associated with marked clinical efficacy in refractory, genetically high-risk chronic lymphocytic leukemia. Blood 2007; 109:399–404.

63. Lin TS, Fischer B, Blum KA, et al. Preliminary results of a phase II study of flavopiridol (alvocidib) in relapsed chronic lymphocytic leukemia (CLL): confirmation of clinical activity in high-risk patients and achievement of complete responses (CR). Blood 2007; 110:3104 (abstr).

64. Heerema NA, Byrd JC, Andritsos LA, et al. Clinical activity of flavopiridol in relapsed and refractory chronic lymphocytic leukemia (CLL) with high-risk cytogenetic abnormalities: updated data on 89 patients (Pts). Blood 2007; 110:3107 (abstr).

65. Andritsos LA, Fischer B, Lin TS, et al. Low incidence of opportunistic infections in CLL patients treated with single agent flavopiridol. Blood 2007; 110:3128 (abstr).

66. O'Brien SM, Cunningham CC, Golenkov AK, et al. Phase I to II multicenter study of oblimersen sodium, a Bcl-2 antisense oligonucleotide, in patients with advanced chronic lymphocytic leukemia. J Clin Oncol 2005; 23:7697–7702.

67. O'Brien S, Moore JO, Boyd TE, et al. Randomized phase III trial of fludarabine plus cyclophosphamide with or without oblimersen sodium (Bcl-2 antisense) in patients with relapsed or refractory chronic lymphocytic leukemia. J Clin Oncol 2007; 25:1114–1120.

68. Jahrsdorfer B, Blackwell SE, Wooldridge JE, et al. B-chronic lymphocytic leukemia cells and other B cells can produce granzyme B and gain cytotoxic potential after interleukin-21-based activation. Blood 2006; 108:2712–2719.

69. di Carlo E, de Totero D, Piazza T, et al. Role of IL-21 in immune-regulation and tumor immunotherapy. Cancer Immunol Immunother 2007; 56:1323–1334.

70. de Totero D, Meazza R, Zupo S, et al. Interleukin-21 receptor (IL-21R) is up-regulated by CD40 triggering and mediates proapoptotic signals in chronic lymphocytic leukemia B cells. Blood 2006; 107:3708–3715.

71. de Totero D, Meazza R, Capaia M, et al. The opposite effects of IL-15 and IL-21 on CLL B cells correlate with differential activation of the JAK/STAT and ERK1/2 pathways. Blood 2008; 111:517–524.

72. Jin H, Carrio R, Yu A, et al. Distinct activation signals determine whether IL-21 induces B cell costimulation, growth arrest, or Bim-dependent apoptosis. J Immunol 2004; 173:657–665.

73. Gowda A, Roda J, Hussain SR, et al. IL-21 mediates apoptosis through up-regulation of the BH3 family member BIM and enhances both direct and antibody dependent cellular cytotoxicity in primary chronic lymphocytic cells. Blood 2008; 111(9): 4723–4730.

74. Timmerman JM, Byrd JC, Andorsky DJ, et al. Recombinant interleukin-21 plus rituximab: clinical activity in a phase 1, dose-finding trial in relapsed low-grade B cell lymphoma. Blood 2007; 110:2577–.
75. Weng WK, Levy R. Two immunoglobulin G fragment C receptor polymorphisms independently predict response to rituximab in patients with follicular lymphoma. J Clin Oncol 2003; 21:3940–3947.
76. Cartron G, Dacheux L, Salles G, et al. Therapeutic activity of humanized anti-CD20 monoclonal antibody and polymorphism in IgG Fc receptor FcgammaRIIIa gene. Blood 2002; 99:754–758.
77. Treon SP, Hansen M, Branagan AR, et al. Polymorphisms in FcgammaRIIIA (CD16) receptor expression are associated with clinical response to rituximab in Waldenstrom's macroglobulinemia. J Clin Oncol 2005; 23:474–481.
78. Lin TS, Flinn IW, Modali R, et al. FCGR3A and FCGR2A polymorphisms may not correlate with response to alemtuzumab in chronic lymphocytic leukemia. Blood 2005; 105:289–291.
79. Zhao X, Lapalombella R, Joshi T, et al. Targeting CD37-positive lymphoid malignancies with a novel engineered small modular immunopharmaceutical. Blood 2007; 110:2569–2577.
80. Moldenhauer G. Cd37. J Biol Regul Homeost Agents 2000; 14:281–283.
81. Schwartz-Albiez R, Dorken B, Hofmann W, et al. The B cell-associated CD37 antigen (gp40-52). Structure and subcellular expression of an extensively glycosylated glycoprotein. J Immunol 1988; 140:905–914.
82. Okochi H, Kato M, Nashiro K, et al. Expression of tetra-spans transmembrane family (CD9, CD37, CD53, CD63, CD81 and CD82) in normal and neoplastic human keratinocytes: an association of CD9 with alpha 3 beta 1 integrin. Br J Dermatol 1997; 137:856–863.
83. Peters RE, Janossy G, Ivory K, et al. Leukemia-associated changes identified by quantitative flow cytometry. III. B-cell gating in CD37/kappa/lambda clonality test. Leukemia 1994; 8:1864–1870.
84. Press OW, Eary JF, Badger CC, et al. Treatment of refractory non-Hodgkin's lymphoma with radiolabeled MB-1 (anti-CD37) antibody. J Clin Oncol 1989; 7:1027–1038.
85. Press OW, Howell-Clark J, Anderson S, et al. Retention of B-cell-specific monoclonal antibodies by human lymphoma cells. Blood 1994; 83:1390–1397.
86. Belov L, de la Vega O, dos Remedios CG, et al. Immunophenotyping of leukemias using a cluster of differentiation antibody microarray. Cancer Res 2001; 61:4483–4489.
87. Marti GE, Zenger V, Brown M, et al. Antigenic expression of B-cell chronic lymphocytic leukemic cell lines. Leuk Lymphoma 1992; 7:497–504.
88. Binsky I, Haran M, Starlets D, et al. IL-8 secreted in a macrophage migration-inhibitory factor- and CD74-dependent manner regulates B cell chronic lymphocytic leukemia survival. Proc Natl Acad Sci U S A 2007; 104:13408–13413.
89. Stein R, Mattes MJ, Cardillo TM, et al. CD74: a new candidate target for the immunotherapy of B-cell neoplasms. Clin Cancer Res 2007; 13:5556s–5563s.
90. Stein R, Qu Z, Cardillo TM, et al. Antiproliferative activity of a humanized anti-CD74 monoclonal antibody, hLL1, on B-cell malignancies. Blood 2004; 104:3705–3711.
91. Lin K, Rockliffe N, Johnson GG, et al. Hsp90 inhibition has opposing effects on wild-type and mutant p53 and induces p21 expression and cytotoxicity irrespective of p53/ATM status in chronic lymphocytic leukaemia cells. Oncogene 2008; 27:2445–2455.
92. Johnson AJ, Wagner AJ, Cheney CM, et al. Rituximab and 17-allylamino-17-demethoxygeldanamycin induce synergistic apoptosis in B-cell chronic lymphocytic leukaemia. Br J Haematol 2007; 139:837–844.
93. Pelicano H, Carew JS, McQueen TJ, et al. Targeting Hsp90 by 17-AAG in leukemia cells: mechanisms for synergistic and antagonistic drug combinations with arsenic trioxide and Ara-C. Leukemia 2006; 20:610–619.
94. Jones DT, Addison E, North JM, et al. Geldanamycin and herbimycin A induce apoptotic killing of B chronic lymphocytic leukemia cells and augment the cells' sensitivity to cytotoxic drugs. Blood 2004; 103:1855–1861.
95. Castro JE, Prada CE, Loria O, et al. ZAP-70 is a novel conditional heat shock protein 90 (Hsp90) client: inhibition of Hsp90 leads to ZAP-70 degradation, apoptosis, and impaired signaling in chronic lymphocytic leukemia. Blood 2005; 106:2506–2512.

96. Contri A, Brunati AM, Trentin L, et al. Chronic lymphocytic leukemia B cells contain anomalous Lyn tyrosine kinase, a putative contribution to defective apoptosis. J Clin Invest 2005; 115:369–378.
97. Aguillon RA, Llanos CA, Suarez CJ, et al. Dasatinib induces apoptosis in chronic lymphocytic leukemia and enhances the activity of rituximab and fludarabine. Blood 2007; 110:1116 (abstr).
98. Veldurthy A, Patz M, Pallasch CP, et al. The Src-Abl kinase inhibitor dasatinib (BMS-354825) shows anti-proliferative and anti-apoptotic effects in chronic lymphocytic leukemia (CLL) cells in vitro. Blood 2007; 110:3101 (abstr).
99. Amrein PC, Attar EC, Takvorian T, et al. A phase II study of dasatinib in relapsed and refractory chronic lymphocytic leukemia (CLL/SLL). Blood 2007; 110:3126–.
100. Bali P, Pranpat M, Bradner J, et al. Inhibition of histone deacetylase 6 acetylates and disrupts the chaperone function of heat shock protein 90: a novel basis for antileukemia activity of histone deacetylase inhibitors. J Biol Chem 2005; 280:26729–26734.
101. Aron JL, Parthun MR, Marcucci G, et al. Depsipeptide (FR901228) induces histone acetylation and inhibition of histone deacetylase in chronic lymphocytic leukemia cells concurrent with activation of caspase 8-mediated apoptosis and down-regulation of c-FLIP protein. Blood 2003; 102:652–658.
102. Byrd JC, Shinn C, Ravi R, et al. Depsipeptide (FR901228): a novel therapeutic agent with selective, in vitro activity against human B-cell chronic lymphocytic leukemia cells. Blood 1999; 94:1401–1408.
103. Inoue S, Walewska R, Dyer MJ, et al. Downregulation of Mcl-1 potentiates HDACi-mediated apoptosis in leukemic cells. Leukemia 2008; 22(4):819–825.
104. Natoni A, MacFarlane M, Inoue S, et al. TRAIL signals to apoptosis in chronic lymphocytic leukaemia cells primarily through TRAIL-R1 whereas cross-linked agonistic TRAIL-R2 antibodies facilitate signalling via TRAIL-R2. Br J Haematol 2007; 139:568–577.
105. Inoue S, Riley J, Gant TW, et al. Apoptosis induced by histone deacetylase inhibitors in leukemic cells is mediated by Bim and Noxa. Leukemia 2007; 21:1773–1782.
106. Inoue S, Mai A, Dyer MJ, et al. Inhibition of histone deacetylase class I but not class II is critical for the sensitization of leukemic cells to tumor necrosis factor-related apoptosis-inducing ligand-induced apoptosis. Cancer Res 2006; 66:6785–6792.
107. MacFarlane M, Inoue S, Kohlhaas SL, et al. Chronic lymphocytic leukemic cells exhibit apoptotic signaling via TRAIL-R1. Cell Death Differ 2005; 12:773–782.
108. Inoue S, MacFarlane M, Harper N, et al. Histone deacetylase inhibitors potentiate TNF-related apoptosis-inducing ligand (TRAIL)-induced apoptosis in lymphoid malignancies. Cell Death Differ 2004; 11(suppl 2):S193–S206.
109. Lucas DM, Davis ME, Parthun MR, et al. The histone deacetylase inhibitor MS-275 induces caspase-dependent apoptosis in B-cell chronic lymphocytic leukemia cells. Leukemia 2004; 18:1207–1214.
110. Byrd JC, Marcucci G, Parthun MR, et al. A phase 1 and pharmacodynamic study of depsipeptide (FK228) in chronic lymphocytic leukemia and acute myeloid leukemia. Blood 2005; 105:959–967.
111. West DA, Lucas DM, Davis ME, et al. The novel histone deacetylase inhibitor OSU-HDAC42 has class I and II histone deacetylase (HDAC) inhibitory activity and represents a novel therapy for chronic lymphocytic leukemia. Blood 2006; 108:2807 (abstr).
112. Castro JE, Loria OJ, Aguillon RA, et al. A phase II, open label study of AT-101 in combination with rituximab in patients with relapsed or refractory chronic lymphocytic leukemia. Evaluation of Two Dose Regimens. Blood 2007; 110:3119 (abstr).
113. O'Brien S, Kipps TJ, Faderl S, et al. A phase I trial of the small molecule pan-Bcl-2 family inhibitor GX15-070 administered intravenously (IV) every 3 weeks to patients with previously treated chronic lymphocytic leukemia (CLL). Blood 2005; 106:446 (abstr).
114. Wilson WH, Tulpule A, Levine AM, et al. A phase 1/2a study evaluating the safety, pharmacokinetics, and efficacy of ABT-263 in subjects with refractory or relapsed lymphoid malignancies. Blood 2007; 110:1371 (abstr).

11

Stem Cell Transplantation in CLL

John G. Gribben
St. Bartholomew's Hospital, CRUK Medical Oncology Unit,
Barts and The London School of Medicine, London, U.K.

INTRODUCTION

CLL is an extremely heterogeneous disease, with clinical course varying from patients who can live with CLL for decades and who never require therapy to those with a rapidly progressive and fatal malignancy. In addition, most patients with CLL are elderly. This means that for the vast majority of patients with CLL, hematopoietic stem cell transplantation (SCT) is not a suitable treatment option. However, younger patients will die of their disease and are better able to tolerate the toxicities associated with this approach. In addition, advances in the understanding of the biology of this disease have led to an increasing ability to identify patients likely to have more rapid disease progression, (1) and such younger patients are suitable candidates for SCT. Although encouraging results have been achieved in phase II clinical trials, there have been no prospective studies evaluating the outcome after SCT compared with conventional therapy unlike other hematological malignancies where the role of SCT for specific risk groups has been established in prospective studies (2–8). The biggest challenge remains identification of which patients with CLL are sufficiently high risk to merit SCT and when in the course of their disease that SCT should be considered.

Most phase II studies of transplantation in CLL have enrolled younger patients with "high-risk" disease, but this term is often loosely defined, and it is difficult to determine precisely the risk factors used in each of the reported studies. In addition, the majority of studies were performed in an era where only clinical risk characteristics were available. Considerable recent work has helped identify a number of clinical and biologic characteristics that allow identification of which patients with CLL may merit consideration for transplant. Newer risk factors such as cytogenetics (9), immunoglobulin heavy chain (IgVH) mutational status (10,11) and zeta-associated protein-70 (ZAP-70) expression (12–14) have been identified. The precise role of these factors in determining risk and which factors should be incorporated within risk assessment remains to be fully determined from ongoing clinical trials. However, there are sufficient data available for the European Bone Marrow Transplant (EBMT) to issue guidelines outlining indications for SCT in CLL (15). The guidelines conclude that there is evidence base for the efficacy of allogeneic SCT in CLL in high-risk patients. High-risk patients, defined as those with p53 deletions or mutations requiring treatment, are considered candidates for SCT in first remission. The results of ongoing studies will be required to assess the impact of biomarkers including IgVh mutational status and cytogenetic abnormalities in identifying other patient groups at sufficiently high risk to merit consideration for transplant in first remission. Other groups for whom allogeneic transplantation is indicated include young patients with CLL who fail to achieve complete remission (CR) or who progress within 12 months after purine analogues and those who relapse within 24 months after having achieved a response with purine analogue–based combination therapy or autologous transplantation. It should be stressed that none of these categories requires assessment of biologic risk factors.

ROLE OF ALLOGENEIC SCT IN CLL

Allogeneic SCT is associated with increased morbidity and mortality and for this reason has been studied even less extensively in CLL than in other leukemias. Nonetheless, it remains a potentially curative procedure that provides a tumor-free source of stem cells and allows exploitation of the graft versus leukemia (GVL) effect, which is evident in this disease. The morbidity and mortality result from regimen-related toxicity, graft versus host disease (GVHD), and infection; in registry data, transplant-related mortality (TRM) following allogeneic SCT in CLL patients was 46%, with mortality from GVHD of 20% (16). However, surviving patients have long-term disease control (16–20). The results of studies of allogeneic SCT in CLL are shown in Table 1.

The major advantage of allogeneic SCT is the potential for a GVL effect. Strong evidence for the presence of a GVL effect in CLL comes from the finding that there is a decreased risk of relapse in patients with chronic GVHD (21), increased risk of relapse with T-cell depletion (20), and response to therapy with donor lymphocyte infusion (DLI) (Fig. 1) (20). Studies from M.D. Anderson Cancer Center have demonstrated improved outcome after allogeneic compared with autologous SCT (22). Among 14 patients with chemorefractory CLL, 13 (87%) achieved CR posttransplant, 9 remained alive and in CR with median follow-up of 36 months (23), suggesting that allogeneic SCT can induce durable remission even in patients with refractory disease. Of 25 patients with CLL who underwent allogeneic SCT at the Fred Hutchinson Cancer Center (19), grade 2 to 4 acute

Table 1 Myeloablative Allogeneic Transplantation for CLL

Reference	No.	TRM	Severe GVHD	Ongoing CR	Median FU (mo)
Michellet et al. 1996 (16)	54	25	18	24	27
Khouri et al. 1997 (23)	15	5	26	8	35
Pavletic et al. 2000 (18)	23	8	47	14	24
Doney et al. 2002 (19)	25	7	56	9	60
Gribben et al. 2005 (20)	25	1 early 5 late	5	13 8 after DLI	78

Abbreviations: CLL, chronic lymphocytic leukemia; TRM, transplant-related mortality; GVHD, graft versus host disease; CR, complete remission; DLI, donor lymphocyte infusion; FU, follow up.

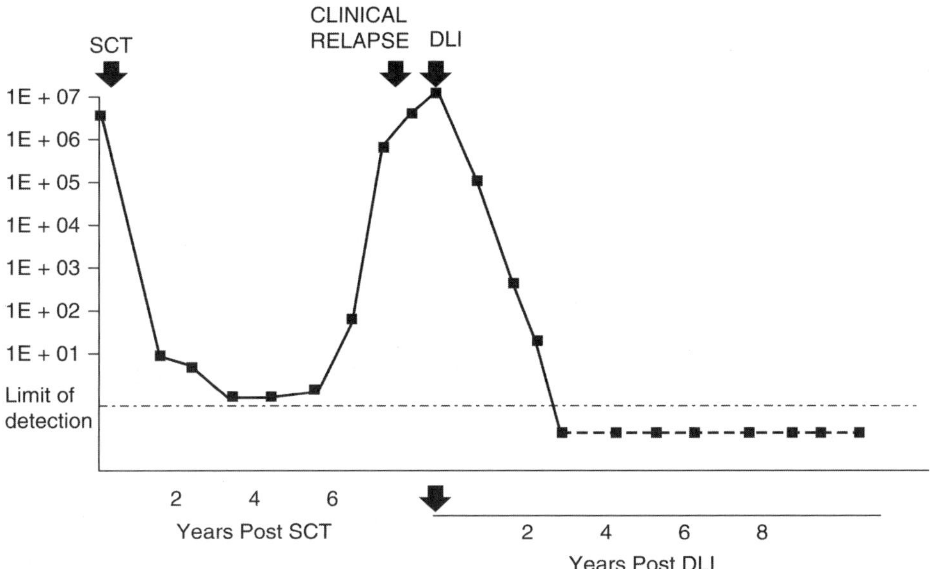

Figure 1 Response to DLI in CLL. Quantitative real-time PCR analysis of levels of disease following T-cell-depleted allogeneic SCT. DLI administered as sole therapy after clinical evidence of relapse induced subsequent achievement of CR and eradication of PCR-detectable disease. *Abbreviation*: DLI, donor lymphocyte infusion; CLL, chronic lymphocytic leukaemia; PCR, polymerase chain reaction. *Source*: From Ref. 20.

GVHD was seen in 14 patients and 10 developed clinical extensive chronic GVHD; the estimated overall survival (OS) at five years was 32%. Nonrelapse mortality at day 100 was unacceptably high at 57% for patients conditioned with busulfan and cyclophosphamide compared with 17% for patients conditioned with total body irradiation (TBI)-containing regimens. Among 30 patients (20 related donors and 10 unrelated donors) transplanted for CLL between 1989 and 2001 in Vancouver with a median follow-up of 4.3 years, 47% were alive in CR. Estimated OS and disease free-survival (DFS) at five years was 39% and a strong GVL effect was noted with those developing acute or chronic GVHD having near complete protection from relapse (21). IgVH mutation status maintains its poor prognostic significance after autologous SCT (24,25), but it would appear that this adverse event can be overcome with the use of allogeneic SCT (26). Among 50 patients who underwent SCT, 34 had unmutated IgVH genes (14 allogeneic SCT and 20 autologous SCT) and 16 had mutated IgVH genes (9 allogeneic SCT and 7 autologous SCT). There was no difference in CR rate between type of transplantation and IgVH mutational status; however, after a median follow-up of five years, there was a significantly higher relapse rate following autologous compared with allogeneic SCT in both mutational groups. Therefore, the GVL effect of allogeneic SCT may overcome the negative impact of unmutated IgVH gene mutation status on outcome.

Although there are no randomized studies comparing the outcome of autologous versus allogeneic SCT, a phase II study at Dana-Farber Cancer Institute enrolled 162 patients with high risk CLL in a "biologic randomization" in which 25 patients with an HLA (human leukocyte antigen)-matched sibling donor underwent T-cell-depleted myeloablative allogeneic SCT, while 137 with no sibling donor underwent B-cell-purged autologous SCT. The 100-day TRM was 4% after autologous or allogeneic SCT, but later, TRM had a major impact on outcome. At the median follow-up of 6.5 years, progression-free survival (PFS) was

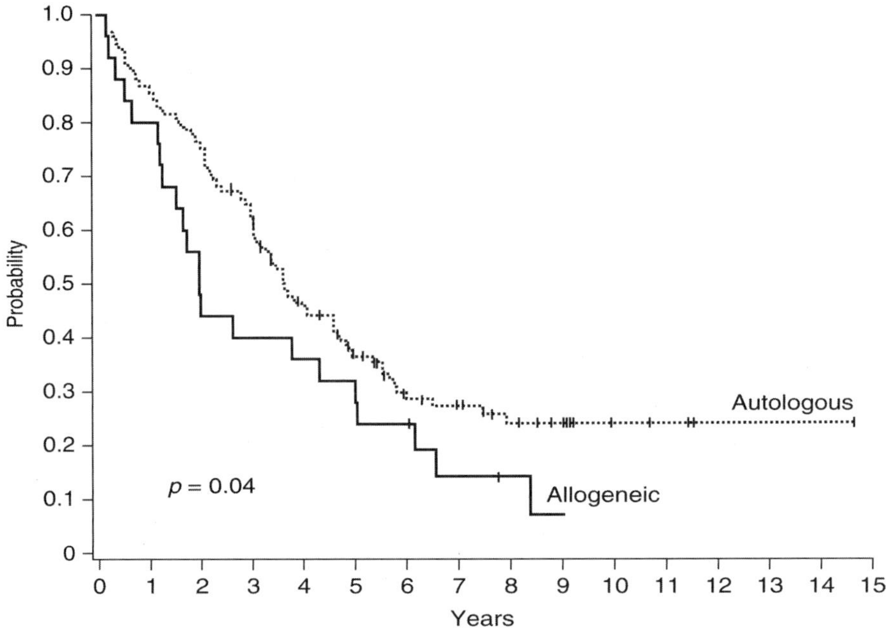

Figure 2 PFS after autologous and T-cell-depleted allogeneic SCT. *Abbreviation*: PFS, progression-free survival; SCT, stem cell transplantation. *Source*: From Ref. 20.

significantly longer following autologous than T-cell-depleted allogeneic SCT, but no significant differences were observed in disease recurrence or deaths without recurrence by type of transplant, and although there was a difference in progression free-survival (PFS) (Fig. 2) there was no difference in OS between the two groups, with OS of 58% after autologous and 55% after allogeneic SCT. Registry data is in support of this finding since the data demonstrated that although durable responses were achieved after allogeneic SCT, survival was worse after allogeneic than after autologous SCT with three years' probability of survival reported as 45% for allogeneic SCT and 87% for autologous SCT (27).

On the basis of these results, myeloablative allogeneic SCT is associated with high morbidity and mortality rates in CLL, and its use should be restricted to young patients with chemorefractory disease. TBI-containing regimens are associated with a lower TRM than chemotherapy-based regimens for this patient population and is the preferred preparative regimen.

REDUCED-INTENSITY CONDITIONING SCT FOR CLL

To improve outcome following allogeneic SCT, it will be necessary to exploit maximal GVL without concomitant GVHD and decrease the TRM. A major advance in reducing the short-term morbidity and mortality of allogeneic SCT has been the introduction of nonmyeloablative or reduced-intensity conditioning (RIC) regimens to allow engraftment of allogeneic stem cells. Although these procedures are commonly known as "mini–stem cell transplantation," this misnomer significantly underestimates the risks of such procedures, mainly due to the high incidence of GVHD. No formal assessment of RIC compared with myeloablative allogeneic SCT has been undertaken, but the outcome after RIC allogeneic SCT of 73 patients who had undergone RIC was compared with that of 82 matched patients who had undergone standard myeloablative conditioning for CLL from the EBMT registry database during the same period. Patients undergoing RIC transplants had significantly reduced TRM, but higher relapse incidence, and there was no significant difference in OS or PFS between these two groups (28). It appears that the results after RIC SCT are improving, and whether this is due to changes in patient selection or improvement in management of the complications following these procedures remains unclear.

Several RIC regimens have been developed, and there is wide variation in the regimen components and intensity, GVHD prophylaxis, and timing of the application of DLIs, which may contribute the subsequent morbidity of the procedure. In addition, there is a marked heterogeneity of patients' specific disease characteristics, and many patients to date have been treated on experimental treatment protocols that allowed enrollment of patients with chemorefractory end-stage disease. In this setting, the majority of the antilymphoma effect results from the graft versus lymphoma effect and not from the chemotherapy (29,30). The truly nonmyeloablative regimens are highly immunosuppressive and include regimens including cyclophosphamide and fludarabine, low-dose TBI with or without fludarabine, and the total lymphoid radiation with thymoglobulin. Median intensity regimens include fludarabine in combination with busulfan. More intense regimens, such as fludarabine and melphalan or the BEAM (Carmustine, etoposide, cytosine arabinoside, and melphalan) combination, allow cytoreduction and donor cell engraftment. To date, there is little evidence that any one of these regimens is associated with any survival advantage over any other, but there is little evidence to support the use of the higher-dose reduced-intensity regimens in patients with chemosensitive disease.

The major advantage of RIC regimens is that they allow transplantation in older patients, making this approach more applicable to increased numbers of CLL patients (29,31–35), which is a disease of the elderly. Results from selected studies are shown in Table 2. At median follow-up of two years, 23 of 30 patients (77%) were alive, with two-year estimated OS of 72%, PFS 67%, and nonrelapse mortality 15% (31). Acute GVHD grade 2 to 4 was seen in 17 patients (56%), with chronic GVHD in 21 patients (75%). Among 28 responding patients, 12 (40%) achieved CR, and late CR occurred up to two years after transplantation. Minimal residual disease (MRD) was monitored using clone-specific polymerase chain reaction. All CR patients analyzed achieved a molecular CR. The use of low-dose TBI with or without the addition of fludarabine has been reported for 64 patients with advanced CLL, using related ($N = 44$) or unrelated donors ($N = 20$) (33), with a median age of 56 (range 44–69) years. The majority of these patients were fludarabine refractory. TRM at 100 days was 11%, and 22% by two years, with significant GVHD remaining a problem. At a median follow-up of 24 months, 39 patients were alive, 25 in CR. Two-year OS was 60%, and DFS was 52%. Although complications were higher in the patients with unrelated donors, there were higher CR and lower relapse rates, suggesting more effective GVL activity with unrelated donors. Excellent results have been obtained at the M. D. Anderson Cancer Center using RIC based on a combination of fludarabine and cyclophosphamide, an approach designed to maximize GVL by early tapering of immune suppression with use of DLI and with the addition of rituximab. Among 39 patients treated, median age was 57 (range 34–70) years, and median time from diagnosis to transplantation was 4.5 years (34). All patients had recurrent advanced disease, were heavily pretreated with a median of 3 (range 2–8) chemotherapy regimens, and all had been previously treated with fludarabine-rituximab-based regimens. At transplant, 34 patients (87%) had active disease, including nine (23%) with evidence of Richter's transformation. In this series, only four of the donors were unrelated. Fourteen patients required immunomodulation with rituximab and DLI for persistent disease after

Table 2 RIC Allogeneic SCT for CLL

Reference	N	Age (yr) (range)	Prior regimens (range)	Chemorefractory (number with prior autologous SCT)	Donor (includes mismatch)	TRM	GVHD acute grade 2–4	Chronic extensive GVHD	Survival
Schetelig et al. 2002 (31)	30	50 (12–63)	3 (0–8)	47%	50% related 50% unrelated	13% overall	56%	21%	OS 72% 2 yr PFS 67%
Dreger et al. 2003 (32)	77	54 (30–66)	3 (0–8)	33% (10)	81% related	18% 12 mo	34%	58%	OS 72% 2 yr PFS 56%
Sorror et al. 2005 (33)	64	56 (44–69)	4	53%	69% related 31% unrelated	11% at 100 day 22% overall	61%	50%	OS 60% 2 yr PFS 52%
Khouri 2006 (34)	39	57 (34–70)	3 (2–8)	Not stated	90% related 10% unrelated	2% at 100 day	45%	58%	OS 48% 4 yr PFS 44%
Brown et al. 2006 (35)	46	53 (35–67)	5 (1–10)	57% (10)	33% related 67% unrelated	17% overall	34%	43%	OS 54% 2 yr PFS 34%
Delgado et al. 2006 (36)	41	54 (37–67)	3 (1–8)	27% (11)	58% related 42% unrelated	5% at 100 day 26% overall	10% (grade 3–4)	33%[a] (after DLI)[a]	OS 51% 2 yr PFS 45%

[a]after donor lymphocyte infusion (DLI).

Abbreviations: SCT, stem cell transplantation; CLL, chronic lymphocytic leukaemia; TRM, transplant-related mortality; GVHD, graft versus host disease; OS, overall survival; PFS, progression-free survival.

SCT. Only one patient died early, and among the 38 evaluable patients, 27 (71%) achieved CR; the estimated OS at four years was 48% with current PFS at 44%. Acute grade 2 to 4 GVHD was observed in 45%, and chronic extensive GVHD was seen in 58%.

Forty-six patients underwent RIC transplantation using fludarabine and busulfan, 67% using unrelated donors (35). These patients were heavily pretreated, with a median of five prior therapies (range 1–10); 10 (22%) had relapsed after prior autologous SCT. At the time of SCT, 26 (57%) had progressive chemoresistant disease, 50% had active progressive disease, 7% were induction failures, and only 17% were in CR. Two-year OS was 54%, and PFS 34% in this refractory patient population. The primary cause of treatment failure was relapse, with a two-year cumulative incidence of 48%. Factors associated with increased risk of relapse include low levels of donor chimerism at day 30, chemorefractory disease, increased number of previous therapies, and adverse cytogenetics (35).

Most reported patients were heavily pretreated and refractory to therapy, but despite this, the majority demonstrated donor engraftment, and there was a high CR rate. The induction of molecular remissions in patients with advanced CLL and the observation of late remissions in patients treated with low doses of chemotherapy provide the strongest direct evidence for a powerful GVL effect that can be exploited in the management of CLL. When immune manipulation is planned, this should be performed early before the tumor becomes too bulky.

It is clear from the results seen in Table 2 that GVHD remains a major concern. The addition of alemtuzumab to the conditioning regimen can decrease the incidence of GVHD, but results in delayed immune reconstitution, increased risk of infective complications, particularly cytomegalovirus (CMV) infections, and impairs the GVL effect. In 41 consecutive CLL patients treated (24 HLA-matched sibling donors and 17 unrelated volunteer donors, including 4 mismatched) the conditioning regimen alemtuzumab, fludarabine and melphalan, had significant antitumor effects with 100% of patients with chemosensitive disease and 86% with chemorefractory disease responding (36). The TRM rate was 26%, OS 51%, and relapse risk 29% at two years. GVHD rates were relatively low with acute GVHD (aGVHD) occurring in 17 (41%) and chronic GVHD (cGVHD) in 13 (33%). The unexpectedly high TRM rate was due to a high incidence of fungal and viral infections.

RISK FACTORS FOR POOR OUTCOME
AFTER RIC ALLOGENEIC SCT

RIC procedures are currently investigational in nature, and although the acute morbidity and mortality appears significantly lower compared to high-dose conditioning regimens with myeloablative allogeneic SCT, longer-term results with regard to morbidity of chronic GVHD and disease control are currently lacking. Further research is required to elucidate the mechanisms of treatment failure after RIC allogeneic SCT. It is not clear whether chemotherapy-refractory disease and adverse cytogenetics predict intrinsic resistance to graft versus CLL activity, since these could be markers of aggressive disease that progresses too rapidly to be controlled even by an active immune response.

High-dose therapy and myeloablative conditioning regimens do not appear to be necessary to overcome the poor prognostic impact of IgV$_H$ mutational status and cytogenetics. Thirty patients with poor prognosis CLL as defined by mutational status of VH genes and cytogenetic abnormalities (11q–, 17p–) who had undergone RIC allogeneic SCT had an OS of 90% and DFS of 92%; this was not significantly different from that seen in the good prognosis group (37).

The impact of ZAP-70 expression on outcome was retrospectively examined in 39 patients with CLL who had undergone RIC allogeneic SCT (38). Using immunohistochemical techniques on bone marrow biopsies, 25 patients were ZAP-70 positive, 13 were ZAP-70 negative, and 1 was of indeterminate status. Patients who were ZAP-70 positive had a median age of 54 years. With a median follow-up time of 41 months (range 4–80 months), their OS and current PFS rates at four years were 56% and 53%, respectively. By multivariate analysis, chemorefractory disease at transplantation ($p = 0.01$) and mixed T-cell chimerism at day 90 ($p = 0.02$) but not ZAP-70 status were correlated with the risk of progression after transplantation.

The fact that even heavily pretreated patients with refractory disease can achieve objective responses suggests some capacity of GVL reaction to control the disease, at least transiently (35). However, on multivariate analysis, chemotherapy-refractory disease at transplantation was associated with a 3.2-fold risk of progression and a 4.6-fold risk of death. Increasing number of previous therapies and increasing bone marrow involvement were also associated with decreased PFS and OS. High–hematopoietic donor chimerism on day 30 was also a significant predictor of two-year PFS. It is not clear whether achieving high–early-donor chimerism is primarily a function of disease status prior to transplant or of GVL activity. In either case, research efforts to enhance early-donor chimerism could include better cytoreduction and bone marrow debulking prior to NST, early taper of immunosuppression, or DLI. Maintaining this initial graft versus CLL response over time would then be the challenge. Relapses tend to reflect the original pattern of disease, suggesting a widespread loss of GVL activity. Consistent with this hypothesis, once relapse occurred in this study, less than 20% responded to DLI infusions alone (31,33,36). Coculture of CLL cells with allogeneic T cells induces changes in gene expression of the donor T cells, suggesting that tumor bulk might have a direct ability to impair effector T-cells' function. Research efforts to promote and sustain the initial GVL reaction are therefore needed and could include transplantation of patients earlier in their disease course while they are still chemoresponsive, planned prophylactic DLI, vaccination with or without cytokine stimulation, or maintenance antibody therapy.

AUTOLOGOUS SCT

The antitumor activity of autologous SCT is dependent upon a dose-response effect in CLL, and there is good evidence for such an effect in CLL (39–41). The role of autologous SCT has not been established since there have been no prospective randomised trials that have compared the outcome following autologous SCT with standard chemotherapy in CLL. However, a retrospective matched-pair analysis suggested a survival advantage for autologous SCT over conventional therapy (25). In this analysis, a risk-matched comparison was made between 66 patients who had undergone a uniform high-dose therapy and autologous SCT with a database of 291 patients treated conventionally. The variables matched included age, Binet stage, IgVH gene mutational status, and lymphocyte count. The study identified 44 pairs who were fully matched for all four variables and who were well balanced for additional risk factors including adverse genomic abnormalities and CD38 expression. With an overall median follow-up time of 70 and 86 months, respectively, survival was significantly longer for the patients who had undergone autologous SCT compared with conventionally treated patients when calculated from diagnosis ($p = 0.03$) or from study entry ($p = 0.006$).

A number of phase II studies have been reported examining the outcome following autologous SCT for CLL (20,22,42–48). These studies have demonstrated that this

Table 3 Autologous Transplantation for CLL

Reference	No. of patients	TRM	Ongoing CR	Median FU (mo)
Rabinowe et al. 1993 (42)	12	1 early	5	12
Khouri et al. 1994 (22)	11	1	2	10
Itala et al. 1997 (43)	5	0	4	9
Pavletic et al. 1998 (44)	16	2	5	37
Dreger et al. 1998 (45)	13	0	12	19
Sutton et al. 1998 (46)	8 20 enrolled 12 stem cells collected	0	5	36
Milligan et al. 2005 (47)	65	1 early 5 MDS/AML	45	36
Gribben et al. 2005 (20)	137	5 early 13 MDS/AML 15 other cancer	67	78
Jantunen et al. 2006 (48)	77	0	50	28

Abbreviations: TRM, transplant-related mortality; CR, complete remission; MDS, myelodysplasia; AML, acute myeloid leukaemia; FU, follow up.

approach is feasible in CLL with a TRM of 1% to 10%, with most toxicity occurring late (Table 3). Encouraging early results were reported in a pilot study in patients with chemosensitive relapsed disease (42). Eligibility criteria for entry into this study included documented chemosensitivity and achievement of a protocol-eligible minimal disease status. Following this pilot study, a total of 137 patients with chemosensitive disease underwent autologous SCT in a phase II study (20).

Patients transplanted in relapse or with chemoresistant disease had poor outcome with autologous SCT (22). These patients were heavily pretreated and underwent autologous SCT not at a time of minimal tumor burden but after subsequent relapse. Seven patients received stem cells purged by immunomagnetic depletion, but residual clonal B cells remained detectable in five patients. The outcome of these patients was poor. Three underwent a Richter's transformation, two died in CR, and two relapsed. Only two patients achieved CR and one achieved a partial remission. Poor results with a high relapse rate after autologous SCT were also observed in a study of 16 CLL patients in whom eight had relapsed and six had died (three from progressive malignancy) at a median follow-up of 41 months (44). Eight heavily pretreated patients received autologous SCT with partially purged CD34+ peripheral blood stem cells, and although four patients remained in CR, the median follow-up was very short at only nine months (43). When autologous SCT is performed early in the course of the disease, outcome appears better. Among 18 such patients enrolled, autologous SCT was performed in 13 patients, only one of whom had relapsed at the time of publication (45).

In a Medical Research Council (MRC) study, only one TRM was seen among 65 patients who underwent autologous SCT, and the CR rate after transplantation was 74% (48 of 65) (47). The five-year estimated OS was 77.5% and PFS was 51.5%. None of the variables examined at study entry were predictive for OS or DFS, but detectable MRD after transplant was highly predictive of disease recurrence. There was no TRM among 72 patients who underwent autologous SCT in five Finnish centers; median age was 57 (range 38–69) years, and transplantation was performed at a median of 32 (range 6–181) months from diagnosis (48). At median follow-up of 28 months, 37% had progressed, with median OS of 95 months and median PFS of 48 months.

FEASIBILITY OF AUTOLOGOUS SCT

In many of the phase II studies, it is not possible to determine the denominator since patients were often referred to the transplant center after having achieved protocol-eligible response to therapy, and patients who failed to achieve this level of response may not have been referred or referred for allogeneic SCT. However, single-center studies have suggested that less than 50% of patients enrolled on an intent-to-treat basis will proceed to autologous SCT (46). Among 20 patients with relapsed CLL enrolled in this study, 13 patients responded to salvage chemotherapy, stem cells were collected from eight patients, but only eight patients proceed to autologous SCT. It is difficult to collect sufficient CD34+ cells in CLL, especially in heavily pretreated CLL patients, and at least three months should be allowed between the last dose of fludarabine and leukapheresis (49). Among 115 previously untreated CLL patients prospectively enrolled in a multicenter pilot study to assess the feasibility of performing autologous SCT, only 65 (56%) proceeded to transplant (47).

EX VIVO AND IN VIVO PURGING OF STEM CELLS

A number of methods including multiparameter flow cytometry analysis (50) and polymerase chain reaction (PCR) (51) are being used to investigate whether persistence of MRD will predict which patients will relapse following transplant in CLL. Molecular remissions can be achieved in more than two-thirds of patients, but these are not durable (47,51–53), and most patients who achieve CR after autologous SCT will eventually relapse. Detectable molecular disease posttransplant is highly predictive of clinical recurrence (47,51). One approach to increase the likelihood of elimination of MRD after autologous SCT is to attempt to eradicate any residual lymphoma cells ex vivo using monoclonal antibodies (20). Ex vivo purging of stem cells results in stem cell loss, which might be overcome by in vivo treatment with alemtuzumab or rituximab. When alemtuzumab was used in the conditioning regimen for autologous SCT in one arm of the German CLL Study Group CLL3 trial, 12 of 16 patients (87%) developed a skin rash between 43 and 601 days post-SCT, and in seven of these patients, a biopsy confirmed GVHD, which persisted for a median duration of 517 (range 60–867) days (54). The trial was discontinued because of the TRM, but addition of alemtuzumab led to improved disease control.

The concept of using alemtuzumab for in vivo purging should perhaps not yet be discarded. When used at a modification from the standard dose (10 mg subcutaneously 3 times per week for 6 weeks) in 34 patients who had had a clinical response to a fludarabine-based regimen, the CR rate improved from 35% to 79.5% with 56% achieving eradication of MRD (55). Peripheral blood stem cell collection was subsequently successfully performed in 92%. Eighteen patients underwent autologous SCT with 17 remaining in CR at a median follow-up of 14.5 months post-SCT.

LATE COMPLICATIONS

Studies reported with short follow-up focus only on the early posttransplant TRM. Of particular concern are the late consequences of high-dose therapy and autologous SCT. Notable among these is the development of secondary myelodysplasia (MDS) and acute myeloid leukaemia (AML) after autologous SCT. Among 65 newly diagnosed patients treated with fludarabine followed by autologous SCT, eight developed MDS/AML (47), with a five-year actuarial risk of developing MDS/AML of 12.4% (95% CI, 2.5–24%) after autologous SCT. No potential risk factor analyzed was predictive. The group postulate that potential causative factors may be exposure to fludarabine, the low stem cell dose infused, and use of TBI in the conditioning regimen. The study with the longest follow up is from the Dana-Farber Cancer Institute (20), which reports not only a high incidence of secondary MDS/AML but also a high incidence of other tumors with longer follow-up. Second (non-CLL) malignancies developed after SCT in 31 (19%) patients. The median time from transplantation to the diagnosis of a hematological second malignancy was 35 months (range 1–138 months). Thirteen patients (9%) have developed MDS at a median of 36 months (range 11–87 months) after autologous SCT. Eight (62%) of the 13 patients diagnosed with MDS developed MDS during remission, whereas five patients developed MDS after progression of their CLL. At eight years after transplantation, the incidence of MDS was 12% (95% CI, 5–19%), and no patients have developed MDS at a later point of time than this. The risk of MDS was not associated with the type of prior therapy ($p = 0.99$). One patient developed diffuse large B-cell lymphoma at 13 months and another a T-cell lymphoma at 138 months after autologous SCT. The B-cell lymphoma was not related to the underlying CLL clone, as assessed by IgH gene rearrangement sequencing from both malignancies. Fifteen patients have developed other cancers at a median time of 41 months (range 23–114 months) after SCT; four nonmelanomatous skin cancers at 26 to 109 months and one melanoma at 25 months after autologous SCT. Nine patients have developed carcinomas at a median of 81 months (range 28–114 months) after autologous SCT (2 colorectal, 2 breast, 3 lung, 1 head and neck, and 1 prostate cancer). Only two of these patients also had CLL progression. It is well recognized that patients with CLL are at greater risk for development of other cancers, but there is concern that the incidence of second malignancies after autologous SCT is higher than might be expected. This finding is not specific for autologous SCT for CLL, and a second cancer is the most common cause of late TRM after autologous SCT (56).

ROLE OF AUTOLOGOUS SCT IN CLL

From the available data, it seems clear that patients have better outcome after autologous SCT when they are treated early in the course of the disease and at a time with low tumor burden, suggesting that high-risk patients should be transplanted early in their disease course (45). However, high-risk patients may also have an adverse outcome after SCT, and IgV_H mutation status maintains its poor prognostic significance after autologous SCT (24,25), although more than 90% of the patients undergoing autologous SCT in one series had unmutated IgV_H genes (20). The major problem after autologous SCT remains relapse of disease, late complications, and no evidence of a plateau in DFS (Fig. 3) (20). On the basis of the results obtained to date, autologous SCT is not recommended in routine clinical practice and should be offered only in the setting of well-designed clinical trials.

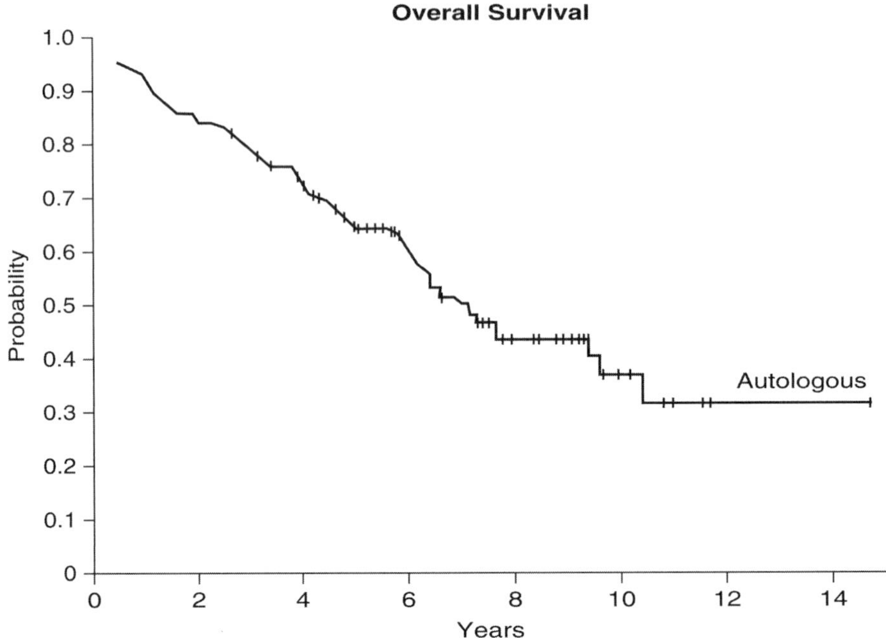

Figure 3 OS after autologous SCT. *Abbreviation*: OS, overall survival; SCT, stem cell transplantation. *Source*: From Ref. 20.

SUMMARY

Despite improvements in outcome achieved using chemoimmunotherapy approaches in chronic lymphocytic leukemia (CLL), the disease remains incurable. Younger patients as well as those with adverse prognostic factors will die from their disease. These patients are therefore candidates to investigate the potential role of hematopoietic stem cell transplantation (SCT) in the management of their disease. Most interest recently has focused on the use of reduced-intensity conditioning allogeneic SCT, which attempts to exploit the graft versus leukemia effect of allogeneic donor cells but to reduce the toxicity. Myeloablative allogeneic SCT is associated with high treatment-related morbidity and mortality but few late relapses. Autologous SCT is feasible and safe, but there is a high incidence of subsequent relapse. With many potential treatments available, appropriate patient selection and the timing of stem cell transplantation in the management of CLL remain controversial and remain the focus of ongoing clinical trials.

CONCLUSIONS

SCT has a role to play only in selected patients with high-risk CLL. Myeloablative allogeneic SCT has high TRM and morbidity and should be restricted to patients with very poor prognosis. Although no direct comparisons of myeloablative and RIC transplants have been performed, given the older age of patients with CLL, it seems most reasonable to consider RIC regimens' transplants as the approach of choice for patients with CLL in whom SCT is being considered. Although RIC SCT appears to result in high response rates and eradication of PCR-detectable MRD, the follow-up of most clinical trials is too short to assess whether SCT can cure CLL. Autologous SCT is feasible in younger patients with poor risk CLL but is not curative, particularly in patients with high-risk disease. Autologous SCT may result in prolongation of OS compared with conventional therapy, but this must always be considered in the context of improved outcome using conventional chemoimmunotherapy.

Future approaches to the management of this disease must take into account the balance between the increased morbidity and mortality of SCT in CLL with the curative potential that these approaches potentially offer in the setting of the improvements in outcome that can now be seen using chemoimmunotherapy. In the absence of any other treatment modalities currently capable of improving outcome in this disease, SCT should be considered as a treatment approach for younger patients with high-risk CLL early in the course of the disease, ideally in the setting of well-designed clinical trials assessing the impact of this treatment on outcome in these patients.

REFERENCES

1. Seiler T, Dohner H, Stilgenbauer S. Risk stratification in chronic lymphocytic leukemia. Semin Oncol 2006; 33(2):186–194.
2. Philip T, Armitage JO, Spitzer G, et al. High-dose therapy and autologous bone marrow transplantation after failure of conventional chemotherapy in adults with intermediate-grade or high-grade non-Hodgkin's lymphoma. N Engl J Med 1987; 316:1493–1498.
3. Schouten HC, Qian W, Kvaloy S, et al. High-dose therapy improves progression-free survival and survival in relapsed follicular non-Hodgkin's lymphoma: results from the randomized European CUP trial. J Clin Oncol 2003; 21(21):3918–3927.
4. Burnett AK, Wheatley K, Goldstone AH, et al. The value of allogeneic bone marrow transplant in patients with acute myeloid leukaemia at differing risk of relapse: results of the UK MRC AML 10 trial. Br J Haematol 2002; 118(2):385–400.
5. Suciu S, Mandelli F, de Witte T, et al. Allogeneic compared with autologous stem cell transplantation in the treatment of patients younger than 46 years with acute myeloid leukemia (AML) in first complete remission (CR1): an intention-to-treat analysis of the EORTC/GIMEMAAML-10 trial. Blood 2003; 102(4):1232–1240.
6. Dombret H, Gabert J, Boiron JM, et al. Outcome of treatment in adults with Philadelphia chromosome-positive acute lymphoblastic leukemia—results of the prospective multicenter LALA-94 trial. Blood 2002; 100(7):2357–2366.
7. Sebban C, Lepage E, Vernant JP, et al. Allogeneic bone marrow transplantation in adult acute lymphoblastic leukemia in first complete remission: a comparative study. French Group of Therapy of Adult Acute Lymphoblastic Leukemia. J Clin Oncol 1994; 12(12):2580–2587.
8. Attal M, Harousseau JL, Stoppa AM, et al. A prospective, randomized trial of autologous bone marrow transplantation and chemotherapy in multiple myeloma. Intergroupe Francais du Myelome. N Engl J Med 1996; 335(2):91–97.
9. Dohner H, Stilgenbauer S, Benner A, et al. Genomic aberrations and survival in chronic lymphocytic leukemia. N Engl J Med 2000; 343(26):1910–1916.
10. Damle RN, Wasil T, Fais F, et al. Ig V gene mutation status and CD38 expression as novel prognostic indicators in chronic lymphocytic leukemia. Blood 1999; 94(6):1840–1847.
11. Hamblin TJ, Davis Z, Gardiner A, et al. Unmutated Ig V(H) genes are associated with a more aggressive form of chronic lymphocytic leukemia. Blood 1999; 94(6):1848–1854.
12. Crespo M, Bosch F, Villamor N, et al. ZAP-70 expression as a surrogate for immunoglobulin-variable-region mutations in chronic lymphocytic leukemia. N Engl J Med 2003; 348(18):1764–1775.
13. Rassenti LZ, Huynh L, Toy TL, et al. ZAP-70 compared with immunoglobulin heavy-chain gene mutation status as a predictor of disease progression in chronic lymphocytic leukemia. N Engl J Med 2004; 351(9):893–901.
14. Orchard JA, Ibbotson RE, Davis Z, et al. ZAP-70 expression and prognosis in chronic lymphocytic leukaemia. Lancet 2004; 363(9403):105–111.

15. Dreger P, Corradini P, Kimby E, et al. Indications for allogeneic stem cell transplantation in chronic lymphocytic leukemia: the EBMT transplant consensus. Leukemia 2007; 21(1):12–17.
16. Michallet M, Archimbaud E, Bandini G, et al. HLA-identical sibling bone marrow transplantation in younger patients with chronic lymphocytic leukemia. European Group for blood and marrow transplantation and the International bone marrow transplant registry. Ann Internal Med 1996; 124:311–315.
17. Khouri I, Champlin R. Allogenic bone marrow transplantation in chronic lymphocytic leukemia. Ann Internal Med 1996; 125(9):780–787.
18. Pavletic ZS, Arrowsmith ER, Bierman PJ, et al. Outcome of allogeneic stem cell transplantation for B cell chronic lymphocytic leukemia. Bone Marrow Transplant 2000; 25(7):717–722.
19. Doney KC, Chauncey T, Appelbaum FR. Allogeneic related donor hematopoietic stem cell transplantation for treatment of chronic lymphocytic leukemia. Bone Marrow Transplant 2002; 29(10):817–823.
20. Gribben JG, Zahrieh D, Stephans K, et al. Autologous and allogeneic stem cell transplantation for poor risk chronic lymphocytic leukemia. Blood 2005; 106(13):4389–4396.
21. Toze CL, Galal A, Barnett MJ, et al. Myeloablative allografting for chronic lymphocytic leukemia: evidence for a potent graft-versus-leukemia effect associated with graft-versus-host disease. Bone Marrow Transplant 2005; 36(9):825–830.
22. Khouri IF, Keating MJ, Vriesendorp HM, et al. Autologous and allogeneic bone marrow transplantation for chronic lymphocytic leukemia: preliminary results. J Clin Oncol 1994; 12(4): 748–758.
23. Khouri IF, Przepiorka D, van Besien K, et al. Allogeneic blood or marrow transplantation for chronic lymphocytic leukaemia: timing of transplantation and potential effect of fludarabine on acute graft-versus-host disease. Br J Haematol 1997; 97(2):466–473.
24. Ritgen M, Lange A, Stilgenbauer S, et al. Unmutated immunoglobulin variable heavy-chain gene status remains an adverse prognostic factor after autologous stem cell transplantation for chronic lymphocytic leukemia. Blood 2003; 101(5):2049–2053.
25. Dreger P, Stilgenbauer S, Benner A, et al. The prognostic impact of autologous stem cell transplantation in patients with chronic lymphocytic leukemia: a risk-matched analysis based on the VH gene mutational status. Blood 2004; 103(7):2850–2858.
26. Moreno C, Villamor N, Colomer D, et al. Allogeneic stem-cell transplantation may overcome the adverse prognosis of unmutated VH gene in patients with chronic lymphocytic leukemia. J Clin Oncol 2005; 23(15):3433–3438.
27. Horowitz M, Montserrat E, Sobocinski K, et al. Haemopoietic stem cell transplantation for chronic lymphocytic leukaemia. Blood 2000; 96(suppl. 1): 2245 (abstr).
28. Dreger P, Brand R, Milligan D, et al. Reduced-intensity conditioning lowers treatment-related mortality of allogeneic stem cell transplantation for chronic lymphocytic leukemia: a population-matched analysis. Leukemia 2005; 19(6):1029–1033.
29. Khouri IF, Keating M, Korbling M, et al. Transplant-lite: induction of graft-versus-malignancy using fludarabine-based nonablative chemotherapy and allogeneic blood progenitor-cell transplantation as treatment for lymphoid malignancies. J Clin Oncol 1998; 16(8):2817–2824.
30. Khouri IF, Saliba RM, Giralt SA, et al. Nonablative allogeneic hematopoietic transplantation as adoptive immunotherapy for indolent lymphoma: low incidence of toxicity, acute graft-versus-host disease, and treatment-related mortality. Blood 2001; 98(13):3595–3599.
31. Schetelig J, Thiede C, Bornhauser M, et al. Evidence of a graft-versus-leukemia effect in chronic lymphocytic leukemia after reduced-intensity conditioning and allogeneic stem-cell transplantation: the Cooperative German Transplant Study Group. J Clin Oncol 2003; 21(14): 2747–2753.
32. Dreger P, Brand R, Hansz J, et al. Treatment-related mortality and graft-versus-leukemia activity after allogeneic stem cell transplantation for chronic lymphocytic leukemia using intensity-reduced conditioning. Leukemia 2003; 17(5):841–848.
33. Sorror ML, Maris MB, Sandmaier BM, et al. Hematopoietic cell transplantation after nonmyeloablative conditioning for advanced chronic lymphocytic leukemia. J Clin Oncol 2005; 23(16):3819–3829.

34. Khouri IF. Reduced-intensity regimens in allogeneic stem-cell transplantation for non-hodgkin lymphoma and chronic lymphocytic leukemia. Hematology Am Soc Hematol Educ Program 2006: 390–397.

35. Brown JR, Kim HT, Li S, et al. Predictors of improved progression-free survival after nonmyeloablative allogeneic stem cell transplantation for advanced chronic lymphocytic leukemia. Biol Blood Marrow Transplant 2006; 12(10):1056–1064.

36. Delgado J, Thomson K, Russell N, et al. Results of alemtuzumab-based reduced-intensity allogeneic transplantation for chronic lymphocytic leukemia: a British Society of Blood and Marrow Transplantation Study. Blood 2006; 107(4):1724–1730.

37. Caballero D, Garcia-Marco JA, Martino R, et al. Allogeneic transplant with reduced intensity conditioning regimens may overcome the poor prognosis of B-cell chronic lymphocytic leukemia with unmutated immunoglobulin variable heavy-chain gene and chromosomal abnormalities (11q- and 17p-). Clin Cancer Res 2005; 11(21):7757–7763.

38. Khouri IF, Saliba RM, Keating MJ. ZAP-70 status may not predict outcome after non-myeloablative allogeneic transplantation (NMT) in patients with chronic lymphocytic leukemia (CLL) who failed conventional chemotherapy. Blood 2005; 106(suppl 1):577a.

39. Eichhorst BF, Busch R, Hopfinger G, et al. Fludarabine plus cyclophosphamide versus fludarabine alone in first-line therapy of younger patients with chronic lymphocytic leukemia. Blood 2006; 107(3):885–891.

40. Keating MJ, O'Brien S, Albitar M, et al. Early results of a chemoimmunotherapy regimen of fludarabine, cyclophosphamide, and rituximab as initial therapy for chronic lymphocytic leukemia. J Clin Oncol 2005; 23(18):4079–4088.

41. Hallek M. Chronic Lymphocytic Leukemia (CLL): First-Line Treatment. Hematology Am Soc Hematol Educ Program 2005: 285–291.

42. Rabinowe SN, Soiffer RJ, Gribben JG, et al. Autologous and allogeneic bone marrow transplantation for poor prognosis patients with B-cell chronic lymphocytic leukemia. Blood 1993; 82(4):1366–1376.

43. Itala M, Pelliniemi TT, Rajamaki A, et al. Autologous blood cell transplantation in B-CLL: response to chemotherapy prior to mobilization predicts the stem cell yield. Bone Marrow Transplant 1997; 19(7):647–651.

44. Pavletic ZS, Bierman PJ, Vose JM, et al. High incidence of relapse after autologous stem-cell transplantation for B-cell chronic lymphocytic leukemia or small lymphocytic lymphoma. Ann Oncol 1998; 9(9):1023–1026.

45. Dreger P, von Neuhoff N, Kuse R, et al. Early stem cell transplantation for chronic lymphocytic leukaemia: a chance for cure? Br J Cancer 1998; 77(12):2291–2297.

46. Sutton L, Maloum K, Gonzalez H, et al. Autologous hematopoietic stem cell transplantation as salvage treatment for advanced B cell chronic lymphocytic leukemia. Leukemia 1998; 12(11): 1699–1707.

47. Milligan DW, Fernandes S, Dasgupta R, et al. Results of the MRC pilot study show autografting for younger patients with chronic lymphocytic leukemia is safe and achieves a high percentage of molecular responses. Blood 2005; 105(1):397–404.

48. Jantunen E, Itala M, Siitonen T, et al. Autologous stem cell transplantation in patients with chronic lymphocytic leukaemia: the Finnish experience. Bone Marrow Transplant 2006; 37(12): 1093–1098.

49. Michallet M, Thiebaut A, Dreger P, et al. Peripheral blood stem cell (PBSC) mobilization and transplantation after fludarabine therapy in chronic lymphocytic leukaemia (CLL): a report of the European Blood and Marrow Transplantation (EBMT) CLL subcommittee on behalf of the EBMT Chronic Leukaemias Working Party (CLWP). Br J Haematol 2000; 108(3):595–601.

50. Rawstron AC, Kennedy B, Evans PA, et al. Quantitation of minimal disease levels in chronic lymphocytic leukemia using a sensitive flow cytometric assay improves the prediction of outcome and can be used to optimize therapy. Blood 2001; 98(1):29–35.

51. Provan D, Bartlett-Pandite L, Zwicky C, et al. Eradication of polymerase chain reaction-detectable chronic lymphocytic leukemia cells is associated with improved outcome after bone marrow transplantation. Blood 1996; 88(6):2228–2235.

52. Schey S, Ahsan G, Jones R. Dose intensification and molecular responses in patients with chronic lymphocytic leukaemia: a phase II single centre study. Bone Marrow Transplant 1999; 24(9):989–993.
53. Schultze JL, Donovan JW, Gribben JG. Minimal residual disease detection after myeloablative chemotherapy in chronic lymphatic leukemia. J Mol Med 1999; 77(2):259–265.
54. Zenz T, Ritgen M, Dreger P, et al. Autologous graft-versus-host disease-like syndrome after an alemtuzumab-containing conditioning regimen and autologous stem cell transplantation for chronic lymphocytic leukemia. Blood 2006; 108(6):2127–2130.
55. Montillo M, Tedeschi A, Miqueleiz S, et al. Alemtuzumab as consolidation after a response to fludarabine is effective in purging residual disease in patients with chronic lymphocytic leukemia. J Clin Oncol 2006; 24(15):2337–2342.
56. Jantunen E, Itala M, Siitonen T, et al. Late non-relapse mortality among adult autologous stem cell transplant recipients: a nation-wide analysis of 1,482 patients transplanted in 1990–2003. Eur J Haematol 2006; 77(2):114–119.

12

Gene Therapy, Vaccines, and Immune Modulation

William G. Wierda
Department of Leukemia, Division of Cancer Medicine, University of Texas M.D. Anderson Cancer Center, Houston, Texas, U.S.A.

INTRODUCTION

Chronic lymphocytic leukemia (CLL) is a malignancy of well-differentiated B lymphocytes that express surface immunoglobulin and a constellation of surface differentiation antigens. CLL cells generally are resistant to apoptosis but maintain some of the physiologic functions of B cells such as the ability to present antigen when appropriately stimulated. Although there are a number of chromosome abnormalities associated with CLL such as trisomy 12 and deletions at 13q, 11q, or 17p, there have not been any genes found responsible for development or progression of the disease. Therefore, gene replacement or knockout strategies have not been considered. Gene therapy approaches for patients with CLL have primarily been directed at modifying autologous leukemia cells to produce antileukemia vaccines. Harnessing and utilizing the immune system as a therapeutic modality could provide a unique and powerful approach, distinct from traditional chemotherapy. Strategies will be reviewed in this chapter.

IMMUNE THERAPY AND CLL ANTIGENS

The objective of vaccine strategies for cancer is to induce cell- and humoral-mediated immune responses against autologous malignant cells to eliminate tumor and provide lasting protection from recurrence. Various vaccine strategies have been studied for patients with CLL, including vaccination with modified autologous leukemia cells and use of antigen-pulsed dendritic cells (Table 1).

Immune recognition of leukemia antigens is the basis for adaptive immunity and developing vaccine strategies. Leukemia antigens also can be a tool to study the interactions between the immune system and leukemia cells to evaluate mechanisms of immune regulation and suppression. There is limited data on leukemia antigens in CLL. Candidate CLL antigens studied to date are reviewed in Table 2. These antigens, or peptide fragments, typically are derived from proteins expressed by the leukemia cell and

Table 1 Active/Adaptive Immune-Based Treatment Strategies for CLL

Treatment	Examples	Target	Clinical trial
Modified autologous leukemia cell vaccine	Ad-CD154-modified autologous CLL cells	Unselected leukemia antigens	Phase I
	Oxidized autologous CLL cells	Unselected leukemia antigens	Phase I
Autologous dendritic cell vaccine	Antigen pulsed autologous dendritic cells	Selected antigen versus unselected leukemia antigens	Phase I/II
Activated autologous T cells	Xcellerate T cells	Unidentified leukemia antigen	Phase I/II
Allogeneic stem cell transplant	Donor hematopoietic cells (myeloablative vs. non-myeloablative conditioning)	Unidentified leukemia antigen	Phase II

Abbreviation: CLL, chronic lymphocytic leukemia.

are intracellular, surface, or secreted proteins. Antibody production (normal B cell mediated) providing humoral immunity is directed at surface proteins. Cellular immune recognition (T cell mediated) requires that antigen be degraded and processed into peptides that are displayed with major histocompatibility complex (MHC) molecules on the cell surface. The pathways to production and the peptides presented are different for MHC class I versus II molecules. Furthermore, MHC haplotype dictates and restricts which peptides are presented for a specific protein in the class I and II molecules. Therefore, the immunogenic antigens may be different between individuals for the same protein. Intracellular, surface, and secreted proteins can all be processed and presented with MHC and can be targets of cellular (T cell) immunity. Help from activated T cells is usually required for antibody production. This makes it difficult to identify a single antigen that applies to all patients for vaccine development and favors strategies with whole cells or cell lysates. Antibody production against antigen-MHC complexes is not a component of humoral antitumor immunity.

Tumor-associated antigen (TAA) and tumor-specific antigen (TSA) can serve as targets for immune recognition in both cellular and humoral responses. TSAs are antigens expressed by tumor cells but not by normal cells or normal tissues. TSAs are ideal candidates for vaccine strategies because they target the immune system to the tumor with little concern for cross-reaction with normal cells or tissues and as such are unlikely to be associated with autoimmunity. Immunoglobulin idiotype expressed by CLL cells is the best example of a TSA. The immunoglobulins expressed by CLL cells have features that distinguish them from antibodies made by normal, nonmalignant B cells, making them potential target antigens (21–23). Cellular proteins that have become mutated in the leukemia to produce unique antigens are also TSAs. TAAs are antigens that can be expressed in normal adult cells or tissues, or through development. The majority of antigens studied are TAAs.

Proteins that are required for survival of the leukemia cells are ideal candidates for vaccines. Leukemia cells must all express the antigen and could not evade immune recognition through loss of the antigen. Immunoglobulin is a good example of such an

Table 2 Potential Tumor Antigens in Patients with CLL

Potential CLL antigen	Reported normal function (location)	Expression in normal adult tissues	Expression in CLL	Immune responses in CLL pts
Idiotype (tumor-specific antigen) (1–3)	Antigen binding portion of immunoglobulin (surface)	None	Patient specific (100% of CLL cells)	T-cell response
Orphan receptor type 1 tyrosine kinase (ROR1) (4,5)	Developmental protein; organogenesis (surface)	None	100%	T cells NT; Ab response
Oncofetal antigen immature laminin receptor protein (OFA-iLRF) (6,7)	Mature form is cofactor to stabilize binding of laminin to integrins (surface)	Immature form not found in adult cells or tissues	Up to 100%; increased expression in advanced stage	T-cell response
Human telomerase reverse transcriptase (hTERT) (8)	Catalytic subunit of telomerase; telomere extension (intracellular)	Not detected in adult tissues	~75%	T-cell response
Fibromodulin (9,10)	Collagen-binding protein (extracellular)	Connective tissue	60–100%	T-cell response
RHAMM/CD168 (peptide R3) (11,12)	Mitotic spindle organization and maintenance; activates erk1 (intracellular)	Thymus; testis; placenta	>75%	T-cell response
Survivin (9,13,14)	IAP and regulates cell division (intracellular)	Thymus, testis, placenta; hormone stimulated hematologic progenitors and endothelial cells	0–75% (induced with CD40 ligation)	T-cell response
MDM2 (9,15)	Regulates cell growth, apoptosis, differentiation, DNA repair, and transcription; interacts with p53 (downstream) (intracellular)	Ubiquitous	75–100%	T-cell response
FMNL1 (9,16,17)	Regulates actin dynamics (intracellular)	PBMC; thymus; lung; spleen	~60%	T-cell response; Ab response
NTB-A (SLAMF6) (18)	Kinase involved in lymphocyte "activation" (surface)	B, T, and NK cells	100%	NT
SLLP1 (19)	Acrosomal c-lysozyme-like protein in spermatozoa	Testis; spermatozoa	~30%	Antibodies demonstrated in CLL patients
Adipophilin (20)	Adipose differentiation–related protein (intracellular)	Adipocytes; monocytes; macrophages;	Unknown	T-cell responses generated

Abbreviations: CLL, chronic lymphocytic leukemia; IAP, inhibitor of apoptosis; NT, not tested; PBMC, peripheral blood mononuclear cells; Pts, patients; Ab, antibody.

antigen in CLL. Ideal candidate vaccine antigens have limited expression in normal cells or tissues. This would be the case for developmental proteins such as ROR1 (4,5). Vaccination with these types of antigens could minimize the possibility of autoimmunity. Vaccines that utilize whole cells, cell lysates, or bulk mRNA do not select a particular tumor antigen but typically include multiple antigens. This has been the most common source of antigens with vaccines under investigation.

IMMUNE GENE THERAPY

Transfer of an immune-stimulatory gene into malignant cells and use of these autologous cells as a vaccine has been the most extensively studied strategy for gene therapy of hematologic malignancies, including B-cell leukemias and lymphomas. With this strategy, there are potentially multiple TSAs and TAAs that can induce an immune response.

Transduction of CLL Cells

Gene therapy typically employs a vector, which mediates transfer of the transgene into the cells being transduced. The ideal vector for development of cellular vaccines in gene therapy of CLL should have high transduction efficiency, allowing for infection of most leukemia cells and high-level expression of the selected transgene. To be considered for clinical use, a virus vector should be replication deficient and not cause active infection. Insertion of the virus genome and transgene (stable transduction) into the infected cells' genome usually requires cell replication, which does not occur with CLL cells; therefore, stable transduction is not usually feasible with CLL. The ideal vector should not induce CLL-cell proliferation or make the neoplastic cells clinically more aggressive. The vector should not be toxic to the CLL cells so that the transduced cells are able to express the transgene and have time to perform their intended function. Finally, the ideal vector should not result in expression of immune-dominant vector antigens that might compete with the development of antileukemia immune responses.

Adenovirus has been the most extensively studied vector for transduction of CLL cells. This virus offers many advantages over other virus vectors for gene transfer. Replication-defective adenovirus is not associated with serious infections, generally cannot transform infected cells, can be produced to high titer, is stable, and can infect post-mitotic, nondividing cells, such as most CLL cells. Serotypes 2 and 5 are the most widely used adenovirus vectors. Adenovirus infection usually occurs through viral attachment to the Coxsakie/adenovirus receptor (CAR). Lymphoid cells, particularly CLL cells, do not express CAR. Therefore, high titers of adenovirus must be used to transduce CLL cells. Viral attachment and entry is achieved via nonspecific uptake of virus. As such, a multiplicity of infection (MOI) of up to 1000 typically is needed to achieve high-level transgene expression in most CLL cells with adenovirus type 5 vectors.

Strategies are being developed to improve the transduction efficiency of adenovirus vectors for patients with CLL. Adenovirus serotype 35 (Ad35) is a group B adenovirus that infects cells by binding to CD46, a surface antigen present on all CLL cells. Studies demonstrated that Ad35-based vectors are more efficient at infecting and transducing CLL cells than standard Ad5-based vectors (24). Adeno-associated virus (AAV) vectors are nonenveloped human parvoviruses that also have been used to transduce CLL cells (25–27). These vectors may be more efficient at transducing CLL cells than Ad5-based vectors (27).

Herpes simplex virus (HSV) has been developed as a vector and evaluated for gene therapy of B-cell leukemias and lymphomas (28,29). CLL cells are highly sensitive to infection by herpes simplex virus-1 via herpesvirus-entry-mediator A (30). Analyses demonstrate that HSV amplicons are efficient vectors for gene transfer to neoplastic B cells, including CLL cells, and are expected to be suitable vectors for clinical gene transfer studies.

Transduction of CLL cells has also been demonstrated using nonviral methods, including electroporation-based delivery (31–33). Electroporation involves exposing the primary leukemia cells to an electrical pulse in appropriate buffer containing plasmid DNA carrying the transgene of interest. In this process, the cells take up the plasmid and subsequently express the transgene. These transduced cells, however, are short lived and can be cryopreserved for future use but cannot be maintained in culture for any significant period of time. Electroporation with mRNA (transgene) may result in longer-lived transduced cells (34).

Transgenes and Mechanisms of Immune Activation

The immune-stimulatory genes used as transgenes include immune cytokines, interleukin (IL)-2 and IL-12, as well as genes encoding immune accessory surface molecules, like CD80 and CD40-ligand (CD154).

Cytokine Genes

Interleukin-2 Transduction of tumor cells with the gene encoding IL-2 generates tumor cells that secrete large amounts of this cytokine, which in turn can stimulate local proliferation and activation of tumor-specific T cells and minimizes systemic toxicity. CLL cells have been transduced to express IL-2 with adenovirus vector. When these cells were combined in vitro with cells expressing CD154, a co-stimulatory molecule, the combined stimulation produced greater T-cell activation than either population alone (35). This combination was subsequently evaluated in clinical trial (see below).

Interleukin-12 Interleukin-12 is a potent cytokine that stimulates T and natural killer (NK) cells. In a preclinical animal model, replication-defective retrovirus encoding IL-12 was used to transduce the murine B lymphoma cell line A20. The IL-12-transduced A20 cells induced T cell–mediated antitumor immunity in vivo more effectively than A20 cells that were transduced with a control vector (36,37). Furthermore, in contrast to A20 cells or A20 cells transduced with a negative control vector, A20 cells made to express IL-12 via gene transfer could not form tumors following injection into syngeneic mice (37).

Surface Function-Associated Molecules

The coordinated expression of molecules on the surface of antigen-presenting cells (APCs) and T cells determine whether cell-cell interactions lead to antigen-specific T-cell activation and proliferation or T-cell anergy and tolerance. Productive T-cell activation requires APCs to present antigen to the T-cell receptor (TCR) via MHC class I or class II molecules (Signal 1) (Fig. 1). Stimulation through the TCR induces rapid T-cell expression of CD40-ligand (CD154), a member of the tumor necrosis factor (TNF) family (38,39). CD154 then binds CD40 on APCs and induces APC expression of co-stimulatory molecules, CD80 and CD86. These co-stimulatory molecules in turn bind to CD28 on

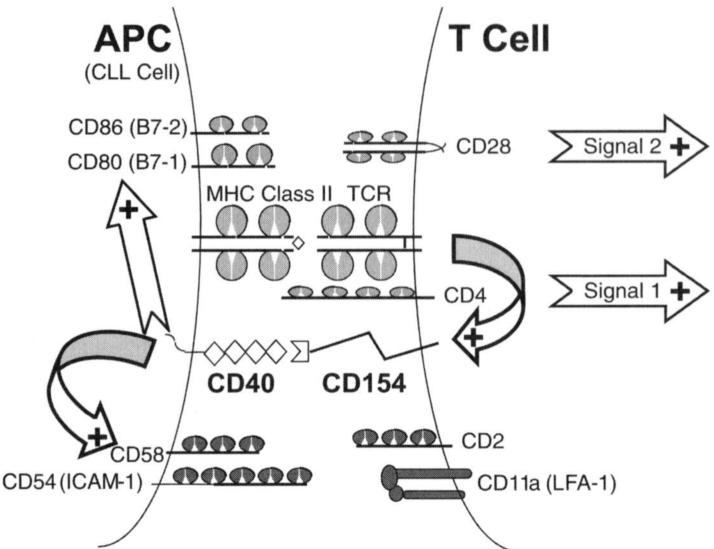

Figure 1 Cognate T cell-antigen presenting cell interactions.

activated T cells, providing a second signal to the T cells leading to their activation and proliferation (40,41).

CD80 and CD86 (B7-1 and B7-2)   The co-stimulatory molecules CD80 and CD86 bind to CD28 on T cells and provide "Signal 2" to T cells for activation and proliferation (Fig. 1). In preclinical studies, AAV was used to induce transient expression of CD80 and CD86 in myeloma cell lines (42). Tumor cell expression of CD80 and CD86 could activate T cells, resulting in high-level production of IL-2, interferon-gamma (INF-γ), and generation of tumor-specific cytotoxic T cells (42).

TRICOM is the name given to a vaccine strategy employing cells transduced to express immune co-stimulatory and adhesion molecules (43–45). TRICOM relies on gene transfer with fowlpox vector to affect expression of a triad of co-stimulatory and adhesion molecules, including CD80, intercellular adhesion molecule-1 (ICAM-1), and leukocyte function–associated antigen-3 (LFA-3). In an animal model, the modified cells could induce antitumor immune responses in vivo more effectively than nonmodified lymphoma cells (43,44). Subsequently, TRICOM was placed in a modified vaccinia virus strain Ankara (MVA) vector that was more efficient at transducing primary CLL cells. CLL cells transduced with this vector efficiently induced production of cytotoxic T lymphocytes (CTLs) against autologous CLL cells in vitro (45). Furthermore, the in vitro-derived CTLs were reactive against uninfected, unmodified CLL cells. It is reasonable to expect that this strategy will be evaluated in phase I clinical trial for patients with CLL.

CD40-ligand (CD154)   Advances in the understanding of how lymphocytes interact with one another provided insight into the mechanisms that contribute to T-cell dysfunction in patients with B-cell CLL (46). Importantly, CLL cells are stealth-like, which enables them to evade immune detection, even by allogeneic T cells from healthy donors. Despite expressing abundant amounts of MHC class II antigens, CLL cells do not stimulate normal allogeneic T cells in mixed lymphocyte reactions, even in the presence of neutralizing antibodies to immunosuppressive cytokines, such as transforming growth factor beta (TGF-β) (47). In addition, CLL cells can downmodulate CD154 expressed on activated T cells (47). Downmodulation of CD154 consequently abrogates expression of co-stimulatory molecules such as CD80 and CD86 on CLL cells and thereby interferes with effective antigen presentation. This mechanism may be, in part, responsible for the observed T-cell tolerance to the leukemia B cells in allogeneic and autologous mixed lymphocyte cultures. Therefore, for vaccine development using whole leukemia cells, it is critical to change the tolerance-inducing phenotype of CLL cells into one that can stimulate T cells to respond to leukemia-associated antigens.

Under certain conditions, the stealth-like phenotype of CLL cells can be reversed. When CLL cells are cultured with activated, CD154-expressing T cells, they express co-stimulatory molecules such as CD80, CD86, and CD54 (ICAM-1), which facilitate effective antigen presentation (46,48). Infection of CLL cells with a replication-defective adenovirus vector encoding recombinant CD40-ligand, Ad-CD154, induces prolonged expression of CD154 by the transduced CLL cells. This, in turn, induces expression of immune co-stimulatory molecules CD80 and CD86, making the modified CLL cells highly effective stimulators in autologous mixed lymphocyte reactions. Moreover, such cells can stimulate and expand CTLs specific for autologous noninfected leukemia cells in vitro (49). Also, factors that potentially render the leukemia B cells tolerogenic, such as expression of CD27, are downmodulated following transduction with Ad-CD154. A study comparing CLL cells stimulated via exogenous CD154 with CLL cells transduced to express CD154 in their relative capacity to stimulate and activate autologous T cells (9) demonstrated that CLL cells transduced to express CD154 were more efficient at stimulating and activating antigen-specific T cells than CLL cells that were stimulated with exogenous CD154.

Through an innate immune mechanism, CD40 activation of CLL cells upregulates expression of death receptors, such as CD95 (Fas) and DR5. Although CLL cells are resistant to CD95-mediated apoptosis immediately following CD40 activation, they become increasingly sensitive to CD95-mediated apoptosis over time, a phenomenon known as *latent sensitivity to Fas-mediated apoptosis* (50). The pro-apoptotic shift is, in part, the result in decline in the amount of FLICE-inhibitory protein (FLIP) and increase in Fas-associated death domain protein (FADD) and DAP3, which facilitate signaling leading to apoptosis following ligation of these death receptors. Also, CD40 activation induces CLL cells to express the BH3-interacting domain death agonist called BID, a pro-apoptotic protein that facilitates cross talk between mitochondria-dependent mediators of apoptosis and death receptors such as CD95 and DR5 (50,51). Non-CD40-activated CLL cells do not express BID. Furthermore, expression of BID has been associated with development of sensitivity to cytotoxic chemotherapy (52). Therefore, CD40 activation could transform CLL cells from resistant to sensitive to antileukemic drugs through induction of BID expression (53,54). Additionally, CD40 activation could be combined with other treatments at optimal time points in order to increase tumor cell killing.

Clinical Trials of Gene Therapy in CLL

A phase I clinical trial was performed with a single dose of autologous Ad-CD154-transduced CLL cells to assess tolerability, toxicities, and activity. The transgene was murine CD154 (mCD154). On average, half of the Ad-CD154-transduced CLL cells expressed the CD154 transgene and all expressed immune co-stimulatory molecules. Three patients received 3×10^8, three received 1×10^9, and three received 3×10^9 autologous Ad-CD154-CLL cells. The transgene-expressing cells could be detected in the blood for up to 24 after infusion. Some patients also received repeated doses of autologous Ad-CD154-transduced cells. The infusion of transduced cells was well tolerated. Patients experienced flu-like symptoms, including fever, fatigue, and anorexia, and some had small reversible elevations in hepatic transaminases and transient thrombocytopenia. None of the treated patients experienced dose-limiting toxicity or autoimmune hemolytic anemia or immune thrombocytopenia.

The biologic effects were encouraging. Within one to two days after receiving the modified cells, virtually all of the patients had measurable increases in plasma cytokines, including IL-12, IFN-γ, and/or IL-6. There was no measurable increase in the levels of TNF-α in the plasma of any of the treated patients. Following the infusion, bystander CLL cells in the blood expressed immune co-stimulatory molecules, CD80 and CD86, consistent with a bystander effect. In addition, they expressed death receptors, CD95 (Fas) and DR5. These phenotypic changes were noted one to two days after treatment, when circulating Ad-CD154-infected cells were no longer detected, and lasted for at least two weeks following the infusion. Incubation in plasma from the treated patients did not induce immune co-stimulatory molecules on noninfected pretreatment CLL cells, suggesting that a soluble factor was not responsible for these changes.

The clinical effects in this trial were also encouraging. Most patients experienced significant acute decreases in leukemia cell counts within a day or two after the infusion. Subsequently, the lymphocyte count tended to gradually return to approximately 60% of pretreatment, prepheresis levels. However, not all the blood lymphocytes that returned were CLL cells. At one to four weeks after treatment, nearly all of the treated patients had significant increases in the absolute number of CD4$^+$ T cells and CD8$^+$ T cells, sometimes to more than four times that of pretreatment levels. The CLL cell counts of most of the patients remained at or below treatment levels for several weeks, if not longer. Nearly all of the patients experienced significant reductions in lymph node size, beginning one to two weeks after treatment and lasting several weeks. The consistent increases in blood T-cell counts were associated with increases in the numbers of autologous, leukemia-specific T cells. This was confirmed by mixed lymphocyte reactions and ELISPOT assays using autologous nontransduced CLL cells to stimulate blood T cells isolated from patients before and after treatment.

The kinetics of leukemia-cell clearance following treatment were faster than would be expected for an adaptive cellular immune response. Instead, the induced expression of the death receptors, CD95 and DR5, and innate immune effector mechanisms previously discussed probably contributed to the acute decreases in leukemic cell counts following Ad-CD154 treatment. Activated blood CD4$^+$ CTLs from patients with CLL express both tumor necrosis factor-related apoptosis-inducing ligand (TRAIL) (DR5 ligand) and CD178 (Fas ligand). Increased DR5 and CD95 expression on bystander CLL cells was noted within 24 hours of infusion with Ad-CD154-transduced autologous CLL cells (51). Simultaneous cross-linking of CD95 and DR5 on CD40-activated CLL cells via CD178 and tumor necrosis factor-related apoptosis-inducing ligand (TRAIL) acted synergistically to induce caspase-dependent apoptosis in vitro and possibly in vivo within one to two days after infusion.

Finally, many cytotoxic drugs, including alkylating agents and purine analogs, induce apoptosis of CLL cells via a metabolic pathway that is dependent on functional p53. As such, loss of functional p53 in CLL cells is associated with resistance to most forms of chemotherapy. However, CD40 activation can induce expression of CD95 and BID and latent sensitivity to Fas-mediated apoptosis even in CLL cells that lack functional p53. This was found secondary, in part, to the capacity of CD40 ligation to induce expression of p73, a p53-related transcription factor regulated by c-Abl kinase that could render p53-deficient CLL cells sensitive to fludarabine (55). Moreover, ligation of CD40 on CLL cells could induce p73 via c-Abl kinase to bypass the resistance of p53-deficient CLL cells to anticancer therapy. Based on this, one must consider evaluating the combined effects of chemotherapy (fludarabine) with Ad-CD154 gene therapy.

Some of the patients in the initial phase I trial received repeated doses of Ad-mCD154-transduced cells. Some developed antibodies against mCD154 but not human CD154 and in some cases these were neutralizing. Subsequently, a chimeric CD154 molecule (ISF35) consisting mostly of human sequence was produced that could be expressed on CLL cells following transduction with adenovirus transduction. We completed a second phase I trial with autologous Ad-ISF35-transduced cells with similar results (56). We are about to initiate a phase II, multiple-dose trial with this strategy.

Additional Clinical Trials with CD154

Primary CLL cells transduced in vitro to express CD154 by electroporation subsequently expressed CD80 and CD86 and increased expression of CD54 and MHC class II (33). Furthermore, these transduced cells could stimulate allogeneic T cells in mixed lymphocyte reactions. This strategy was evaluated in a clinical trial in which CLL cells were subjected to electroporation in the presence of DNA plasmids encoding human CD154 or human IL-2, then cryopreserved (57). Subsequently, a fixed dose of autologous CLL cells expressing IL-2 was administered with increasing doses of cells expressing CD154. Seven patients received a total of six subcutaneous injections of autologous transduced cells. Subsequent to vaccination, all patients had stable leukemia counts and one patient had approximately 50% decrease in adenopathy. No complete or partial responses by NCI criteria were noted for the patients treated on this trial. In another study, subcutaneous administration of autologous CLL cells modified to express CD154 and IL-2 was evaluated as a vaccine strategy (58). There were eight patients who received treatment with autologous modified leukemia cells on this phase I clinical trial. Several of these patients had enhanced T-cell reactivity against autologous CLL cells.

In another strategy, leukemia cells from patients with CLL were cocultured with a human embryonic lung fibroblast cell line that was transduced with an adenovirus vector to express human CD154 (35). Coculture resulted in passive transfer of CD154 from the transduced fibroblasts to the leukemia cells, which in turn expressed surface CD154, CD80, CD86, and increased levels of CD54 (59). In parallel, CLL cells cultured with nonmanipulated lung fibroblast cells were transduced with adenovirus vector encoding human IL-2. Patients received a fixed dose of irradiated IL-2-secreting autologous CLL cells and increasing doses of CD154-expressing leukemia cells (2×10^5 to 2×10^7 transduced cells). A total of nine patients were treated on this clinical trial and all patients received from three to eight subcutaneous vaccinations (60). The vaccines were well tolerated with no significant local or systemic toxicities. Seven of the nine patients had T-cell responses against autologous leukemia cells; three patients produced leukemia-specific antibodies. Three patients had a transient >50% reduction in affected lymph nodes. The authors reported high levels of regulatory T cells, which they speculated might have limited the magnitude and duration of the induced antileukemia immune response. Alternatively, the transient expression of CD154 that was passively acquired by the leukemia B cells using this approach might have been responsible for the limited effects of such treatment. Further work is required to define the optimal approach for CD154 gene therapy in this disease.

OTHER VACCINE STRATEGIES AND CELLULAR THERAPY

Chimeric Receptors

Recent in vitro and preclinical studies evaluated the activity of autologous T cells genetically engineered to target the immunoglobulin light chain of leukemia B cells (61). This strategy uses a chimeric receptor for immunoglobulin kappa light chains composed of a single-chain monoclonal antibody (scFv) with the IgG1-CH2CH3 domain, the CD28 endodomain, and the zeta chain of the TCR complex. The gene encoding this receptor was cloned into a retrovirus for stable transduction of human T cells. T cells transduced with this retrovirus were cytotoxic against human kappa light chain–expressing tumor cells, but not lambda light chain–expressing target cells or cells that did not express human immunoglobulin light chains. Furthermore, the genetically engineered T cells could specifically control the growth of transplanted human kappa light chain–expressing tumor cells in a xenogeneic mouse model system. Because B cells expressing lambda light chain are spared, there is potential for continued antibody production.

In a similar strategy, $CD8^+$ T cells were transduced with an scFvFc:ζ chimeric TCR specific for human CD20. The transduced T cells specifically were cytotoxic for tumor cells that expressed CD20. This strategy is being considered for use in clinical trials involving patients with CD20-positive B-cell malignancies, including follicular lymphoma, small lymphocytic lymphoma, splenic marginal zone lymphoma, diffuse large B-cell lymphoma, and CLL (62).

In another strategy, NK cells are transduced to express an engineered chimeric receptor linked to CD3-ζ that was specific for human CD19, a pan-B cell surface antigen that is expressed by most B-cell malignancies, including CLL (63). The growth and activation of such NK cells with cytokines and 4-1BB ligand generated large numbers of such cells that specifically were cytotoxic for CD19-bearing tumor cells. This approach is also being considered for clinical trials involving patients with a variety of different B-cell malignancies.

Xcellerated T Cells

The T cells of patients with CLL display phenotypic and functional defects that are brought about by the presence of leukemic B cells. These defects result in dysregulation of T-cell immunity and overall immunosuppression. Current treatments for CLL, including purine analogues, exacerbate immune deficiency by depleting already dysfunctional T cells.

A process was developed in which T cells can be activated and expanded up to 100- to 1000-fold ex vivo by the Xcellerate process (64). With this process, T cells are obtained by leukapheresis and cultured with magnetic beads coated with monoclonal antibodies against CD3 and CD28 in the presence of IL-2. During expansion, T cells also may regain their capacity to respond to antigen.

A phase I/II dose escalation clinical trial with Xcellerated T cells for patients with CLL was recently reported (65). Doses up to 100×10^9 autologous Xcellerated T cells were administered as a single infusion to patients with CLL. Xcellerated T cells were well tolerated with no dose-limiting toxicities reported. The treatment resulted in consistent dose-dependent increases in blood T-cell counts and reduction in the lymph nodes and spleen. Unexpectedly, there were improvements in absolute neutrophil counts, hemoglobin, and platelet counts, suggesting overall clinical improvement. Disappointingly, reductions in blood leukemia cell counts were not observed. However, this may offer a future strategy for immune reconstitution for patients with CLL.

Oxidized Autologous Leukemia Cell Vaccine

Oxidizing radiation potentially makes cells more immunogenic (66). In another study, early-stage, "watch and wait" patients were vaccinated with oxidized autologous leukemia cells (67). Clinical partial responses were noted in 5 of 18 patients that were associated with enhanced T-cell antitumor activity. Six patients had stable disease and 6 of the 18 patients had progression. No significant toxicities were observed.

Dendritic Cell Vaccines

Dendritic cells are highly effective antigen-presenting cell. They can be activated to take up antigen and present it to T cells, resulting in potent T-cell activation and proliferation. Several in vitro studies confirmed the rationale for and feasibility of dendritic cell vaccines in CLL. In a recent clinical trial, dendritic cells generated from unrelated donors were pulsed ex vivo with patient CLL cell lysate or apoptotic bodies (11). In this trial with nine early-stage, previously untreated patients with CLL, the allogeneic APCs (3×10^6 cells) were administered as five repeated subcutaneous doses. There was no autoimmunity and some patients had reductions in blood leukemia cell counts during vaccination. Importantly, patients demonstrated increases in T-cell counts that reacted against a potential CLL antigen, RHAMM (Table 2). Subsequently, these investigators did a clinical with autologous dendritic cells pulsed with CLL cell lysates in 12 previously untreated, early-stage patients (68). Autologous APCs (7×10^6 cells) were administered intradermally eight times. There were significant increases in RHAMM-specific or fibromodulin-specific CTLs in four patients after vaccination, and some patients had reductions in leukemia cell counts.

CONCLUSIONS

Immune therapy and gene therapy for patients with CLL have been investigated for more than 10 years. Although our understanding has advanced, much work needs to be done in order to make further progress in this field. There is limited knowledge of the leukemia antigens expressed in CLL, and further identification and characterization will provide tools for advances. A variety of vaccine strategies have been studied, confirming mechanisms of immunization and demonstrating antileukemia immune responses, but with limited clinical benefit to patients. Nevertheless, these studies provide very encouraging results to continue work to develop this modality for significant clinical advances.

REFERENCES

1. Harig S, Witzens M, Krackhardt AM, et al. Induction of cytotoxic T-cell responses against immunoglobulin V region-derived peptides modified at human leukocyte antigen-A2 binding residues. Blood 2001; 98(10):2999–3005.
2. Trojan A, Schultze JL, Witzens M, et al. Immunoglobulin framework-derived peptides function as cytotoxic T-cell epitopes commonly expressed in B-cell malignancies. Nat Med 2000; 6(6):667–672.
3. Zirlik KM, Zahrieh D, Neuberg D, et al. Cytotoxic T cells generated against heteroclitic peptides kill primary tumor cells independent of the binding affinity of the native tumor antigen peptide. Blood 2006; 108(12):3865–3870.
4. Baskar S, Kwong KY, Hofer T, et al. Unique cell surface expression of receptor tyrosine kinase ROR1 in human B-cell chronic lymphocytic leukemia. Clin Cancer Res 2008; 14(2):396–404.

5. Fukuda T, Chen L, Endo T, et al. Antisera induced by infusions of autologous Ad-CD154-leukemia B cells identify ROR1 as an oncofetal antigen and receptor for Wnt5a. Proc Natl Acad Sci U S A 2008; 105(8):3047–3052.
6. Siegel S, Wagner A, Friedrichs B, et al. Identification of HLA-A*0201-presented T cell epitopes derived from the oncofetal antigen-immature laminin receptor protein in patients with hematological malignancies. J Immunol 2006; 176(11):6935–6944.
7. Siegel S, Wagner A, Kabelitz D, et al. Induction of cytotoxic T-cell responses against the oncofetal antigen-immature laminin receptor for the treatment of hematologic malignancies. Blood 2003; 102(13):4416–4423.
8. Kokhaei P, Palma M, Hansson L, et al. Telomerase (hTERT 611-626) serves as a tumor antigen in B-cell chronic lymphocytic leukemia and generates spontaneously antileukemic, cytotoxic T cells. Exp Hematol 2007; 35(2):297–304.
9. Mayr C, Kofler DM, Buning H, et al. Transduction of CLL cells by CD40 ligand enhances an antigen-specific immune recognition by autologous T cells. Blood 2005; 106(9):3223–3226.
10. Mayr C, Bund D, Schlee M, et al. Fibromodulin as a novel tumor-associated antigen (TAA) in chronic lymphocytic leukemia (CLL), which allows expansion of specific CD8+ autologous T lymphocytes. Blood 2005; 105(4):1566–1573.
11. Hus I, Rolinski J, Tabarkiewicz J, et al. Allogeneic dendritic cells pulsed with tumor lysates or apoptotic bodies as immunotherapy for patients with early-stage B-cell chronic lymphocytic leukemia. Leukemia 2005; 19(9):1621–1627.
12. Giannopoulos K, Li L, Bojarska-Junak A, et al. Expression of RHAMM/CD168 and other tumor-associated antigens in patients with B-cell chronic lymphocytic leukemia. Int J Oncol 2006; 29(1):95–103.
13. Reker S, Meier A, Holten-Andersen L, et al. Identification of novel survivin-derived CTL epitopes. Cancer Biol Ther 2004; 3(2):173–179.
14. Schmidt SM, Schag K, Muller MR, et al. Survivin is a shared tumor-associated antigen expressed in a broad variety of malignancies and recognized by specific cytotoxic T cells. Blood 2003; 102(2):571–576.
15. Mayr C, Bund D, Schlee M, et al. MDM2 is recognized as a tumor-associated antigen in chronic lymphocytic leukemia by CD8+ autologous T lymphocytes. Exp Hematol 2006; 34(1):44–53.
16. Favaro PM, de Souza Medina S, Traina F, et al. Human leukocyte formin: a novel protein expressed in lymphoid malignancies and associated with Akt. Biochem Biophys Res Commun 2003; 311(2):365–371.
17. Schuster IG, Busch DH, Eppinger E, et al. Allorestricted T cells with specificity for the FMNL1-derived peptide PP2 have potent antitumor activity against hematologic and other malignancies. Blood 2007; 110(8):2931–2939.
18. Korver W, Singh S, Liu S, et al. The lymphoid cell surface receptor NTB-A: a novel monoclonal antibody target for leukaemia and lymphoma therapeutics. Br J Haematol 2007; 137(4):307–318.
19. Wang Z, Zhang Y, Mandal A, et al. The spermatozoa protein, SLLP1, is a novel cancer-testis antigen in hematologic malignancies. Clin Cancer Res 2004; 10(19):6544–6550.
20. Schmidt SM, Schag K, Muller MR, et al. Induction of adipophilin-specific cytotoxic T lymphocytes using a novel HLA-A2-binding peptide that mediates tumor cell lysis. Cancer Res 2004; 64(3):1164–1170.
21. Johnson TA, Rassenti LZ, Kipps TJ. Ig VH1 genes expressed in B-cell chronic lymphocytic leukemia exhibit distinctive molecular features. J Immunol 1997; 158:235–246.
22. Rassenti LZ, Kipps TJ. Lack of allelic exclusion in B cell chronic lymphocytic leukemia. J Exp Med 1997; 185:1435–1445.
23. Fais F, Ghiotto F, Hashimoto S, et al. Chronic lymphocytic leukemia B cells express restricted sets of mutated and unmutated antigen receptors. J Clin Invest 1998; 102(8):1515–1525.
24. Whitacre DC, Hedjran F, Schmidt-Wolf I, et al. Highly efficient gene-transfer into chronic lymphocytic leukemia cells using adenovirus type 35 genetic vectors. Blood 2005; 106(11):596a (abstr #2109).

25. Wendtner CM, Kofler DM, Theiss HD, et al. Efficient gene transfer of CD40 ligand into primary B-CLL cells using recombinant adeno-associated virus (rAAV) vectors. Blood 2002; 100(5):1655–1661.
26. Kofler DM, Buning H, Mayr C, et al. Engagement of the B-cell antigen receptor (BCR) allows efficient transduction of ZAP-70-positive primary B-CLL cells by recombinant adeno-associated virus (rAAV) vectors. Gene Ther 2004; 11(18):1416–1424.
27. Jewell AP, Cochrane M, McIntosh J, et al. Comparison of viral vectors for gene transfer into CLL cells: efficient transduction with adeno-associated virus-8 (AAV-8). Blood 2005; 106(11): 837a (abstr #2985).
28. Tolba KA, Bowers WJ, Hilchey SP, et al. Development of herpes simplex virus-1 amplicon-based immunotherapy for chronic lymphocytic leukemia. Blood 2001; 98(2):287–295.
29. Tolba KA, Bowers WJ, Eling DJ, et al. HSV amplicon-mediated delivery of LIGHT enhances the antigen-presenting capacity of chronic lymphocytic leukemia. Mol Ther 2002; 6(4): 455–463.
30. Eling DJ, Johnson PA, Sharma S, et al. Chronic lymphocytic leukemia B cells are highly sensitive to infection by herpes simplex virus-1 via herpesvirus-entry-mediator A. Gene Ther 2000; 7(14):1210–1216.
31. Fratantoni JC, Dzekunov S, Singh V, et al. A non-viral gene delivery system designed for clinical use. Cytotherapy 2003; 5(3):208–210.
32. Gresch O, Engel FB, Nesic D, et al. New non-viral method for gene transfer into primary cells. Methods 2004; 33(2):151–163.
33. Li LH, Biagi E, Allen C, et al. Rapid and efficient nonviral gene delivery of CD154 to primary chronic lymphocytic leukemia cells. Cancer Gene Ther 2006; 13(2):215–224.
34. Van Bockstaele F, Pede V, Naessens E, et al. Efficient gene transfer in CLL by mRNA electroporation. Leukemia 2008; 22(2):323–329.
35. Takahashi S, Rousseau RF, Yotnda P, et al. Autologous antileukemic immune response induced by chronic lymphocytic leukemia B cells expressing the CD40 ligand and interleukin 2 transgenes. Hum Gene Ther 2001; 12(6):659–670.
36. Nishimura T, Watanabe K, Yahata T, et al. The application of IL-12 to cytokine therapy and gene therapy for tumors. Ann N Y Acad Sci 1996; 795:375–378.
37. Nishimura T, Watanabe K, Yahata T, et al. Application of interleukin 12 to antitumor cytokine and gene therapy. Cancer Chemother Pharmacol 1996; 38(suppl):S27–S34.
38. van Kooten C, Banchereau J. CD40-CD40 ligand: a multifunctional receptor-ligand pair. Adv Immunol 1996; 61:1–77.
39. Grewal IS, Flavell RA. CD40 and CD154 in cell-mediated immunity. Annu Rev Immunol 1998; 16(6):111–135.
40. Lanier LL, O'Fallon S, Somoza C, et al. CD80 (B7) and CD86 (B70) provide similar costimulatory signals for T cell proliferation, cytokine production, and generation of CTL. J Immunol 1995; 154:97–105.
41. Matulonis U, Dosiou C, Freeman G, et al. B7-1 is superior to B7-2 costimulation in the induction and maintenance of T cell-mediated antileukemia immunity. Further evidence that B7-1 and B7-2 are functionally distinct. J Immunol 1996; 156:1126–1131.
42. Wendtner CM, Nolte A, Mangold E, et al. Gene transfer of the costimulatory molecules B7-1 and B7-2 into human multiple myeloma cells by recombinant adeno-associated virus enhances the cytolytic T cell response. Gene Ther 1997; 4(7):726–735.
43. Briones J, Timmerman J, Levy R. In vivo antitumor effect of CD40L-transduced tumor cells as a vaccine for B-cell lymphoma. Cancer Res 2002; 62(11):3195–3199.
44. Briones J, Timmerman JM, Panicalli DL, et al. Antitumor immunity after vaccination with B lymphoma cells overexpressing a triad of costimulatory molecules. J Natl Cancer Inst 2003; 95(7):548–555.
45. Palena C, Foon KA, Panicali D, et al. Potential approach to immunotherapy of chronic lymphocytic leukemia (CLL): enhanced immunogenicity of CLL cells via infection with vectors encoding for multiple costimulatory molecules. Blood 2005; 106(10):3515–3523.

46. Ranheim EA, Kipps TJ. Activated T cells induce expression of B7/BB1 on normal or leukemic B cells through a CD40-dependent signal. J Exp Med 1993; 177:925–935.
47. Cantwell MJ, Hua T, Pappas J, et al. Acquired CD40-ligand deficiency in chronic lymphocytic leukemia. Nat Med 1997; 3:984–989.
48. Ranheim EA, Kipps TJ. Tumor necrosis factor-alpha facilitates induction of CD80 (B7-1) and CD54 on human B cells by activated T cells: complex regulation by IL-4, IL-10, and CD40L. Cell Immunol 1995; 161:226–235.
49. Kato K, Cantwell MJ, Sharma S, Kipps TJ. Gene transfer of CD40-ligand induces autologous immune recognition of chronic lymphocytic leukemia B cells. J Clin Invest 1998; 101: 1133–1141.
50. Chu P, Deforce D, Pedersen IM, et al. Latent sensitivity to Fas-mediated apoptosis after CD40 ligation may explain activity of CD154 gene therapy in chronic lymphocytic leukemia. Proc Natl Acad Sci U S A 2002; 99(6):3854–3859.
51. Dicker F, Kater AP, Fukuda T, et al. Fas-ligand (CD178) and TRAIL synergistically induce apoptosis of CD40-activated chronic lymphocytic leukemia B cells. Blood 2005; 105(8): 3193–3198.
52. Sax JK, Fei P, Murphy ME, et al. BID regulation by p53 contributes to chemosensitivity. Nat Cell Biol 2002; 4(11):842–849.
53. de Totero D, Tazzari PL, Capaia M, et al. CD40 triggering enhances fludarabine-induced apoptosis of chronic lymphocytic leukemia B-cells through autocrine release of tumor necrosis factor-alpha and interferon-gama and tumor necrosis factor receptor-I-II upregulation. Haematologica 2003; 88(2):148–158.
54. Romano MF, Lamberti A, Tassone P, et al. Triggering of CD40 antigen inhibits fludarabine-induced apoptosis in B chronic lymphocytic leukemia cells. Blood 1998; 92(3):990–995.
55. Dicker F, Kater AP, Prada CE, et al. CD154 induces P73 to overcome the resistance to apoptosis of chronic lymphocytic leukemia cells lacking functional P53. Blood 2006; 108(10): 3450–3457.
56. Wierda WG, Castro J, Aguillon R, et al. A phase I study of immune gene therapy for patients with CLL using a membrane-stable, humanized CD154. Blood 2007; 110(11):607a (abstr #2040).
57. Fratantoni JC, Li L, Liu LN, et al. A practical approach for achieving clinical immunotherapy of CLL with hCD40L- and hIL-2-expressing autologous tumor cells. Blood 2005; 106(11):136a (abstr #450).
58. Biagi E, Popat U, Raphael R, et al. Immunotherapy of chronic lymphocytic leukemia using CD40L and IL-2 expressing autologous tumor cells. Blood 2004; 104(11):220a (abstr #768).
59. Biagi E, Dotti G, Yvon E, et al. Molecular transfer of CD40 and OX40 ligands to leukemic human B cells induces expansion of autologous tumor-reactive cytotoxic T lymphocytes. Blood 2005; 105(6):2436–2442.
60. Biagi E, Rousseau R, Yvon E, et al. Responses to human CD40 ligand/human interleukin-2 autologous cell vaccine in patients with B-cell chronic lymphocytic leukemia. Clin Cancer Res 2005; 11(19 pt 1):6916–6923.
61. Vera J, Savoldo B, Vigouroux S, et al. T lymphocytes redirected against the kappa light chain of human immunoglobulin efficiently kill mature B lymphocyte-derived malignant cells. Blood 2006; 108(12):3890–3897.
62. Wang J, Press OW, Lindgren CG, et al. Cellular immunotherapy for follicular lymphoma using genetically modified CD20-specific CD8+ cytotoxic T lymphocytes. Mol Ther 2004; 9(4): 577–586.
63. Imai C, Iwamoto S, Campana D. Genetic modification of primary natural killer cells overcomes inhibitory signals and induces specific killing of leukemic cells. Blood 2005; 106(1):376–383.
64. Hami LS, Green C, Leshinsky N, et al. GMP production and testing of Xcellerated T cells for the treatment of patients with CLL. Cytotherapy 2004; 6(6):554–562.
65. Castro JE, Wierda WG, Kipps TJ, et al. A phase I/II trial of Xcellerated T Cells™ in patients with chronic lymphocytic leukemia. Blood 2004; 104(11):687a (abstr #2508).

66. Demaria S, Ng B, Devitt ML, et al. Ionizing radiation inhibition of distant untreated tumors (abscopal effect) is immune mediated. Int J Radiat Oncol Biol Phys 2004; 58(3):862–870.
67. Spaner DE, Hammond C, Mena J, et al. A phase I/II trial of oxidized autologous tumor vaccines during the "watch and wait" phase of chronic lymphocytic leukemia. Cancer Immunol Immunother 2005; 54(7):635–646.
68. Hus I, Schmitt M, Tabarkiewicz J, et al. Vaccination of B-CLL patients with autologous dendritic cells can change the frequency of leukemia antigen-specific CD8+ T cells as well as CD4+CD25+FoxP3+ regulatory T cells toward an antileukemia response. Leukemia 2008; 22(5):1007–1017.

13
Prolymphocytic Leukemias

Claire E. Dearden
Department of Haemato-Oncology, The Royal Marsden Hospital and Institute of Cancer Research, London, United Kingdom

INTRODUCTION

Prolymphocytic leukemias (PLLs) of B- and T-cell subtype are rare diseases, which together account for around 2% of all mature lymphoid leukemias. When first described in the 1970s (1), the different cells of origin were not appreciated, and the disease was called a variant of chronic lymphocytic leukemia (CLL). Advances in immunophenotyping and molecular cytogenetics have significantly contributed to a more precise classification of the mature lymphoid leukemias, and this has resulted in better management of patients with these conditions. Recent studies have highlighted the role of specific oncogenes such as *TCL1*, *MTCP-1*, and *ATM* in T-cell prolymphocytic leukemia (T-PLL) and *TP53* mutations in the case of B-cell prolymphocytic leukemia (B-PLL). However, despite better understanding of the underlying cell biology, prognosis for these patients remains poor with no curative therapy and shortened survival. The advent of monoclonal antibody therapy and the wider application of nonmyeloablative allogeneic transplantation have increased the treatment options for this group of patients. Table 1 summarizes the characteristic features of the PLLs.

B-CELL PROLYMPHOCYTIC LEUKEMIA

There has been considerable debate regarding the distinction between CLL (with an increase in prolymphocytes), mantle cell lymphoma in leukemic phase, and "true" B-PLL. Certainly, these cases can present a diagnostic challenge but with careful morphological, immunophenotypical, and genetic analysis, it is usually possible to discriminate between these disorders, which are all currently recognized as separate entities in the World Health Organization (WHO) classification (2).

Pathogenesis

The primary B-cell leukemias include a number of disease entities arising from mature B lymphocytes and primarily involve the bone marrow, blood, and other lymphoid organs

Table 1 Clinical and Laboratory Characteristics of the PLLs

Characteristic findings	B-PLL	T-PLL
Clinical features	Median age 70 yr	Median age 65 yr
	M:F = 1.6:1	M:F = 1.2:1
	Splenomegaly	Splenomegaly, lymphadenopathy, skin rash, edema, and serous effusions
	High WBC	Very high WBC
Morphology	>55% PLs	Basophilic PLs with cytoplasmic blebs
		Small cell (20%) and Sezary variants (5%)
Immunophenotyping	CD19, CD20, CD22, CD79a+	CD2, CD3, CD5, CD7+
	CD23–, CD5–/+	CD4/8 variable
	FMC7+	CD1a–, TdT–, CD25 –/+
Cytogenetics	13q del, 11q del, 17p del	t(14,14); inversion 14; t(X,14); idec8q; complex
Oncogenes	*TP53, c-myc*	*TCL-1, MTCP-1, ATM*
Prognosis	Median survival—3 yr	Median survival < 1yr
Treatment	Purine analogue combination	Alemtuzumab alone or in combination
	MoAb (alemtuzumab, rituximab)	Consolidation with SCT
	SCT if eligible	

Abbreviations: PLL, prolymphocytic leukemias; B-PLL, B-cell prolymphocytic leukemia; T-PLL, T-cell prolymphocytic leukemia; WBC, white blood cell; SCT, stem cell transplant; PLs, prolymphocytes.

such as the spleen. While CLL is common, B-PLL is rare. Initially, when first described by Galton et al. in 1974, B-PLL was considered a variant of CLL (1). However, more recently it has become apparent that B-PLL is a distinct disorder with important clinical and laboratory differences from CLL and does not simply evolve from it (3). Recent studies in CLL based on gene expression profiling (4) have confirmed that CLL derives from an activated, antigen-experienced B cell, which resembles memory B cells and has a common pathogenetic pathway distinct from other B-cell lymphoproliferative disorders such as B-PLL. Little is known of the underlying molecular mechanisms in B-PLL. The overall frequency of *TP53* mutations in B-PLL is high. Deletions of 13q14 and 11q23 are also common in B-PLL, and in contrast to CLL, there is a preferential loss of RB1 with respect to the D13S25 locus, suggesting that allelic loss of the RB1 gene may play a role in the pathogenesis of B-PLL (5).

Clinical and Laboratory Features

B-PLL is a distinct clinical entity with different physical signs, morphology, cell markers, and clinical evolution compared with CLL. B-PLL mainly affects the elderly, and the median age of patients at presentation is 69 years with a male to female ratio of 1.6:1. Typically, patients present with splenomegaly without significant lymphadenopathy. The white blood cell (WBC) count is high, usually over 100×10^9/L, and the majority of these cells are prolymphocytes. Anemia and thrombocytopenia are seen in at least 50% of cases reflecting the degree of bone marrow infiltration present. A serum monoclonal band is also seen more commonly than in CLL. Central nervous system (CNS) involvement or serous effusions are rare, and skin involvement, in contrast to T-PLL, is not seen.

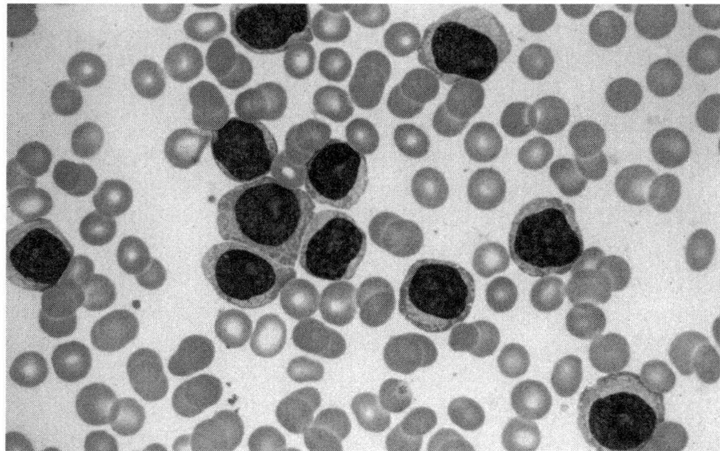

Figure 1 May-Grumwald-Giemsa stained peripheral blood film from a patient with B-PLL showing prolymphocytes with a regular nuclear outline, single nucleolus, and a relatively abundant pale cytoplasm. *Abbreviation*: B-PLL, B-cell prolymphocytic leukaemia (*See Color Insert*).

Morphology

The key criterion for the diagnosis of B-PLL is the recognition of a prolymphocyte count greater than 55% in the peripheral blood. The prolymphocyte has a characteristic larger size, one-and-a-half-to-two times that of a CLL lymphocyte. The nuclear chromatin is moderately condensed but not clumped; there is often a prominent single central nucleolus (Fig. 1), and the nuclear outline is typically more uniform than that in CLL/PL. Cytoplasm is abundant, clear, and only weakly basophilic in contrast to that in T-PLL. The nuclear to cytoplasmic ratio is lower than it is in CLL or T-PLL. In contrast to hairy cell leukemia variant, the cytoplasm is generally smooth.

Bone marrow trephine biopsies show diffuse intertrabecular infiltration by cells similar to those seen in the peripheral blood. When the WBC count is high and the blood smear shows unequivocal features of B-PLL, lymph node histology is rarely necessary. When available, histology shows diffuse or nodular infiltration and distinction from mantle cell lymphoma and marginal zone lymphoma, and CLL may be difficult. In cases presenting with a massively enlarged spleen, spleen histology can often be of diagnostic value showing extensive white and red pulp involvement. The prolymphocytoid morphology is particularly seen in the red pulp.

Immunophenotyping

The circulating prolymphocytes have a mature clonal B-cell phenotype with strong expression of pan-B antigens such as CD20, CD22, CD24, CD79b, and FMC7. Surface immunoglobulins [immunoglobulin M (IgM) and/or immunoglobulin D (IgD)] show light chain restriction and are strongly expressed, in contrast to the weak expression in CLL. The cells are usually, but not always, CD23 and CD5 negative. Up to a third of cases may express CD5, making the distinction from mantle cell lymphoma in leukemic phase more difficult. The "CLL score" (6) is <3, usually 0 to 1. The expression of markers such as FMC7 and CD11c suggests that the cells are at a late stage of maturation. CD38 and ZAP-70 are expressed in a proportion of cases; in more than half of 19 B-PLL cases ZAP-70 expression was >20% in 57% (7). Expression of these two markers has not yet been shown to correlate with prognosis.

Cytogenetics

There are difficulties in eliciting metaphases for conventional cytogenetic analysis in small lymphocytic disorders such as CLL and B-PLL, and the use of B-cell mitogens might increase the detection rate of cytogenetic changes (8). B-PLL has no distinct genetic marker, which is diagnostic for the disease. The most frequent aberrations involve chromosomes 14, 6, and 1. Florescence in situ hybridization (FISH) studies are valuable as they can be assessed on interphase cells. Lens et al. evaluated 18 patients with B-PLL and described 13q14 deletions in 55% and mono-allelic 11q23 deletions in 39% (5). Other abnormalities included 6q–, t(6;12), and structural aberrations of 1p and 1q(9). Although t(11;14) (q13;q32) has previously been described in B-PLL, it is becoming apparent that most of these cases represent a leukemic phase of mantle cell lymphoma, for which this is the "hallmark" translocation (9). This also highlights the importance of tissue staining for cyclin D1 in such cases, as peripheral blood morphology and immunophenotyping are not always discriminatory. In contrast to B-PLL, mantle cell lymphoma is also more commonly associated with extranodal disease and positive CD5 expression (81% vs. 31%).

There have been sporadic cases of B-PLL in which translocations involving the c-myc locus on chromosome 8 have been described [t(8,14) and t(8,22)] (10,11). This oncogene may therefore be involved in the pathogenesis of a subset of B-PLL.

Abnormalities of the *TP53* gene (loss of heterozygosity, p53 protein expression and mutations) have been documented in 50% to 75% of cases (12). This incidence is the highest reported among all the subtypes of B-cell malignancies and is comparable to that seen in solid tumors. This abnormality is likely to be associated with the aggressive clinical course and relative chemoresistance seen in B-PLL. Interestingly, the pattern of *TP53* mutations consists of insertions and deletions of this gene different from those seen in CLL and other hematological malignancies, implying that distinct pathogenetic mechanisms may be operating in B-PLL.

In one series, 9 of 17 cases (53%) had unmutated immunoglobulin heavy chain variable region (IgVH) genes, with preferential usage of V3-23 and V4-34 in a third(7). The majority of *TP53* deleted cases were unmutated.

Differential Diagnosis

The differential diagnosis of B-PLL includes CLL/PL, leukemic mantle cell lymphoma, the variant form of hairy cell leukemia (HCL-V) and T-PLL. Immunophenotyping and morphology will distinguish B-PLL from T-PLL and CLL/PL. In the latter, morphological examination shows a mixture of small mature CLL lymphocytes and prolymphocytes in contrast to the monomorphic prolymphocytic population seen in B-PLL (13). In addition, histology and cytogenetic analyses allow distinction between B-PLL, HCL variant, and mantle cell lymphoma.

Management and Prognosis

B-PLL is associated with a poorer prognosis than CLL, has a median survival of three years, and is often difficult to treat. Poor prognostic variables include age, anemia, and the presence of *TP53* deletion. Unlike CLL, IgVH mutation status and CD38 and ZAP-70 expression do not appear to have prognostic value in the small number of cases tested.

Treatment may not be indicated in asymptomatic patients with no or slow progression, but the majority of patients will require therapy. Alkylating agents such as chlorambucil are of little value in the management of B-PLL (14). Combination regimens such as cyclophosphamide, doxorubicin, vincristine, and prednisolone (CHOP) have

Table 2 Purine Analogue Therapy in B-PLL

Study	Regimen	CR	PR	ORR
Kantarjian (16)	Fludarabine +/− pred	18%	18%	35%
Dohner (17)	Pentostatin	0%	50%	50%
Saven (18)	Cladribine	63%	37%	100%
Herold (19)	FC	19%	50%	69%

Abbreviations: B-PLL, B-cell prolymphocytic leukemia; CR, complete remission; pred, prednisolone; FC, fludarabine and cyclophosphamide; ORR, overall response rate.

recorded responses [partial responses and rare complete remissions (CRs)] in up to one-third of cases (15). Preliminary data suggest that purine analogues such as fludarabine, cladribine, and pentostatin may achieve responses in up to 50% of patients, including CRs (Table 2). Some patients may achieve prolonged periods of progression-free survival with fludarabine. Kantarjian et al. described the results of fludarabine therapy in 16 patients with B-PLL (16). Twelve patients received fludarabine as a single agent at a dose of 30 mg/m^2 daily for five days every four weeks, and in five patients, fludarabine was given in combination with prednisolone. The overall response rate was 35% with three patients (18%) achieving a CR and three (18%) a PR (partial remission). The responses lasted from 5+ to 23+ months. A prospective phase II trial performed by the Leukemia Cooperative Group of the European Organization for Research into Treatment of Cancer (EORTC) assessed the activity and toxicity of pentostatin at a dosage of 4 mg/m^2 intravenously once a week for three weeks, then every other week for three courses (17). Responders received maintenance therapy once a month for a maximum of six months. Seven of the 14 patients with B-PLL achieved a PR with median duration of response of nine months (range 2–30 months). No CRs were observed. Saven et al. treated eight patients with de novo B-PLL using cladribine 0.1 mg/kg/day for seven days by continuous infusion or 0.14 mg/kg/day over two hours for five days every 28 days for a median of three courses (18). Five patients achieved a CR with a median duration of 14 months, and three achieved a PR. There is still insufficient data on the use of fludarabine in combinations with cyclophosphamide (FC) plus mitoxantrone (FCM) or rituximab (FCR) in B-PLL. A phase II trial using FC showed an overall response rate of 50% with a median survival of 32 months (19).

Monoclonal antibodies have also been used in B-PLL. There are case reports documenting the successful treatment of B-PLL with both the anti-CD52 monoclonal antibody alemtuzumab (20) and the anti-CD20 monoclonal antibody rituximab (21). A pilot study has also investigated the combination of bendamustine/mitoxantrone/rituximab (22). Alemtuzumab has considerable potential in the treatment of B-PLL; it is effective in patients with CLL who have p53 abnormalities and is also most active in blood, bone marrow, and spleen, which are the main sites involved in B-PLL. Further studies investigating the role of alemtuzumab and rituximab in B-PLL are warranted.

Patients presenting with massive splenomegaly may be effectively palliated with splenectomy. Not only does splenectomy remove a major proliferative focus and considerable tumor bulk in this disease, but it can also relieve hypersplenism and facilitate further treatment. Indeed, some patients have been reported to have normalization of blood counts following splenectomy without any chemotherapy. In elderly patients, splenectomy may not be feasible, and splenic irradiation may be a suitable option (23).

Stem cell transplantation should also be considered in young, fit patients who have responded to their initial therapy, as disease progression is inevitable (24). Allogeneic stem cell transplantation gives patients the possibility of a long-term cure by harnessing a graft versus leukemia effect. However, the morbidity and mortality associated with this procedure is significant, and often it is not a feasible option due to patient's age or comorbidities.

T-CELL PROLYMPHOCYTIC LEUKEMIA

T-PLL was first documented in a patient presenting with clinical features similar to B-PLL but in whom the cells had a T-cell phenotype (25). T-PLL is recognized in the WHO classification as having three morphological variants: typical, small cell, and cerebriform, all of which have a similar clinical course and identical molecular genetics (2).

Pathogenesis

Mature T-cell malignancies are rare (26). The maturation of T cells is strictly controlled by the thymic cellular microenvironment and depends on the presence of a complex mix of cytokines and growth factors (27). Unlike B cells, which rely on immunoglobulin rearrangement to present a specific antibody to bind to a foreign antigen, T cells rely on the T-cell receptor (TCR)-CD3 complex. Mutations in any of the TCR subunits lead to T-lymphoproliferative diseases derived from postthymic immunocompetent lymphoid cells such as in T-PLL. There is no evidence that radiation, carcinogenic agents, or viruses play a role in the pathogenesis of T-PLL (28).

Overexpression of two proto-oncogenes of similar structure: *TCL1a* (14q32.1) and p13 *MTCP1* (Xq28) have been implicated in the pathogenesis of T-PLL (29,30). The *TCL-1* oncoprotein is expressed in approximately 70% of T-PLL cases (20) and has been shown to associate with protein kinase B (Akt) resulting in the promotion of Akt-induced cell proliferation and survival (31).

In adults, T-PLL arises sporadically. There is a close relationship between this sporadic form of T-PLL and the leukemia that occurs in patients with the hereditary debilitating neurological disease ataxia telengectasia (A-T) (32). Patients with A-T have bi-allelic inactivation of the A-T mutated gene (*ATM*) located at the 11q23 locus (33). Approximately 10% of A-T homozygotes develop cancer, mostly of the lymphoid system and in particular of the T-cell type (34). Some of these patients develop abnormal clonal proliferation of T cells with morphological, immunological, cytogenetic, and molecular features (e.g., overexpression of the *TCL-1* oncogene) identical to T-PLL. Genetic abnormalities (mutations and deletions) of *ATM* are well documented in T-PLL (35–38). *ATM* is therefore a candidate gene likely to be involved in the pathogenesis of both sporadic and A-T-associated T-PLL, possibly through its role as a tumor suppressor.

Clinical and Laboratory Features

T-PLL affects adults, with a median age at presentation of 65 years, and is slightly more frequent in males. It has been described in the West and East without a geographical or racial clustering. Patients typically present with widespread disease at diagnosis characterized by hepatosplenomegaly, lymphadenopathy, and a high WBC count (39). Skin lesions are found in up to one-third of such cases. Serous effusions are seen in 15% at diagnosis but are common in relapsed or refractory disease. Not infrequently, patients present with periorbital edema. CNS involvement is rare. Occasionally, patients are asymptomatic and present with a peripheral blood lymphocytosis, which insidiously rises, mimicking stage A CLL (40). Although this "smouldering" T-PLL may have a prolonged indolent phase, progression is inevitable and may arise acutely. A rapidly rising peripheral blood lymphocyte count is more typical, and peripheral blood lymphocyte counts can range from 35 to 1000 $\times$ 10^9/L. Bone marrow failure with anemia and thrombocytopenia is also present in a third of cases.

Morphology

As with B-PLL, the morphology of prolymphocytes in the peripheral blood and cell markers is the vital requirement to make the diagnosis of T-PLL and distinguish it from other mature lymphoid leukemias.

T-PLL has a broad morphological spectrum (41). In half of the cases, the cells have a round-to-oval nucleus, while in the remainder, the nuclei are irregular, often with convolutions. The degree of nuclear irregularity, however, is less pronounced than that seen in Sézary or adult T-cell leukemia/lymphoma (ATLL) cells. In three quarters of cases, the morphology is "typical" with prolymphocytes of medium size with condensed nuclear chromatin, a single prominent nucleolus, intensely basophilic agranular cytoplasm with cytoplasmic protrusions or "blebs" in most of the cases. Approximately 20% of T-PLL cases are much smaller in size with a rather inconspicuous nucleolus under light microscopy. Electron microscopy has confirmed the presence of a nucleolus in such cases, which are referred to as "small cell variant" of T-PLL. Rarely, the T-PLL cells have a cerebriform nucleus resembling Sézary cells (cerebriform variant, 5%). Both these variants are otherwise similar to the typical T-PLL, including immunophenotype and cytogenetics, and thus it is justified that all three are grouped together in a single category (2).

Tissue histology is not essential for diagnosis. Diffuse and interstitial infiltration of the bone marrow is seen in the majority of cases, and reticulin fibrosis is almost always present. Lymph nodes and skin may be diffusely infiltrated. The skin histology differs from that seen in mycosis fungoides and Sezary syndrome (SS), showing dermal infiltration preferentially around the appendages and without epidermotropism. Spleen histology differs from that seen in T-cell large granular lymphocytic leukemia, showing expansion of both the red and white pulp with atrophy of the follicular centers.

Immunophenotype

Immunophenotyping demonstrates that T prolymphocytes have membrane markers consistent with a postthymic phenotype: negative for terminal deoxynucleotidyl transferase (TdT) and the cortical thymic marker CD1a, while expressing CD2, CD3, CD5, and CD7. CD7 is usually expressed with strong intensity in contrast to other mature T-cell malignancies where this marker may be weak or negative. CD3 and anti-TCR-α/βmay be negative in the cell membrane but are always expressed in the cytoplasm, and the TCR-β and/or γ chain genes are rearranged in all cases. In most patients, 65%, the cells are CD4+/CD8–, but cells alternatively may coexpress CD4 and CD8 (21%), or be CD4–/CD8+ (13%) (39). Cell surface antigens linked to T-cell activation such as CD25, CD38, and class II HLA-DR are variably expressed, and monoclonal antibodies against natural killer cells and TIA-1 are negative. T prolymphocytes strongly express the CD52 antigen at a high density (42), which can be targeted by the monoclonal antibody, alemtuzumab. In most cases, patients with T-PLL express the TCR-α/β phenotype, although rare instances of TCRγδ have been reported (43).

Cytogenetics

T-PLL is characterised by complex chromosomal abnormalities (Fig. 2), and this suggests that chromosomal aberrations may occur progressively during the course of the disease

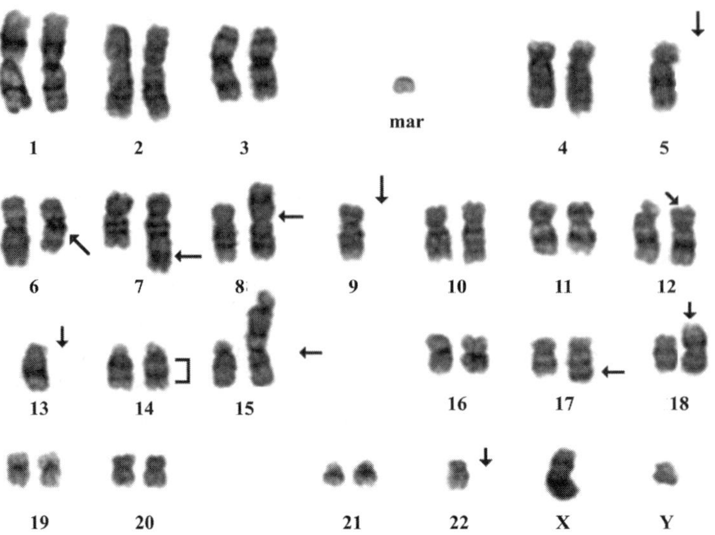

Figure 2   Karyotype of peripheral blood cells from a patient with T-PLL showing a complex clone that included isochromosome for 8q and inversion of chromosome 14. *Abbreviation*: T-PLL, T-cell prolymphocytic leukemia.

explaining the aggressive nature of this condition. Recurrent changes mainly affect chromosomes 14, 8, 11, and X (44). Inversion (14)(q11;q32) is characteristic of T-PLL and is detected in over two-thirds of cases. Tandem translocations between the two chromosomes 14, t(14;14) are also present in some cases. These two rearrangements involve the 14q11 and 14q32.1 loci where the genes coding for the TCR-α and the proto-oncogene *TCL-1* are localized, respectively. The rearrangements result in juxtaposition of these two genes and lead to activation of *TCL-1*. About 20% of patients have the translocation t(X;14) (q28;q11) resulting in rearrangement of the *MTCP-1* gene with *TCR-α*. Abnormalities involving both arms of chromosome 8 are frequent and overexpression of the c-myc protein is found in cases with iso8q. While the 14q abnormality and trisomy 8q are common in western countries, they are rarely seen in Japan (45). Although 11q23 abnormalities are seldom detected on cytogenetics, molecular analysis frequently detects mutations of the *ATM* gene. In addition, studies have demonstrated that T-PLL is associated with recurrent regions of chromosomal loss at 22q11, 13q, 6q, 9p, 12p, 11p11–p14, and 17p as well as chromosomal gain at 8q, 14q32, 22q21, and 6p (46). Recent single nucleotide polymorphism–based genomic mapping and global gene expression profiling has identified differential expression of a number of genes in T-PLL compared with normal CD3+ T-cells (47). These include functionally important genes involved in lymphomagenesis, cell cycle regulation, apoptosis and DNA repair, which clustered in regions affected by known recurrent chromosomal aberrations in T-PLL. This information may help to clarify the mechanisms involved in disease progression.

Differential Diagnosis

T-PLL can be distinguished from B-PLL by immunological markers. Furthermore, skin infiltration and lymphadenopathy are unusual in B-PLL, while they are present in a substantial proportion of T-PLL patients. Morphology, histology, and immunological markers help to differentiate T-PLL from other mature T-cell malignancies such as T-cell large granular lymphocytic leukemia (T-LGL), ATLL and SS. The predominant population in T-cell LGL leukemia is a granular lymphocyte, often with a CD8+, CD57+, CD16+/– phenotype, with or without expression of natural killer (NK) cell markers. The distinct geographical background, the clinical features (e.g., hypercalcemia), and HTLV-I serology distinguishes T-PLL from ATLL. SS has distinct clinical features, skin histology, and cell morphology.

Management and Prognosis

T-PLL is an aggressive disease, which is often resistant to therapy. Overall prognosis is poor with a median overall survival of approximately seven months in an historic cohort of patients treated with conventional combination regimens. More recent data show that median survival has been extended to more than two years following the introduction of new therapies. The M. D. Anderson Cancer Center reported a five-year overall survival rate of 21% (48). Poorer outcome in their series correlated with high WBC, short lymphocyte doubling time, older age, and high expression of TCL-1 protein.

Alkylating agents and combination chemotherapies such as CHOP provide low response rates of short duration. 2-deoxycoformycin (DCF) has been shown to be effective, particularly in patients who are CD25+, CD38+, and CD103+ (49). A study performed in 1994 reported an overall response rate of 45% (9% CR) using a dose of 4 mg/m^2 weekly for four weeks and then every two weeks until maximum response (50). This also resulted in an improvement in overall survival. More recently the anti-CD52 monoclonal antibody, alemtuzumab, has been used to target the CD52 antigen, which is expressed at high density on the surface of T prolymphocytes. An early study of 14 patients reported a response rate of 73% (51). More recently, a European study of 39 patients with relapsed/refractory T-PLL, who received alemtuzumab intravenously three times a week after initial dose escalation, reported a remarkable overall response rate of 76% with a CR rate of 60% (52). Nine of the 39 patients were refractory to DCF. The median overall survival was 10 months, but was 16 months in those patients who achieved complete responses. Responses were poor in patients who had serous effusions and hepatic or CNS involvement. In the United States, a retrospective analysis of 76 patients with T-PLL treated on a compassionate use with standard alemtuzumab therapy reported an OR rate of 50% with 37.5% CR (53). These patients, who had received one or more lines of treatment and had progressive and/or refractory disease, had a superior quality and duration of response to alemtuzumab compared to prior therapy. Alemtuzumab has subsequently been investigated in treatment-naive patients. In a preliminary study of 11 patients, 100% achieved a CR with 7 of 11 patients still alive at median follow up of 12 months (range 4–17 months) (54).

The successful use of chemoimmunotherapy in B-cell malignancies has prompted similar studies in T-PLL. The German CLL Study Group (GCLLSG) initiated the T-PLL-1 protocol and prospectively studied nine newly diagnosed cases (55). The combination of fludarabine, mitoxantrone, and cyclophosphamide (FMC) was given and repeated every four weeks for up to four cycles. Responding patients proceeded to consolidation with intravenous alemtuzumab three times a week, one to three months after completion of chemotherapy. Responses post-FMC were CR ($N = 4$), PR ($N = 3$), and stable disease ($N = 1$). Five of these patients received alemtuzumab. A patient with stable disease achieved CR, one patient achieved PR with only minimal residual disease in the marrow, and three patients were in CR at the time of consolidation. Weidmann et al. have used a regimen consisting of fludarabine (days 1–4), cyclophosphamide (day 3), doxorubicin (day 4) together with alemtuzumab in escalating doses (days 1–4) to treat 23 patients with a range of peripheral T-cell malignancies (56). Overall response rate in this series was 61% with a CR rate of 78% in the newly diagnosed patients. However, this cohort only had a single case of T-PLL.

Although monoclonal antibody therapy with alemtuzumab has improved outcome in T-PLL, responses are still transient, and further disease progression is inevitable. Hence, all patients who achieve a response to therapy should be considered for consolidation with a stem cell transplant (SCT) to prolong disease-free and overall survival. In a recent study, 22 patients with T-PLL received an SCT in first CR, second CR, or with a good partial response following alemtuzumab therapy. Thirteen were consolidated with an autologous SCT and nine with an allogeneic SCT (5 siblings and 4 unrelated donor) (57). In the patients who were autografted, 38% remain alive with median disease-free survival of 20 months (range 8–78 months). Of the nine patients who had an allograft, four had full intensity conditioning, and five reduced intensity conditioning. Fifty-six percent remain alive, one patient in continued CR seven years post-SCT. Two patients died from transplant-related mortality, and both had received full intensity conditioning. Two patients relapsed. These results demonstrate that autologous SCT can increase disease-free survival, but two-thirds of patients still relapse. While allogeneic SCT is an attractive option, transplant-related mortality with full intensity conditioning is high. There are other case reports of successful outcome with reduced intensity conditioning (58,59), and this is a strategy that merits further study.

Better understanding of the molecular pathogenesis may also lead to the introduction of new therapeutic approaches targeting specific pathways such as Akt activation.

CONCLUSION

Despite advances in immunophenotyping and molecular cytogenetics, leading to a better understanding of the underlying cell biology of the PLLs, prognosis for these patients remains poor. Alkylating agents either alone or in combination with other drugs are of little value. Purine analogues and monoclonal antibodies have shown efficacy in B-PLL, although further studies are warranted. Monoclonal antibody therapy with alemtuzumab has significantly improved outcome in T-PLL, but responses are still transient and further disease progression is inevitable. While allogeneic SCT is an attractive option, the older age group of PLL patients means that the morbidity and mortality associated with the procedure is significant. The role of reduced intensity conditioning in these aggressive diseases requires further investigation.

REFERENCES

1. Galton DAG, Goldman JM, Wiltshaw E, et al. Prolymphocytic leukaemia. Br J Haematol 1974; 27:7–23.
2. Jaffe ES, Harris NL, Stein H, et al. Pathology and genetics of tumours of haemopoietic and lymphoid tissues. World Health Organisation Classification of Tumours. Lyon: IARC Press, 2001.
3. Bennett JM, Catovsky D, Daniel MT, et alProposals for the classification of chronic (mature) B and T lymphoid leukaemias. French-American-British (FAB) Cooperative Group. J Clin Pathol 1989; 42(6):567–584.
4. Houlston RS, Sellick G, Yuille M, et al Causation of chronic lymphocytic leukaemia—insights from familial disease. Leuk Res 2003; 27:871–876.
5. Lens D, Matutes E, Catovsky D, et al. Frequent deletions at 11q23 and 13ql4 in B-cell prolymphocytic leukemia (B-PLL). Leukemia 2000; 14(3):427–430.

6. Matutes E, Owusu-Ankomah K, Morilla R, et al. The immunological profile of B-cell disorders and proposal of a scoring system for the diagnosis of CLL. Leukaemia 1994; 8:1640–1645.

7. Del Giudice I, Davis Z, Matutes E, et al. IgVH genes mutation and usage, ZAP-7- and CD38 expression provide new insights on B-cell prolymphocytic leukaemia (B-PLL). Leukaemia 2006; 20(7):1231–1237.

8. Pittman S, Catovsky D. Chromosome abnormalities in B-cell prolymphocytic leukemia: a study of nine cases. Cancer Genet Cytogenet 1983; 9(4):355–365.

9. Ruchlemer R, Parry-Jones N, Brito-Babapulle V, et al. B-prolymphocytic leukaemia with t(11;14) revisited: a splenomegalic form of mantle cell lymphoma evolving with leukaemia. Br J Haematol 2004; 125(3):330–336.

10. Kuriakose P, Perveen N, Maeda K, et al. Translocation (8;14)(q24;q32) as the sole cytogenetic abnormality in B-cell prolymphocytic leukaemia. Cancer Genet Cytogenet 2004; 150(2):156–158.

11. Crisostomo RH, Fernandez JA, Caceres W. Complex karyotype including chromosomal translocation (8;14)(q24;q32) in one case with B-cell prolymphocytid leukaemia. Leuk Res 2007; 31(5):699–701.

12. Lens D, De Schouwer PJ, Hamoudi RA, et al. p53 abnormalities in B-cell prolymphocytic leukaemia. Blood 1997; 89(6):2015–2023.

13. Melo JV, Catovsky D, Galton DA, et al. The relationship between chronic lymphatic leukaemia and prolymphocytic leukaemia. I clinical and laboratory features of 300 patients and characterization of an intermediate group. Br J Haematol 1986; 63:377–387.

14. Fava S, De Paoli A, Grimi E, et al. Prolymphocytic leukemia: the therapeutic strategy. Recenti Prog Med 1994; 85(10):496–501.

15. Shvidel L, Shtalrid M, Bassous L, et al. B-cell prolymphocytic leukemia: a survey of 35 patients emphasizing heterogeneity, prognostic factors and evidence for a group with an indolent course. Leuk Lymphoma 1999; 33(1-2):169–179.

16. Kantarjian HM, Childs C, O'Brien S, et al. Efficacy of fludarabine, a new adenine nucleoside analogue, in patients with prolymphocytic leukaemia and the prolymphocytoid variant of chronic lymhocytic leukaemia. Am J Med 1991; 90:223–228.

17. Döhner H, Ho AD, Thaler J, et al. Pentostatin in prolymphocytic leukemia: phase II trial of the European Organization for Research and Treatment of Cancer Leukemia Cooperative Study Group. J Natl Cancer Inst 1993; 85(8):658–662.

18. Saven A, Lee T, Schlutz M, et al. Major activity of cladribine in patients with de novo B-cell prolymphocytic leukemia. J Clin Oncol 1997; 15(1):37–43.

19. Herold M, Spohn C, Schlag R, et al. Fludarabine/Cyclophosphamide chemotherapy for B-prolymphocytic leukemia [abstract 2499]. Blood 2003; 102(11):675a.

20. Bowen AL, Zomas A, Emmett E, et al. Subcutaneous CAMPATH-1H in fludarabine-resistant/relapsed chronic lymphocytic and B-prolymphocytic leukaemia. Br J Haematol 1997; 96(3): 617–619.

21. Mourad YA, Taher A, Chehal A, et al. Successful treatment of B-cell prolymphocytic leukemia with monoclonal anti-CD20 antibody. Ann Hematol 2004; 83(5):319–321.[Epub 2003, Nov 27].

22. Weide R, Pandorf A, Heymanns J, et al. Bendamustine / Mitoxantrone / Rituximab (BMR): a very effective, well tolerated outpatient chemo-immunotherapy for relapsed and refractory CD20-positive indolent malignancies. Final results of a pilot study. Leuk Lymphoma 2004; 45(12): 2445–2449.

23. Oscier DG, Catovsky D, Errington D, et al. Splenic irradiation in B-prolymphocytic leukaemia. Br J Haematol 1981; 48:577–584.

24. Shvidel L, Shtalrid M, Klepfish A, et al. Successful autologous stem cell transplantation in aggressive prolymphocytic leukaemia. Am J Hematol 2000; 63(4):230–231.

25. Catovsky D, Galetto J, Okas A, et al. Prolymphocytic leukaemia of B and T cell type. Lancet 1973; 2:232–234.

26. Jaffe ES, Krenacs L, Raffeld M. Classification of cytotoxic T-cell and natural killer cell lymphomas. Semin Hematol 2003; 40:175–184.

27. Bommhardt U, Beyer M, Hunig T, et al. Molecular and cellular mechanisms of T cell development. Cell Mol Life Sci 2004; 61:263–280.

28. Pawson R, Schulz TF, Matutes E, et al, The human T-cell lymphotropic viruses type 1/11 are not involved in T prolymphocytic luek and large granular lymphocytic leukaemia. Leukaemia 1997; 11:1305–1311.

29. Virgilio L, Narducci MG, Isobe M, et al. Identification of the TCL1 gene involved in T-cell malignancies. Proc Natl Acad Sci U S A 1994; 91:12530–12534.

30. Madani A, Choukroun V, Soulier J, et al. Expression of p13MTCP1 is restricted to mature T-cell proliferations with t(X;14) translocations. Blood 1996; 87:1923–1927.

31. Laine J, Kunstle G, Obata T, et al. The proto-oncogene TCL1 is an Akt kinase coactivator. Mol Cell 2000; 6:395–407.

32. Brito-Babapulle V, Catovsky D. Inversions and tandem translocations involving chromosome 14q11 and 14q32 in T-prolymphocytic leukemia and T-cell leukemias in patients with ataxia telangiectasia. Cancer Genet Cytogenet 1991; 55:1–9.

33. Xu Y, Ashley T, Brainerd E, et al. Targeted disruption of ATM leads to growth retardation, chromosomal fragmentation during meiosis, immune defects and thymic lymphoma. Genes Dev 1996; 10:2411–2422.

34. Taylor AM, Metcalfe JA, Thick M, et al. Leukaemia and lymphoma in ataxia telangiectasia. Blood 1996; 87:423–438.

35. Stilgenbauer S, Schaffner C, Litterst A, et al. Biallelic mutations in the ATM gene in T-prolymphocytic leukemia. Nat Med 1997; 3:1155–1159.

36. Stoppa-Lyonnet D, Soulier J, Lauge A, et al. Inactivation of the ATM gene in T-cell prolymphocytic leukemias. Blood 1998; 91:3920–3926.

37. Yuille MA, Coignet LJ. The ataxia telangiectasia gene in familial and sporadic cancer. Recent Results Cancer Res 1998; 154:156–173.

38. Yamaguchi M, Yamamoto K, Miki T, et al. T-cell prolymphocytic leukemia with der(11)t(1;11) (q21;q23) and ATM deficiency. Cancer Genet Cytogenet 2003; 146:22–26.

39. Matutes E, Brito-Babapulle V, Swansbury J, et al. Clinical and laboratory features of 78 cases of T-prolymphocytic leukemia. Blood 1991; 78:3269–3274.

40. Garand R, Goasguen J, Brizard A, et al. Indolent course as a relatively frequent presentation in T-prolymphocytic leuk. Groupe Francais d'Haematologie Cellularie. Br J Haematol 1998; 103:488–494.

41. Matutes E, Talavera GJ, O'Brien M, et al. The morphological spectrum of T-prolymphocytic leuk. Br J Haematol 1986; 64:111–124.

42. Ginaldi L, De Martinis M, Matutes E, et al. Levels of expression of CD52 in normal and leukemic B and T cells: correlation with in vivo therapeutic responses to Campath-1H. Leuk Res 1998; 22:185–191.

43. Sugimoto T, Imoto S, Matsuo Y, et al. T-cell receptor gamma delta T-cell leukemia with the morphology of T-cell prolymphocytic leukemia and a postthymic immunophenotype. Ann Hematol 2001; 80:749–751.

44. Malajei SH, Brito-Babapulle V, Hirons LR, et al. Abnormalities of chromosomes 8,11,14 and X in T-prolymphocytic leukaemia studied by fluorescence in situ hybridization. Cancer Genet Cytogenet 1998; 103:110–116.

45. Kojima K, Kobayashi H, Imoto S, et al. 14q11 abnormality and trisomy 8q are not common in Japanese T-cell prolymphocytic leukemia. Int J Hematol 1998; 68:291–296.

46. Soulier J, Pierron G, Vecchione D, et al. A complex pattern of recurrent chromosomal losses and gains in T-cell prolymphocytic leukemia. Genes Chromosomes Cancer 2001; 31:248–254.

47. Durig J, Bug S, Klein-Hitpass L, et al. Combined single nucleotide polymorphism-based genomic mapping and global gene expression profiling identifies novel chromosomal imbalances, mechanisms and candidate genes important in the pathogenesis of T-cell prolymphocytic leukaemia with inv (14)(q11q32). Leukaemia 2007; 21(10):2153–2163.

48. Herling M, Patek KA, Teitell MA, et al. High TCL1 expression and intact T-cell receptor signalling define a hyperproliferative subset of T-cell prolymphocytic leukemia. Blood 2008; 111(1):328–337.[Epub 2007 Sep 21].

49. Delgado J, Bustos JG, Jimenez MC, et al. Are activation markers (CD25, CD38 and CD103) predictive of sensitivity to purine analogues in patients with T-cell prolymphocytic leukemia and other lymphoproliferative disorders? Leuk Lymphoma 2002; 43:2331–2334.
50. Mercieca J, Matutes E, Dearden C, et al. The role of pentostatin in the treatment of T-cell malignancies: analysis of response rate in 145 patients according to disease subtype. J Clin Oncol 1994; 12:2588–2593.
51. Pawson R, Dyer MJ, Barge R, et al. Treatment of T-cell prolymphocytic leukemia with human CD52 antibody. J Clin Oncol 1997; 15:2667–2672.
52. Dearden CE, Matutes E, Cazin B, et al. High remission rate in T-cell prolymphocytic leukemia with Campath-1H. Blood 2001; 98:1721–1726.
53. Keating MJ, Cazin B, Coutre S, et al. Campath-1H treatment of T-cell prolymphocytic leukaemia in patients for whom at least one prior chemotherapy regimen has failed. J Clin Oncol 2002; 20:205–213.
54. Dearden C, Matutes E, Cazin B, et al. Very high response rates in previously untreated T-cell Prolymphocytic leukaemia patients receiving alemtuzumab (Campath-1H) therapy. Blood 2003; 102(abstr 2378).
55. Hopfinger G, Kandler G, Koller E, et al. T-PLL 1 protocol of the German CLL Study Group (GCLLSG)-A prospective phase 2 trial of fludarabine phosphate, mitoxantrone and cyclophosphamide (FCM) followed by alemtuzumab consolidation as first line treatment in T-PLL. Blood 2003; 102: (abstr 2495).
56. Weidmann E, Hess G, Krause SW, et al. Combination chemoimmunotherapy using alemtuzumab, fludarabine, cyclophosphomide and doxorubicin (FCD) is an effective first line regimen in peripheral T-cell lymphoma (PTCL). Blood 2004; 104:2460 (abstr).
57. Krishnan B, Cazin B, Ireland R, et al. Improved survival for patients with T-cell prolymphocytic leuk receiving alemtuzumab therapy followed by stem cell transplantation. IWCLL. Leuk Lymphoma 2007; 48(suppl 1):S180.
58. Garderet L, Bittencourt H, Kaliski A, et al. Treatment of T-prolymphocytic leukaemia with nommyeloablative allogeneic stem cell transplantation. Eur J Haematol 2001; 66:137–139.
59. De Lavallade H, Faucher C, Furst S, et al. Allogeneic stem cell transplantation after reduced-intennsity conditioning in a patient with T-cell prolymphocytic leukaemia: graft-versus-tumor effect and long-term remission. Bone Marrow Transplant 2006; 37:709–710.
60. Sole F, Woessner S, Espinet B, et al. Cytogeneic abnormalities in three patients with B-cell prolymphocytic leukemia. Cancer Genet Cytogenet 1998; 103:43–45.

14

CLL-Specific Complications: Autoimmunity and Richter's Transformation

Dennis A. Carney
Department of Haematology, Peter MacCallum Cancer Centre, East Melbourne, Victoria, Australia

John F. Seymour
Department of Haematology, Peter MacCallum Cancer Centre, and University of Melbourne, Melbourne, Victoria, Australia

INTRODUCTION

The highly variable clinical course of chronic lymphocytic leukemia (CLL) may be further complicated by the development of autoimmunity or a histologically distinct aggressive lymphoma (Richter's syndrome). Although there has been significant progress in our understanding of the pathogenesis of these complications, they continue to present major management challenges.

AUTOIMMUNITY

CLL is associated with immune dysregulation involving aspects of both immunodeficiency and autoimmunity (1,2). The autoimmunity is predominantly directed against mature blood cells, although disorders targeting other self-antigens have also been reported (3). CLL cells have autoreactive characteristics, but are usually not the source of pathogenic autoantibody.

CLL Cells Are Autoreactive

The origin of the CLL cell remains in debate, although there is growing evidence for the pathogenic role of antigenic stimulation (4). The expression of CD5 has been central to the search for the normal counterpart of the CLL B cell (5). It is a distinguishing feature in CLL that prompted comparisons with the murine B1 cells that are known to produce polyreactive antibodies (6). However, the use of CD5 as a marker of cellular origin is complicated because its expression can be induced by cellular activation (7). Nevertheless, CLL cells are antigen-experienced B cells capable of producing natural polyreactive autoantibodies (8–10). IgM expressed on CLL cells frequently shows reactivity against self-antigen, including IgG, cardiolipin, actin, thyroglobulin, and DNA (11).

The characteristic proliferation centers in lymph nodes and bone marrow support a role for antigen and possibly autoantigen stimulation in CLL (5). These aggregates of proliferating cells are not found in other B-cell malignancies, but are seen in rheumatoid arthritis and multiple sclerosis (12). Chronic antigen stimulation has been implicated in malignant transformation and particularly in the development of marginal zone lymphomas (13,14). Furthermore, autoantigen stimulation in Sjogren's syndrome and Hashimoto's thyroiditis may be involved in the development of lymphomas in these autoimmune diseases (15,16). Such an association between a preceding autoimmune disease and the development of CLL has yet to be established, but a recent study demonstrated a significantly increased risk of CLL in subjects with a personal history of pernicious anemia (17). No associations with other autoimmune disease and CLL were found in this population-based case-control study involving 7764 CLL patients from Sweden and Denmark.

The immunoglobulin heavy chain gene expressed by a CLL cell can be further characterized according to the presence or absence of somatic gene mutations that define mutated and unmutated subgroups of CLL with contrasting clinical courses (18,19). These mutations affect the reactivity of the resultant antibody with unmutated CLL expressing highly polyreactive antibodies, while antibodies from mutated CLL are more specific (20). The biased use of particular V genes in CLL also favors autoimmunity. Genes commonly expressed in unmutated cases include VH 1-69 associated with anti-IgG/ rheumatoid factor activity (21,22) and VH 4-34 associated with anti-red blood cell or anti-DNA activity (23–26). Furthermore, the germ line counterparts of the mutated antibody sequences also encode polyreactive autoantibody, indicating both CLL subgroups originate from self-reactive B cells (20).

Autoreactivity is an important component of normal immune function (27,28). The innate and adaptive immune responses provide different levels of defence against invading microbes (29). Innate (natural) responses use polyreactive antibodies that have not been subject to somatic hypermutation. These antibodies are generally IgM antibodies with low antigen affinity reactive with a wide range of epitopes and therefore active against multiple pathogens (30). They are often autoreactive and produced in a relatively T-cell independent manner. The adaptive immune response is more specific with somatically mutated antibodies providing higher antigen affinity (29). CLL cells may therefore be derived from B cells that function in both the innate and adaptive immune systems (31).

Autoimmune Cytopenias

Autoimmune complications are a hallmark of CLL and mainly directed against red cells and platelets. Cytopenias are also associated with bone marrow failure and define advanced stages of CLL under both the Rai and Binet staging systems (32,33). In this setting, the cytopenias are an indication for treatment of the underlying CLL, but the National Cancer Institute-sponsored Working Group (NCI-WG) guidelines suggest that autoimmune cytopenias are initially managed independently (34,35). They also recommend that a bone marrow biopsy may be valuable to distinguish the cause of cytopenias. The three main autoimmune diseases in CLL are autoimmune hemolytic anemia (AIHA), immune thrombocytopenia (ITP), and pure red cell aplasia (PRCA) (36).

Prevalence

CLL is the most common cause of AIHA (37,38). Conversely, AIHA is estimated to occur in 10% to 25% of CLL patients during their disease course (39). However, the prevalence of AIHA depends on the disease stage, and more recent studies of large populations of CLL patients representing all disease stages have reported rates of about 5% (38,40,41). The frequency of positive direct antiglobulin tests (DATs) also depends on the stage and activity of CLL, with one series demonstrating a prevalence of 2.9% in stable stage A disease, 10.5% in stages B and C, and 18.2% in progressive stage A (1). Recent trials in CLL patients requiring treatment for the first time have reported positive DAT rates of 7% to 14% (42–44). Hemolysis is more likely in the setting of a positive DAT, but can also occur with a negative DAT. More sensitive tests may be able to detect red cell antibodies in such cases (45,46). The mitogen-stimulated DAT may also uncover the potential for autoantibody production (47). In a study of 69 CLL patients, this test was positive in 28.9% compared with 4.3% with standard DAT.

ITP occurs in approximately 2% to 3% of CLL cases (1,38,48). However, ITP is often a diagnosis of exclusion. The real prevalence of ITP in CLL remains uncertain with platelet antibody tests and bone marrow examinations not always conclusive (3). It may occur early and even be a presenting feature of CLL (36,38). A positive DAT or other evidence of AIHA is also seen in approximately one-third of CLL patients with ITP (36).

PRCA is an isolated failure of erythropoiesis, resulting in severe anemia with an absence of erythroid precursors in the bone marrow and low reticulocyte count (36,49). It is a rare complication of CLL with a prevalence of about 1% and may also develop in early-stage disease (1,36,38). A number of causes of PRCA have been identified with suppression of erythroid activity by large granular lymphocytes (LGLs) favored in CLL (50,51).

Pathogenesis

Autoreactive B and T cells are part of the normal immune repertoire, but are normally quiescent (52,53). Regulatory T-cells (T-reg cells) suppress autoreactive T cells to maintain self-tolerance (54,55). The reason autoreactivity becomes pathological is multifactorial and involves defects in cellular immune function and aberrant cytokine networks (56).

The role of the CLL cell in autoimmune disease and particularly AIHA continues to be explored. CLL cells are capable of secreting autoantibodies, but these are rarely responsible for the AIHA (10). Most hemolysis-complicating CLL is associated with polyclonal IgG warm-reactive autoantibody directed against Rh (rhesus) family antigens (1,36,39,41). Cold hemagglutinin disease is uncommon in CLL (3). IgM autoantibodies were responsible for hemolysis in 11% and 13% of cases in two studies of CLL-associated AIHA, although they were shown to be warm-reactive rather than cold agglutinins in one of the studies (40,41).

The Role of the CLL Cell in Antigen Presentation

The production of IgG antibody is usually a T-cell-dependent process, and AIHA, due to IgG autoantibodies, also appears to require specific T-cell help (57,58). Activated helper T-cells specific for Rh protein epitopes have been found in patients with CLL-associated AIHA and in some CLL patients without AIHA but low levels of red cell autoantibody (46). These autoreactive T-cells require activation by antigen–presenting cells (APCs). B-cells can present autoantigen to T-cells, but CLL cells function poorly as APCs in vitro (59). However, fractionation of putative APC populations from the peripheral blood of CLL patients demonstrated CLL cells were the most efficient cell type to present Rh protein to autoreactive T-helper cells (46). Tolerance may be overcome if there are changes to autoantigen presentation (52,56). AIHA may be stimulated if CLL cells process Rh protein to present novel (cryptic) epitopes to the autoreactive T cells (46). This potential role is further supported by the finding of an increased frequency of CLL phenotype lymphocytes in cases of primary AIHA and ITP (60).

The function of the CLL cell as an APC may be enhanced by ligation of CD40 expressed on the surface of the cell with T-cell expressed CD154 (61,62). This results in upregulation of costimulatory antigens such as CD80 and CD86 and more efficient antigen presentation. This mechanism is the basis of a vaccine strategy to treat CLL (63). CLL cells are modified to express CD154 so that CD40 is activated and CLL antigen presented to autologous T-cells. Furthermore, a subset of CLL cases has been shown to express CD154, which may promote antigen presentation through autoligation of CD40 or directly stimulate nonmalignant B cells, including autoreactive B cells (64). Costimulation of toll-like receptors (TLRs) with the B-cell receptor (BCR) also enhances activation of autoreactive B cells and may play a role in the autoimmune complications of CLL (31,65).

Blood Cell Specificity

The reason for autoimmunity predominantly targeting blood cells is still unclear. This specificity may be related to the coexistence of CLL and blood cell breakdown products at sites such as the spleen (46,66). In addition, red cells and platelets express complement receptors and play an important part in the clearance of immune complexes (29). Perhaps this function also makes them more susceptible to immune-mediated consumption.

Autoimmunity directed against blood cells is also a common feature of autoimmune lymphoproliferative syndrome (ALPS) (67). This syndrome is caused by mutations in the Fas gene, resulting in defective apoptosis of autoreactive lymphocytes. Defects in the Fas-signaling pathway have also been identified in CLL and may contribute to an associated breakdown of self-tolerance (41,68,69).

T-Cell Defects

T-cell numbers are often increased in CLL, but abnormalities in T-cell subsets and function are well described (70–72). Autoimmune complications in CLL are associated with an imbalance toward a type 2 (Th2) helper T-cell cytokine profile involved in humoral immunity rather than a type 1 (Th1) helper T-cell profile involved in cell-mediated immunity (29,47). T-reg cells expressing $CD4^+$ and $CD25^+$ are increased in CLL, particularly in more advanced stages (73). Autoimmune disease has been associated with low numbers of these cells, which suppress autoreactive T-cells (74–76). In contrast, increased numbers of T-reg cells have been reported in solid cancers and are postulated to reduce antitumor immunity in this setting (77–79). T-reg cells may suppress autoreactive T-cells by inhibiting interleukin-2 production (80). They also express cytotoxic T-lymphocyte-associated protein 4 (CTLA-4), which has a key role in inhibiting T-cell activation (81). A particular polymorphism of CTLA-4 is associated with susceptibility to a number of autoimmune diseases and has been shown to correlate with the development of AIHA in CLL (82). The polymorphism was detected in 73% (22/30) of CLL patients with AIHA compared with 47% (47/100) of CLL patients without evidence of autoimmune disease.

Treatment-Related Autoimmune Complications

Another important feature of T-reg cells is a relative sensitivity to the effects of cytotoxic therapy, particularly fludarabine (73). The $CD4^+$ T-cell depletion that occurs with fludarabine appears to preferentially affect CD25$^+$ cells. Furthermore, T-reg cells from CLL patients previously treated with fludarabine have reduced inhibitory function (73). These effects may contribute to the autoimmunity associated with fludarabine treatment of CLL (83–87). AIHA in this setting can be severe and sometimes fatal. Fludarabine-related ITP and PRCA have also been reported (3,88,89). Other purine analogs can also trigger autoimmune complications (90–92). Furthermore, this complication of treatment was recognized with radiotherapy and alkylators before the use of purine analogs (93). Results from the U.K. CLL4 study demonstrated a similar rate of AIHA with chlorambucil (12%) and fludarabine (11%) (87). The rate was lower with the combination of fludarabine and cyclophosphamide (5%), which also resulted in the highest CLL response rate. Of the three treatment arms, fludarabine was most often associated with the DAT remaining positive or changing from negative to positive (94). The German CLL Study Group trial comparing fludarabine (F) with fludarabine and cyclophosphamide (FC) also showed a lower rate of AIHA with the FC combination (2.8% vs. 7.7%; $p = 0.06$), but no difference was observed in the U.S. Intergroup trial comparing F and FC (43,95). It is possible that more effective CLL treatments are more effective at depleting autoreactive B cells. The combination of FC and rituximab (FCR) may provide further protection against the development of AIHA, as it has the highest reported response rates in previously untreated CLL (44). This regimen was associated with 16 cases of AIHA in 224 patients (7.1%), suggesting that the addition of rituximab does not have a major impact on the risk of AIHA, but this awaits further assessment in the setting of a randomized comparative study. A further update suggested the FCR regimen may mask DAT positivity, as most of the cases of hemolysis were DAT-negative (96).

Risk Factors

Risk factors for the development of AIHA include male gender, older age, and higher lymphocyte counts (41). Other associated factors include advanced stage and previous treatment (40,94). A high β_2-microglobulin level is also associated with a positive DAT and is a predictor of AIHA in patients treated with FCR (94,96). The mechanism may involve the role of serum β_2-microglobulin in promoting antigen presentation (97). In a recent study of predominantly early-stage CLL patients, ZAP70 expression was strongly correlated with the development of autoimmune cytopenias with age, gender, stage, lymphocyte count, and previous treatment having no significant association (98). Preliminary analysis of genetic markers in the U.K. CLL4 study indicates mutation status of the immunoglobulin heavy chain gene, and FISH results (deletion at 11q23) were associated with a positive DAT ($p = 0.05$) (94). However, genetic markers were not significant independent predictors of AIHA in multivariate analysis.

Prognostic Significance

The prognostic significance of AIHA in CLL is controversial. It is generally associated with a poor prognosis, but this may be due to its correlation with a number of other adverse prognostic factors (99). Several studies have failed to demonstrate an independent effect on survival (38,40,41). Furthermore, the presence of cytopenias due to autoimmunity is associated with a better prognosis when compared with cytopenias due to CLL-related bone marrow failure (38). However, results from the U.K. CLL4 study indicate that the development of AIHA is associated with a less-favorable response of CLL to treatment and a shorter overall survival (37 vs. 58%) at five years (94). Indeed, both AIHA and a positive DAT emerged as independent prognostic factors for overall survival. The minority of patients with AIHA due to IgM autoantibody appear to have a particularly poor survival (41).

Other Autoimmune Phenomena in CLL

Autoimmune diseases other than AIHA, ITP, and PRCA are rarely associated with CLL and usually limited to case reports (36). Paraneoplastic pemphigus is a rare autoimmune blistering skin disease associated with lymphoid malignancies including CLL (100,101). Lesions occur in the oropharynx and conjunctiva as well as the skin and are associated with epithelial autoantibodies. CLL has also been associated with glomerulonephritis and nephrotic syndrome (3,102). Fludarabine may precipitate this complication and cryoglobulin deposition, and antineutrophil cytoplasmic antibodies have been implicated in the pathogenesis (3,103,104). Acquired angioedema is caused by a deficiency in the complement C1-esterase inhibitor (C1-INH) as a result of inactivation by monoclonal autoantibodies often associated with lymphoid malignancies, including CLL (3,105,106). The syndrome features recurrent episodes of angioedema and abdominal pain. Case reports also link CLL with the development of coagulopathies due to autoantibodies against clotting proteins, including factors VIII and IX and von Willebrand factor (107–110).

A multicenter GIMEMA study of 3150 CLL patients identified 194 cases (5%) with autoimmune complications (40). Non-hematological disease accounted for 30 of 194 (16%) of the autoimmune complications. These included bullous pemphigus (9 cases), Hashimoto's thyroiditis (8 cases), rheumatoid arthritis (4 cases), systemic lupus erythematosus, autoimmune glomerulonephritis, autoimmune gastritis, Sjogren's syndrome, polymyositis-dermatomyositis, vasculitis, autoimmune polyneuropathy, ulcerative colitis, and Raynaud's disease (each 1 case) (40). In addition, 93 of 227 (41%) of CLL patients without autoimmune complications had at least one positive test for an antibody marker of autoimmunity: 36 antinuclear (ANA), 25 anticardiolipin, 23 rheumatoid factor, 23 antithyroid peroxidase/antithyroglobulin, 20 anti-smooth muscle, and 10 miscellaneous (antimitochondrial, anti-DNA, antiparietal cell). In contrast to AIHA and ITP, the non-hematological autoimmune complications and the presence of autoantibodies in patients without autoimmune complications were more prevalent in early-stage CLL (40). Another retrospective study found the frequency of autoimmune complications in 637 patients with lymphoproliferative diseases to be 8% compared with 1.7% in 346 patients with myeloproliferative diseases (48). AIHA and ITP were increased in frequency in CLL when compared with other lymphoproliferative diseases but not the non-hematological autoimmune complications. Indeed, the significance of serological evidence of non-hematological autoimmunity in CLL has been questioned (1,36). A study of the prevalence of autoantibodies in CLL found non-hematological autoantibodies not only in 42 of 195 (21.5%) CLL patients but also in 42 of 194 age and sex-matched controls and concluded that the autoimmune phenomena in CLL are largely confined to autoantibodies directed against the formed elements of blood (1).

Treatment of Autoimmune Complications

Autoimmune complications of CLL are generally treated in the same way as their primary counterparts. Steroids are the mainstay of treatment, with most patients responding to prednisolone 1mg/kg/day given over 10 to 14 days and then slowly tapered (111). Alternatives for patients who have an unsatisfactory response include other immunosuppressive agents, intravenous immunoglobulin (IVIg), splenectomy or splenic irradiation, and the monoclonal antibodies rituximab and alemtuzumab.

The sequence of treatments for AIHA is usually steroids followed by IVIg and cyclosporine as a third-line option (36). Relapses are common when steroid treatment is stopped. IVIg induces responses in approximately 40% of AIHA (112). It is usually administered in combination with steroids, but responses are often transient (113). Cyclosporine can be an effective alternative treatment. In a series of 16 CLL patients with immune-mediated anemia, cyclosporine resulted in an increase in hemoglobin of more than 30g/L in 10 patients (63%) (114). A similar response rate was observed for ITP with 18 of 29 (62%) patients achieving an increase in platelet count of 50×10^9/L or more. Cyclosporine is also recommended for PRCA not responding to steroids (36). In contrast to AIHA and ITP, PRCA may be an indication to institute treatment for the associated CLL.

Splenectomy can be a successful treatment for cytopenias associated with CLL (115). Although AIHA is not a common indication for splenectomy, cases associated with IgG and no complement respond better (116). It is more effective as a treatment for ITP with responses in over 70% of cases unresponsive to steroids (117). Splenic irradiation may be an alternative in patients unable to tolerate splenectomy (118).

Rituximab is a chimeric monoclonal antibody targeting the CD20 antigen on B-cells, with activity in a variety of autoimmune diseases (119–124). Responses are achieved in approximately 75% of patients with autoimmune cytopenias (125). Rituximab has also been effective in CLL-associated autoimmune disease. It achieved responses in four of seven patients with CLL-associated autoimmune disease refractory to conventional immunosuppressive treatment (126). This included one of four patients with AIHA, one cold agglutinin disease, one ITP, and one axonal degenerating neuropathy. Other studies of refractory CLL-associated AIHA have reported responses in three of four patients with rituximab alone and all eight patients treated with a combination of rituximab, cyclophosphamide, and dexamethasone (127,128). In addition, CLL-associated PRCA has been successfully treated with rituximab (129).

Alemtuzumab is another treatment option in refractory CLL-associated autoimmune cytopenias. This monoclonal antibody is directed against the CD52 antigen and has potent immunosuppressive effects (130). Durable remissions were reported in five patients with CLL-associated AIHA refractory to conventional therapy (131). Remission of CLL-related PRCA has also been reported with alemtuzumab (132). The anti-CLL activity of alemtuzumab may provide additional benefit in cases where the CLL requires treatment (131).

Autoimmune complications are often diagnosed when the underlying CLL is progressive or advanced and therefore requires treatment. CLL treatment can either improve or exacerbate the autoimmune complication. In a review of 300 CLL patients treated with FCR (fludarabine, cyclophosphamide, and rituximab), eight patients had AIHA and one had PRCA prior to FCR treatment (96). Two patients had AIHA that responded to FCR alone, four including the patient with PRCA required immunosuppression (steroids $\pm$ cyclosporine $\pm$ growth factors) in addition to FCR, and one had worsening anemia after FCR but responded to steroids, and FCR was ceased. In the U.K. CLL4 study, patients with a positive DAT could commence CLL treatment, but those with AIHA or ITP received specific treatment for their autoimmune complication beforehand (87). In this study, the fludarabine arm was associated with an increase in the percentage of DAT-positive patients, whereas, in the fludarabine and cyclophosphamide arm, there was a decrease in the percentage of DAT-positive cases after therapy. In the CAM307 study, alemtuzumab was associated with four (33%) of 12 patients with a positive baseline DAT converting to negative during treatment and four (3%) of 132 patients with a negative DAT becoming positive (133). These studies were all for previously untreated patients and indicate that autoimmune complications should not preclude treatment of CLL, although careful monitoring for exacerbation is needed. However, the autoimmune complications that develop with the treatment of CLL can be more difficult to manage. In the FCR study, 17 patients developed AIHA during or after FCR treatment, with 7 of 17 (41.2%) responding to steroids alone (96). The other 10 needed additional treatment including cyclosporine, IVIg, rituximab, erythropoietin, and splenectomy (96). Four patients who responded to the addition of cyclosporine remained dependent on steroids and/or cyclosporine for over one year.

Patients with a history of treatment-related autoimmunity who require further treatment are at particular risk of recurrent autoimmune complications (86,92,134). Although the risk is most commonly described for retreatment with purine analogs such as fludarabine, subsequent alkylator treatment may also precipitate recurrent autoimmunity (134). One approach to this dilemma is to preemptively treat the complication. Fludarabine retreatment in a small number of patients with previous fludarabine-associated AIHA was tolerated while they were maintained on cyclosporine (114). Rituximab and alemtuzumab may also have roles in this situation (128,131).

Conclusions

CLL is often complicated by autoimmune complications particularly affecting blood cells. Although the CLL cell has autoreactive characteristics, it is rarely responsible for production of pathogenic autoantibody. Several mechanisms may be involved to overcome self-tolerance, with the CLL cell possibly playing a role as an antigen-presenting cell. Autoimmune complications are usually treated separately from the underlying CLL with a growing repertoire of options, including monoclonal antibodies. The management of cases precipitated by CLL-specific treatment can be particularly challenging and highlight the complex immune dysregulation associated with CLL.

RICHTER'S SYNDROME

Richter's syndrome is a complication associated with a significant adverse prognosis and, similar to autoimmunity, it requires a specific treatment strategy.

History and Scope

The term "Richter's syndrome" usually refers to the secondary development of a histologically aggressive lymphoproliferative disorder typically diffuse large B-cell lymphoma (DLBCL) in a patient with preexisting CLL. The popularization of the term is attributed to Lortholary et al. (135), acknowledging Maurice Richter's original description of the simultaneous occurrence of a "reticulum-cell sarcoma" and CLL in 1928 (136). There remains an ongoing debate regarding the relative frequency of clonal progression of the underlying CLL versus development of a clonally unrelated second tumor, perhaps related to immunosuppression.

While some authors have used the term Richter's syndrome to include instances of prolymphocytic leukemia (137,138), acute lymphoblastic leukemia (139), or multiple myeloma (140), this chapter will be restricted to DLBCL and Hodgkin lymphoma, the most common manifestations of Richter's syndrome.

Clinical, Laboratory, and Radiological Features

It is both scientifically and clinically important to attempt to obtain repeat biopsies of discordantly responding lesions, "dominant" or "disproportionately bulky" disease sites at

Table 1 Indicative Clinical and Laboratory Features of Patients with Richter's Syndrome (DLBCL)

Feature	Relative frequency
Median time from diagnosis of CLL	24–48 mo
Median age at transformation	60–70 yr
Impaired performance status (>1 on ECOG scale)	20–25%
Fever +/− weight loss	50–65%
Progressive lymphadenopathy	60–90%
Symptomatic abdominal mass	20–30%
Involvement of extranodal sites	30–40%
Elevated serum LDH ($\geq$1.5 × ULN)	40–80%
Elevated serum β_2-microglobulin (>3 × ULN)	40%
Hypercalcemia	~5%
Median survival	3–8 mo

Note: Figures are estimated on the basis of available data—see text for references. *Abbreviations*: DLBCL, diffuse large B-cell lymphoma; CLL, chronic lymphocytic leukemia; ECOCT, Eastern Co-operative Oncology Group; LDH, lactate dehydrogenase; ULN, upper limit of normal.

relapse, and any "unusual" extranodal sites apparently involved by CLL. These situations should raise the suspicion of development of Richter's syndrome. The practice of more frequent tissue rebiopsy will provide a more representative profile of the clinical manifestations of this syndrome, as well as a more accurate estimate of its true incidence.

Diffuse Large B-Cell Non-Hodgkin Lymphoma

The development of DLBCL either during the course of the underlying CLL or at the time of diagnosis is the most frequently reported form of Richter's syndrome, constituting 67% of all transformation events in the U.S. Intergroup study cohort (141), 89% of cases from the large database of the MD Anderson Cancer Center (142,143), and 87% of those from the Polish cooperative group (144). The clinical features at the time of recognition have generally been similar across the larger case series and reviews (Table 1) (145–150).

Trump et al. (149) described five cases from Johns Hopkins in 1980 and thoroughly reviewed the features of 41 previously reported cases of Richter's syndrome. They found a male/female ratio of 2:1, a median interval of 24 months from the diagnosis of CLL, fever in 65%, rapidly progressive adenopathy in 46%, weight loss in 29%, and abdominal pain in 26% of patients. Some earlier case reports had noted the phenomenon of a progressive reduction in lymphocytic counts preceding transformation (151), but this has not been confirmed to be a reproducible feature (149). A very substantial male predominance (2.3:1) was also observed by Tsimberidou (143) and Mao (152) and likely reflects the gender imbalance of other biological risk factors for the development of Richter's syndrome (see below). The largest published experience has come from the MD Anderson Group who initially reported 39 patients in 1993 and recently updated their experience with 204 "suspected" cases, including 148 pathologically confirmed (143). The median time from diagnosis of CLL was 48 months, with progressive lymphadenopathy noted in 64%, the systemic symptoms of fever and weight loss in 54%, and a symptomatic abdominal mass evident in 23% (150).

Extranodal manifestations of lymphoma are common, occurring in 38% of patients, with involved sites including the pleura, oropharynx, skin, gastrointestinal tract, bone, and pulmonary parenchyma (145,147,149,150). Infiltration of the bone marrow by frank DLBCL is uncommon, being reported in less than 10% of cases (145–147,149,150), the finding of an increased proportion of "large" lymphoid cells in the marrow biopsy (>7%) was predictive of subsequent development of Richter's syndrome (153). While all tissues are at risk for involvement, some of the less-frequent extranodal sites reported to be involved by Richter's syndrome include the liver, spleen, and peritoneum (145,147,154–156), isolated cutaneous lymphomatous deposits (157,158), and the central nervous system (CNS) (150,159–161) or dura mater (162). Osteolytic bone lesions may be the first manifestation of Richter's syndrome (163) and are associated with hypercalcemia (164). Localized gastric DLBCL associated with *Helicobacter pylori* infection likely represents a separate secondary process, given the confirmed independent clonal origin of the lymphoma in the three cases described (165), although discrete bowel lesions or widespread gastrointestinal tract infiltration are also reported (145,147,149).

Laboratory abnormalities associated with the development of aggressive NHL are common; approximately 50% to 80% of patients have marked elevations of serum LDH (lactate dehydrogenase) disproportionate to that anticipated in uncomplicated CLL in the absence of hemolysis (143,150). The serum β_2-microglobulin was noted to be markedly elevated [>3 × ULN (upper limit of normal)] in 40% of patients in the recent MD Anderson series (143). Serum or urine paraproteins are found in a significant minority of patients (~40%), but this frequency does not appear to differ from a well-studied population of patients with uncomplicated CLL (166). Hypercalcemia has been reported to herald the onset of transformation (145,164,167), because this complication is extremely uncommon in uncomplicated CLL (168), in contrast to its frequency of up to 15% in patients with non-Hodgkin lymphoma (NHL) (169). While the above laboratory features are more common in patients with Richter's syndrome than those with uncomplicated CLL, none are specific, but the new onset of such abnormalities should prompt consideration of possible development of this complication.

Peripheral blood cytopenias, predominantly anemia and thrombocytopenia, are common as may be expected in a similar cohort of patients with progressive CLL. Robertson et al. (150) noted a median $CD4_+$ T-lymphocyte count of 224/μL at the time of transformation in their series, but it is unknown whether this differs from that which would be found in a similar group of heavily pretreated patients in the absence of histological transformation.

While the new development of lesions in any of the uncommon sites described above should mandate investigation and biopsy, the investigation for possible Richter's transformation is more difficult in suspected cases without such specific lesions and widespread lymphadenopathy. There have been a few reports describing the use of functional imaging modalities, initially, high-dose gallium-67 citrate and, more recently, 18-F fluoro-deoxy-glucose (FDG) positron emission tomography (PET) scanning to both identify patients with Richter's syndrome and guide the most appropriate site for biopsy in such cases. While the initial report of gallium described a high sensitivity (78%) and specificity (also 78%) for Richter's syndrome in a cohort of 29 patients (170), a subsequent smaller series of 13 patients described poor discriminatory ability. Given that "indolent" lymphoproliferative disorders such as follicular lymphoma or diffuse small lymphocytic lymphoma typically have low- to moderate-intensity tracer uptake with FDG-PET and more rapidly proliferative processes such as DLBCL, or those associated with a greater degree of associated inflammatory-cell infiltration (such as Hodgkin lymphoma) have more intensive tracer uptake [typically a standardized uptake value (SUV) of >5], there is interest in using FDG-PET to investigate patients suspected of having possible Richter's syndrome. Bruzzi et al. (171) investigated 37 patients with 57 combined FDG-PET/CT scans and, using a "cut-point" of an SUV of 5, reported a sensitivity for Richter's transformation of 91%, but a lower specificity of 80% and importantly a modest positive-predictive value of 50%. The low positive-predictive value was due to the finding of a number of other highly clinically important processes, which were also FDG-avid, including secondary malignancies or pneumonia (171). The cut-point of an SUV of 5 had the greatest use in this cohort, with a median uptake value in patients with confirmed Richter's syndrome of 17.6 (range 7.4–39.4). Thus, FDG-PET scanning has substantial use in the management of patients with CLL and its symptoms and laboratory or structural radiological abnormalities suggestive of Richter's syndrome. While only 50% of patients with intense tracer uptake (an SUV >5) on scanning will ultimately be shown to have Richter's syndrome, all such abnormalities mandate further investigation and biopsy, as other clinical processes, predominantly other malignancies, are very common.

Hodgkin Lymphoma

Hodgkin lymphoma is one of the most frequent "second malignancies" in patients with CLL. Travis et al. (172) reported a relative risk of 7.69. Although most early reports of Richter's syndrome included cases of Hodgkin lymphoma together with those of DLBCL (135,147), the features of patients developing Hodgkin lymphoma as their manifestation of Richter's syndrome do appear to have some differences from those with DLBCL. From the U.S. Intergroup study described earlier, just 1% of all CLL patients developed Hodgkin lymphoma, and these constituted 15% of all cases of Richter's syndrome. Similar proportions were reported from the MD Anderson (0.4% of patients, 11% of Richter's syndrome) (142) and Polish cooperative group (0.15% and 13%, respectively) (144). Typical features, summarized from the larger recent series (142,173–178) describing a total of more than 50 cases, are presented in Table 2.

The largest series have been reported by the MD Anderson group, with a recent analysis including 18 cases (142). The median age at diagnosis of Hodgkin lymphoma was 72 years, and similar to patients with DLBCL, 78% were male (male: female ratio 3.5:1.0). While a small proportion of patients may have both processes present at diagnosis (142), the median time from diagnosis of CLL was slightly longer than for DLBCL at 4.6 years. The Hodgkin lymphoma is typically widespread when recognized, with bone marrow infiltration

Table 2 Indicative Clinical and Laboratory Features of Patients with Richter's Syndrome Manifest as Hodgkin Lymphoma

Feature	Relative frequency
Median time from diagnosis of CLL	4–5 yr
Median age at transformation	65–70 yr
Impaired performance status (>1 on ECOG scale)	25%
Fever +/− weight loss	~70%
Progressive lymphadenopathy	50–75%
Dominant splenomegaly	10–20%
Bone marrow infiltration	30–40%
Involvement of other extranodal sites	~10%
Elevated serum LDH (>ULN)	45%
Elevated serum β_2-microglobulin (>2 × ULN)	65%
Hypercalcemia	6%
Autoimmune hemolytic anemia	~10%
Median survival	10–18 mo

Figures are estimated on the basis of available data—see text for references.
Abbreviations: CLL, chronic lymphocytic leukemia; ECOCT, Eastern Co-operative Oncology Group; LDH, lactate dehydrogenase; ULN, upper limit of normal.

more frequent ($\sim 35\%$) and other extranodal sites somewhat less-frequently involved ($\sim 10\%$) than seen with DLBCL. Characteristically, persistent unexplained high fevers, often with significant weight loss, are presenting features in the majority. Marked elevations of serum LDH ($>2 \times$ ULN) or β_2-microglobulin ($>3 \times$ ULN) are less frequent than in patients with DLBCL-complicating CLL. Similarly, anemia and thrombocytopenia are also somewhat less frequent at the diagnosis of Hodgkin lymphoma, than DLBCL. On occasion, the new development of either AIHA or hypercalcemia may herald the development of Hodgkin lymphoma (142,175).

Histological Features of Richter's Syndrome

Non-Hodgkin Lymphoma

The predominant histopathology is that of DLBCL, however, T-cell lymphomas have also been described, including cutaneous T-cell lymphoma, "pleomorphic" T-cell lymphoma, peripheral T-cell lymphoma, and T-cell anaplastic large cell lymphoma (179–183). The histological and immunophenotypical features of Richter's syndrome manifest as DLBCL have been reviewed by Nakamura et al. (184) and Mao et al. (152). The cellular features are similar to those of de novo DLBCL of either centroblastic ($\sim 80\%$) or immunoblastic types ($\sim 20\%$) (152). In some cases, there can be a more pleomorphic cell population admixed with the background CLL cells (145,147,185). In node biopsies, there may be total effacement by DLBCL, or DLBCL may coexist as a "composite lymphoma" with CLL in the same specimen.

Detailed immunophenotypic studies comparing antigen expression profiles of the CLL cells and their transformed NHL counterparts are infrequent (152). However, most analyzed cases report that the DLBCL retain a number of elements of the phenotype of the original CLL (152,184,186–188). Where differential antigen expression is noted, it most commonly comprises loss of CD5 (68%), CD23 (86%), or surface IgD expression (152,156,160,184,189). In 78% of cases of DLBCL-complicating Zap-70$^+$ CLL, expression of this antigen was lost (152).

Using immunohistochemical profiling to classify DLBCL cases into either "germinal-center B cell" or "activated B cell" subtypes Mao et al. (152) categorized 83% of cases as activated B cell.

Hodgkin Lymphoma

The pathological features of Richter's syndrome manifest as Hodgkin lymphoma can be broadly divided into two groups. In the first group, Reed–Sternberg-like cells are present within a background of CLL. In the second, the appearances are those of typical Hodgkin lymphoma (190).

The presence of scattered Reed–Sternberg-like cells in otherwise typical CLL had been recognized morphologically for many years (147,191,192), but only in more recent years have the pathogenetic role of Epstein–Barr virus (EBV) and the substantial risk of progression to frank Hodgkin lymphoma been realized (176,177,190–192). Momose and colleagues described 13 cases of Reed–Sternberg-like cells in CLL (191). In five cases, the Reed–Sternberg-like cells were CD20-positive and CD15-negative. In two cases, CD20 and CD15 were coexpressed, whereas in six cases, the cells were CD15-positive and CD20-negative. Three patients in the latter group subsequently developed disseminated Hodgkin lymphoma. Similar findings were reported by Williams et al. (192) and Ohno et al. (190) in three additional patients with Richter's syndrome manifest as Hodgkin lymphoma.

While formal histological subclassification is often difficult, all subtypes of classical Hodgkin lymphoma have been reported, with mixed cellularity and nodular sclerosis occurring in approximately 60% and 25% of published cases, respectively (175–177,193). Nodular lymphocyte-predominant Hodgkin lymphoma has also been reported, including one case in which DLBCL later developed (176).

Frequency of Clonal Relatedness

DLBCL

It is apparent from the studies cited earlier that Richter's syndrome may arise either from the same clonal population as the antecedent CLL or as an independent second malignancy. In their review of 27 cases of Richter's syndrome examined for IgH rearrangement, Bessudo and Kipps (185) reported evidence for a common clonal origin of the CLL and DLBCL in 22 patients (81%). Matolcsy and coworkers used direct nucleic acid sequencing of the unique complementary determinant region 3 (CDR3) of the IgH gene to demonstrate clonal evolution of DLBCL from CLL/SLL in seven of nine cases (78%), including one case with disparate IgH gene rearrangements (188,194,195). In two of their nine cases, the CDR3 sequence differed in the CLL and DLBCL cell populations, indicating their independent clonal origins. Similarly, Mao et al. demonstrated identical clonal origins of 78% of the 23 evaluable cases with DLBCL Richter's syndrome, using IgV$_H$ gene sequencing (152). Identical clonal origins were reported in smaller series by Timar et al. (196) in five of eight cases (63%), one of three (33%) by Nakamura et al. (197), and nine of nine by Smits (198). Overall, on the basis of substantial numbers of cases analyzed and the broad consistency of results across series, approximately three-quarters of cases of DLBCL Richter's syndrome occur as a consequence of clonal evolution from the underlying CLL cells.

Hodgkin Lymphoma

In a recent paper, de Leval et al. (199) analyzed two cases of EBV-positive Hodgkin lymphoma-complicating CLL and unequivocally established distinct clonal origins. They carefully reviewed the 13 previously published cases and found that among the nine cases where robust conclusions were possible, the Hodgkin cells arose from the CLL clone in five (55%) and a distinct clone in four (45%). Subsequent publications are consistent with such mixed pathogenesis (152,178), with approximately equal proportions of related and independent clonal origins.

Incidence, Risk Factors, and Epidemiology

Most retrospective series of Richter's syndrome suggested an overall incidence rate of 3% to 5.4% at 10 or more years beyond the diagnosis of CLL (135,143,145,148). However, with more careful scrutiny of relapsing patients and more frequent performance of repeat biopsies, the incidence may be somewhat higher. Prospectively analyzed series have described estimated cumulative incidence rates of 8% (200), approximately 10% (201), and 19% (202). The single-center series of Rossi et al. from the University of Eastern Piedmont, Italy reported an actuarial five-year rate of 13.6% and a 10-year rate of 16.2%, with the frequency steadily increasing with each subsequent relapse (e.g., 28.5% of CLL patients at fourth progression were found to have Richter's transformation) (203). Notably, the larger prospectively analyzed cohorts from multicenter trials, such as the 544 U.S. Intergroup study patients (141), and the aggregated 1379 patients from the MRC (Medical

Research Council) CLL-1, -2, and -3 trials (204) have each reported crude incidences rates of 1% to 2%, perhaps reflecting lesser degrees of scrutiny across multiple centers.

Biological Risk Factors

As discussed in detail elsewhere (205,206), CLL may be classified according to the mutational status of the immunoglobulin heavy chain variable region gene (IgV$_H$) as either "mutated" or "unmutated" with marked demographic, clinical, immunophenotypical, and biological differences between these subgroups. CLL cases with unmutated IgV$_H$ genes have greater genetic instability and manifest a higher rate of clonal evolution on the basis of serial cytogenetic analyses. A greater risk of transformation to Richter's syndrome was seen for patients with unmutated IgV$_H$ genes by Rossi et al. (203) (40% vs. 7% at 10 years for mutated IgV$_H$ cases). However, the significance of this was no longer evident in multivariate analysis, where CD38 expression (a strong surrogate marker for unmutated IgV$_H$ status) was now statistically significantly associated with transformation [hazard ratio (HR) 4.26; $p = 0.018$], along with the specific IgV$_H$4-39 gene usage (HR 4.29; $p = 0.018$).

Early studies of IgV$_H$ mutational status in very small numbers of Richter's cases clearly demonstrated that transformation can occur in cases where the CLL is classified as mutated, such as the two cases reported by Aoki et al. (207), and Nakamura (197), who analyzed four cases, finding three mutated. However, these small samples were somewhat misleading, and a consistent picture has emerged with recent larger studies. Smits et al. (198) evaluated nine cases of Richter's syndrome, finding unmutated IgV$_H$ genes in all nine. Similarly, Timar et al. (196) studied eight cases of Richter's syndrome, finding six to have unmutated IgV$_H$ genes, and five of these showed a shared clonal origin with the underlying CLL. Both cases of Richter's syndrome in patients with mutated IgV$_H$ genes were of independent clonal origin. The most definitive study is that of Mao et al. (152) who presented comprehensive data on 19 evaluable patients with DLBCL Richter's syndrome. There was no apparent predominance for any particular VH gene family usage among the cases with Richter's syndrome (152). However, they noted that 16 (84%) of the 19 cases harbored unmutated IgV$_H$ genes, a proportion substantially in excess of that expected in an unselected group of patients with CLL, even those with clinically progressive disease. These findings substantiate an increased risk of transformation among patients with unmutated IgV$_H$ genes.

Further, of 12 cases with unmutated IgV$_H$ genes, 11 (92%) showed identical clonal origins of the underlying CLL and the DLBCL, confirming clonal evolution in these cases. Conversely, among eight cases of Richter's syndrome emerging in patients with mutated IgV$_H$ genes, only four (50%) showed clonal identity with the emergent DLBCL (152). Thus, in addition to a greater risk of transformation among patients with CLL carrying unmutated IgV$_H$ genes, where such transformation does occur, it is highly likely to arise as a result of clonal evolution of the underlying CLL. Conversely, Richter's syndrome transformation is less likely to occur in patients with CLL carrying hypermutated IgV$_H$ genes, and where such transformation does arise, equal proportions are due to clonal evolution and independent disease origins.

Clinical and Treatment-Related Risk Factors

Despite numerous concerns expressed by a number of authors, as well as summarized by Hamblin (208), the available evidence does not demonstrate any difference in the incidence of Richter's transformation according to initial treatment with alkylating agents or nucleoside analogs, whether fludarabine (141,150) or cladribine (144). Some series have reported a number of cases of transformation occurring soon after the use of nucleoside analogs for relapsed or refractory disease (204), but it is not possible to separate the role of the biological features of the disease that led to the requirement for retreatment as opposed to specific effects of the therapy, per se. Age or gender are not independently predictive of risk of transformation (141,203), although a number of proposed biological risk factors are more common in males (see above). In univariate analysis, Rossi et al. found that at the time of diagnosis an elevated serum LDH, involvement of greater than or equal to three nodal areas and nodal diameter greater than or equal to 3 cm were associated with increased risk of transformation, but when both clinical and biological factors were included in multivariate analysis, only nodal diameter greater than or equal to 3 cm retained statistical significance (HR $= 6.51$; $p = 0.001$).

Prognostic Factors After Development of Richter's Syndrome

Tsimberidou et al. from MD Anderson used their cohort of 130 patients with pathologically confirmed DLBCL Richter syndrome who received treatment to develop a prognostic score for overall survival (143). Including 18 patients who did not receive therapy, the median overall survival was just eight months, with less than 20% of patients surviving beyond two years. In multivariate analysis, there were five factors that remained independently significant in predicting death; performance status ($\geq$2), serum LDH greater than or equal to 1.5 $\times$ ULN, thrombocytopenia ($<$100 $\times$ 10^9/L), maximal tumor diameter greater than 5 cm, and more than one prior systemic therapy (each $p \leq 0.024$). As each of these parameters had a similar magnitude of effect on the HR for death (relative risk approximately 2), a prognostic score was developed, summing the number of the above risk factors present. Patients with zero to two risk factors had a median survival of approximately one year with approximately 25% surviving beyond two years, whereas those with three to five risk factors had a median survival of three to six months, and fewer than 10% survived beyond two years. While this "Richter's syndrome score" can stratify patient outcome in a highly statistically significant fashion ($p < 0.001$), there are no truly "good" prognostic groups identified, and the outcome for all strata remains highly unsatisfactory.

The small number of patients with Hodgkin lymphoma has precluded meaningful exploration of prognostic factors, although neither the Hodgkin prognostic score of Hasenclever, nor the Richter's syndrome score (above) are strongly predictive of outcome (142).

Treatment Options

DLBCL

Broadly, four approaches are reportedly used for the treatment of DLBCL Richter's syndrome. None of these are satisfactory, and outcomes remain very poor with median survival times of less than a year and fewer than 20% of patients surviving beyond one to two years. These dismal outcomes are due to predominantly inadequate disease control; however, treatment intensification is also limited by substantial rates of treatment-related mortality from more intensive regimens. Each of these approaches in turn are discussed below.

"Standard" aggressive lymphoma salvage regimens: The available series has most frequently described the use of anthracycline-based combination chemotherapy such as CHOP after transformation (145,149,209). However, in these series, up to 20% of patients have not been treated, presumably because of severe debilitation at the time of diagnosis.

With such therapies, approximately 40% of patients will obtain an objective response (150), but these responses are transient, with reported median survival figures remarkably consistent at two to five months (145–147,149,150). The small series of seven patients from Yugoslavia (148) is somewhat more optimistic, with three patients surviving at 32 plus, 36 plus, and 120 plus months, which they attribute to the use of more intensive chemotherapy containing both ara-C and methotrexate. The largest series of Robertson et al. reported only 1 of 39 patients alive beyond two years despite the use of MACOP–B or DHAP therapy in a significant proportion of cases (150). The incorporation of the anti-CD20 monoclonal antibody rituximab is a reasonable strategy; however, the available data suggest a modest benefit if any (overall response rate 47% with rituximab compared with 34% without; $p = 0.2$) (143).

The second treatment strategy explored is the use of the more intensive hyper-CVAD regimen (+/– rituximab) alternating with ara-C/methotrexate, a regimen initially developed for the treatment of acute lymphoblastic leukemia (210). The initial study in Richter's syndrome substituted lipsomal daunorubicin for the adriamycin in the standard regimen (211). This was associated with significant myelosuppression, moderate infectious complications, and a 24% treatment-related death rate among a group of 29 patients. In addition to the difficulties of safely delivering the therapy, efficacy was modest, with an overall response rate of 41% [38% CR (complete remission)], and a very disappointing median nine-month overall survival even for those who did achieve a CR. Attempts to optimize this regimen with the addition of rituximab and granulocyte-macrophage colony-stimulating factor (GM-CSF) did not ameliorate the toxicity (212) with 18% of patients dying during the first cycle, and a further 4% during the second. Responses did not appear to be greatly enhanced (overall response rate 43%; 27% CR). Although associated with very substantial toxicity, such aggressive therapies may be justifiable in selected young and fit patients, if subsequent consolidative high-dose therapy and allogeneic transplant are available (see below).

A third approach to therapy has been the use of regimens attempting to exploit the pharmacological synergy between cytarabine and platinum analogs, and the capacity of fludarabine to enhance the cytotoxicity of both of these agents through inhibition of repair of treatment-induced DNA adducts. Such regimens include fludarabine, cisplatin and cytarabine or cyclophosphamide, fludarabine, and cytarabine (213), which produced the promising results of a 45% remission rate and a median survival of 17 months in initial pilot study of 11 patients. However, a subsequent larger follow-on trial using all the four agents (fludarabine, cyclophosphamide, cisplatin, and cytarabine) together with GM-CSF (214) in 22 patients was disappointing with just 5% complete remission rate, 23% of patients progressing on therapy and a median survival of just 2.2 months. The most recent investigational regimen based on this pharmacological strategy is oxalipaltin, fludarabine, cytarabine and rituximab (OFAR) (215). The phase I/II study in 50 patients (20 with Richter's syndrome) achieved a 50% response rate (20% CR), with little evidence of a dose-response relationship for oxaliplatin doses between 17.5 and 25 mg/m^2/day. Responses were achieved in 35% of patients with proven chromosome 17p deletions. Disappointingly, the median response duration was only 10 months, and median survival for patients with Richter's syndrome was less than eight months. The regimen is also markedly myelosuppressive with 85% of patients developing grade 3/4 neutropenia, lasting a median of 12 days (even with growth factor support), and approximately 60% of patients requiring platelet transfusions. While response rates are encouraging, the duration of responses is brief, and all responding patients should be considered for consolidative high-dose therapy if available and appropriate.

While the proportion of patients with CLL and Richter's syndrome ultimately suitable for high-dose therapy and allogeneic transplantation will be small, based on patient age, the requirement to obtain some degree of relatively stable disease control, performance status, organ function, and donor availability criteria; the procedure shows substantial promise and is the only currently available therapy to offer the prospect of durable disease control (216). The potential "immunoresponsiveness" of Richter's syndrome was established by the case report of Espanol et al. (217). They described development of Richter's syndrome four months after allogeneic transplantation, which regressed after withdrawal of immunosuppression and donor lymphocyte infusion and remained in ongoing remission at 18 plus months. A similarly successful case was reported by Milojkovic et al. (218). However, the small series of donor lymphocyte infusions for disease relapse following allografting reported by Russell et al. (219) suggested that such immunotherapy is less effective against Richter's cases than nontransformed CLL. The only series of allogeneic transplantation for patients with Richter's syndrome is from Rodriguez et al. (216), which analyzed eight patients, aged 38 to 59 years, who received sibling or unrelated donor transplants, five of eight were in resistant relapse. Despite such resistant disease and a median of four prior treatment regimens, three patients (38%) remain alive and event-free at 14 to 67 months posttransplant, with two of these three long-term survivors having received non-myeloablative transplants. However, even in this selected young group of patients, toxicity was substantial with five treatment-related deaths, mainly because of infectious complications. An updated analysis from the same group (143) described a 75% three-year progression-free survival for seven patients with Richter's syndrome responding to treatment (CR or PR) who underwent allogeneic transplant during remission, compared with a 27% three-year progression-free survival for responders who did not undergo such consolidation. Transplant in remission is preferred to delaying until the inevitable disease progression, as the three-year progression-free survival was only 21% for those undergoing allografting at relapse. The outcome of autografting subsequent to Richter's transformation was poor (143).

As discussed earlier, transformed disease is usually widespread at the time of recognition. In such circumstances, radiation therapy has no major role when the goal of treatment is durable systemic disease control. However, its local application can provide palliative benefit if individual nodal masses or extranodal disease sites are symptomatic. No accurate data are available on the level of CNS risk in patients with Richter's syndrome, although anecdotal reports clearly demonstrate the risk is present (159,160); the series of Robertson et al. (150) noted CNS involvement at diagnosis in 13% of patients. Given the dominant risk of systemic failure in most cases, it may be reasonable to reserve CNS prophylaxis for those patients believed to be at high risk on the basis of conventional predictive indices (220) and who attain a systemic CR with their initial treatment.

Hodgkin Lymphoma

The natural history and optimal treatment of Hodgkin-type Richter's syndrome is difficult to determine accurately, as the literature is limited to case reports and small series. The largest series of Tsimberidou et al., with 18 patients, described a median survival of approximately 10 months (142). Most reports have used conventional Hodgkin-type combination chemotherapy (MOPP, ABVD, or variants thereof), and there are no prospective studies to guide the choice of a particular regimen. There are no data available on the efficacy and tolerance of more intensive regimens such as BEACOPP-esc or Stanford V, although these merit consideration in younger and fitter patients. When disease has been localized, radiation therapy has usually been incorporated into treatment strategies. Given the role of EBV-infected B cells in the pathogenesis of Hodgkin lymphoma-complicating CLL, incorporation of the anti-CD20 antibody rituximab into the treatment paradigm in patients with CD20-positive disease has a reasonable rationale, although there are no data to support its efficacy in this setting.

Pathogenesis and Molecular Features of Richter's Syndrome

EBV

The B-lymphotropic human herpes virus EBV is implicated in the pathogenesis of a number of lymphoproliferative disorders, including endemic Burkitt lymphoma, posttransplant lymphoproliferative disease, X-linked lymphoproliferative disease, AIDS-related NHL, peripheral T-cell lymphoma, and Hodgkin lymphoma (221). In patients with CLL, EBV has been associated with transformation to both DLBCL and Hodgkin lymphoma (183,204).

While involved in a small proportion of cases of DLBCL-complicating CLL, EBV appears to be of particular pathogenic importance in the development of Hodgkin-type Richter's syndrome, with viral RNA present in the Reed–Sternberg-like cells in 12 of 13 patients, three of whom subsequently developed frank Hodgkin lymphoma (191). In contrast, in a study of 25 patients with DLBCL transformation of CLL, EBV RNA and/or latent membrane protein (LMP) was detected in just four patients (16%), one of whom had T-lineage DLCL (183). Similarly, a recent study (203) found none of 17 cases of DLBCL Richter's to harbor EBV.

Emerging data suggest that those cases of Hodgkin lymphoma harboring EBV that develop in patients with CLL are relatively less frequently clonally related to the underlying CLL. For example, of the three cases studied by Kanzler et al. (222), the two with evidence of EBV infection harbored different immunoglobulin V-region gene rearrangements to the CLL clone. Overall, from 17 evaluable EBV-positive Hodgkin-type Richter cases analyzed, 11 (65%) were clonally unrelated to the underlying CLL (152,178,199,204,222,223), suggesting that this likely represents opportunistic infection, and subsequent malignant transformation of bystander B cells, possibly facilitated by either intrinsic or treatment-related impaired immunity in the host (see chapter "Infections in CLL").

Molecular Abnormalities

The underlying molecular defects and perturbations in cellular control, which are deterministic in the transformation of CLL, remain poorly elucidated. While there is a growing body of literature describing and profiling abnormalities in cells from patients with Richter's syndrome, the direct causative role of these abnormalities remain unproven. Excellent reviews evaluating the frequency of involvement of the broad spectrum of putatively pathogenetic molecular and cell biological abnormalities in DLBCL or Hodgkin–Reed–Sternberg cells developing in patients with CLL have recently been published (184,224). This broad, complex, and dynamic field is only briefly explored here, with the more frequently reported molecular abnormalities summarized in Table 3 (224).

Cytogenetics

Serial cytogenetic analyses comparing karotypes of CLL and Richter's syndrome are very uncommon. Available data from comparative genomic hybridization have shown

Table 3 Overview of Reported Molecular Defects in Richter Syndrome

Pathway and target	Mechanism	Frequency
Apoptosis:		
BCL-2	Chromosomal rearrangement	0/10
	↑protein expression	3/4
Cell cycle regulation:		
P16^{INK4a}	Gene deletions	4/13
	Mutations	0/11
P21$^{Cip1/Waf1}$	Loss of protein expression	4/7
P27^{kip1}	Loss of protein expression	7/7
Rb	Gene rearrangement	0/6
Cyclin D1	Gene rearrangement	0/13
P53 pathway:		
ATM	Loss of heterozygosity	7/15
P53	Loss of heterozygosity	11/30
	↑protein expression	8/15
Chk2	Deletions or mutations	0/8
p14^{ARF}	Loss of heterozygosity	2/14
Microsatellite instability		7/15

Note: Data are aggregated and summarized from Ref. 224.

conservation of the common gains of chromosome 12 and losses of chromosome 13q in Richter's syndrome, but with a higher number of chromosomal gains, losses (most frequently chromosome 8p or 9), and total alterations in Richter's compared with CLL (225). Classical "Burkitt" translocations involving c-myc are uncommon (226).

P53

P53 is one of the more frequently implicated genetic abnormalities in Richter's syndrome. As discussed in detail elsewhere, less than 10% of unselected CLL cases will harbor p53 abnormalities, whereas approximately 40% to 60% of cases of Richter's syndrome have p53 mutations or loss of heterozygosity (225,227,228). The critical role of the acquisition of p53 mutations is supported by the recent study of Rossi et al. (203), which found such mutations in 53% of cases of Richter's transformation, but in just 11% of these patients during their course of nontransformed CLL.

Conclusions

There has been a great fascination with the pathogenesis of Richter's syndrome over the years, which is out of proportion to the frequency of the events. Exploring the clonal relatedness of these disorders has shed a great deal of light on the process of lymphoid cell development and regulation of the immunoglobulin gene cluster. It is now clear that most instances of Richter's transformation are truly manifestations of clonal progression of the underlying CLL, with data emerging that different precipitating events may contribute to the various histological manifestations of such transformation.

Although there has been significant progress in the treatment of the "indolent" phase of CLL, the efficacy of treatment of the various manifestations of Richter's syndrome remains inadequate. The focused work of the MD Anderson group and others in developing specific therapeutic strategies for patients with Richter's syndrome is beginning to show promise that improvements are likely to emerge from rationally designed treatments, likely incorporating B-cell-directed monoclonal antibodies. Tolerance of treatment is a critical issue in these often frail and immunocompromised older patients. Where feasible, allogeneic transplant, including reduced intensity-preparative regimens, should be strongly considered, as it is the only treatment approach with possibly curative potential. Until more effective and better-tolerated treatments are developed, clinicians must remain wary of any apparent changes in the natural history of the disease in their patients, with a high index of suspicion and a willingness to obtain adequate tissue biopsy specimens from atypical sites or other areas of concern due to their dominant bulk or disproportionately rapid growth. FDG-PET scanning will likely prove useful in screening patients and guiding sites for biopsy.

In summary, both autoimmune complications and Richter's syndrome can have a profound effect on the management of a patient with CLL. Our understanding of the pathogenesis of these complications continues to evolve and provides the basis for the development of more effective treatments. Further research should also focus on the prevention of these complications and particularly study their nature and incidence with the various new CLL-treatment strategies.

REFERENCES

1. Hamblin TJ, Oscier DG, Young BJ. Autoimmunity in chronic lymphocytic leukaemia. J Clin Pathol 1986; 39(7):713–716.
2. Rozman C, Montserrat E. Chronic lymphocytic leukemia. N Engl J Med 1995; 333(16): 1052–1057.
3. Hamblin TJ. Autoimmune complications of chronic lymphocytic leukemia. Semin Oncol 2006; 33(2):230–239.
4. Ghia P, Caligaris-Cappio F. The origin of B-cell chronic lymphocytic leukemia. Semin Oncol 2006; 33(2):150–156.
5. Caligaris-Cappio F, Ghia P. The normal counterpart to the chronic lymphocytic leukemia B cell. Best Pract Res Clin Haematol 2007; 20(3):385–397.
6. Kantor A. A new nomenclature for B cells. Immunol Today 1991; 12(11):388.
7. Morikawa K, Oseko F, Morikawa S. Induction of CD5 antigen on human CD5- B cells by stimulation with Staphylococcus aureus Cowan strain I. Int Immunol 1993; 5(8):809–816.
8. Broker BM, Klajman A, Youinou P, et al. Chronic lymphocytic leukemic (CLL) cells secrete multispecific autoantibodies. J Autoimmun 1988; 1(5):469–481.
9. Borche L, Lim A, Binet JL, et al. Evidence that chronic lymphocytic leukemia B lymphocytes are frequently committed to production of natural autoantibodies. Blood 1990; 76(3):562–569.
10. Sthoeger ZM, Wakai M, Tse DB, et al. Production of autoantibodies by CD5-expressing B lymphocytes from patients with chronic lymphocytic leukemia. J Exp Med 1989; 169(1): 255–268.
11. Stamatopoulos K, Belessi C, Moreno C, et al. Over 20% of patients with chronic lymphocytic leukemia carry stereotyped receptors: Pathogenetic implications and clinical correlations. Blood 2007; 109(1):259–270.
12. Corcione A, Aloisi F, Serafini B, et al. B-cell differentiation in the CNS of patients with multiple sclerosis. Autoimmun Rev 2005; 4(8):549–554.
13. Mackay IR, Rose NR. Autoimmunity and lymphoma: tribulations of B cells. Nat Immunol 2001; 2(9):793–795.
14. Suarez F, Lortholary O, Hermine O, et al. Infection-associated lymphomas derived from marginal zone B cells: a model of antigen-driven lymphoproliferation. Blood 2006; 107(8): 3034–3044.
15. Kassan SS, Thomas TL, Moutsopoulos HM, et al. Increased risk of lymphoma in sicca syndrome. Ann Intern Med 1978; 89(6):888–892.

16. Lindsay S, Dailey ME. Malignant lymphoma of the thyroid gland and its relation to Hashimoto disease: a clinical and pathologic study of 8 patients. J Clin Endocrinol Metab 1955; 15(11):1332–1353.

17. Landgren O, Engels EA, Caporaso NE, et al. Patterns of autoimmunity and subsequent chronic lymphocytic leukemia in Nordic countries. Blood 2006; 108(1):292–296.

18. Hamblin TJ, Davis Z, Gardiner A, et al. Unmutated Ig V(H) genes are associated with a more aggressive form of chronic lymphocytic leukemia. Blood 1999; 94(6):1848–1854.

19. Damle RN, Wasil T, Fais F, et al. Ig V gene mutation status and CD38 expression as novel prognostic indicators in chronic lymphocytic leukemia. Blood. 1999; 94(6):1840–1847 (comment).

20. Herve M, Xu K, Ng YS, et al. Unmutated and mutated chronic lymphocytic leukemias derive from self-reactive B cell precursors despite expressing different antibody reactivity. J Clin Invest 2005; 115(6):1636–1643.

21. Silverman GJ, Goldfien RD, Chen P, et al. Idiotypic and subgroup analysis of human monoclonal rheumatoid factors. Implications for structural and genetic basis of autoantibodies in humans. J Clin Invest 1988; 82(2):469–475.

22. Silverman GJ, Schrohenloher RE, Accavitti MA, et al. Structural characterization of the second major cross-reactive idiotype group of human rheumatoid factors. Association with the VH4 gene family. Arthritis Rheum 1990; 33(9):1347–1360.

23. Thompson KM, Sutherland J, Barden G, et al. Human monoclonal antibodies against blood group antigens preferentially express a VH4-21 variable region gene-associated epitope. Scand J Immunol 1991; 34(4):509–518.

24. Silberstein LE, Jefferies LC, Goldman J, et al. Variable region gene analysis of pathologic human autoantibodies to the related i and I red blood cell antigens. Blood 1991; 78(9): 2372–2386.

25. Stevenson FK, Longhurst C, Chapman CJ, et al. Utilization of the VH4-21 gene segment by anti-DNA antibodies from patients with systemic lupus erythematosus. J Autoimmun 1993; 6(6): 809–825.

26. Pascual V, Victor K, Spellerberg M, et al. VH restriction among human cold agglutinins. The VH4-21 gene segment is required to encode anti-I and anti-i specificities. J Immunol 1992; 149(7):2337–2344.

27. Dighiero G, Rose NR. Critical self-epitopes are key to the understanding of self-tolerance and autoimmunity. Immunol Today 1999; 20(9):423–428.

28. Pritsch O, Maloum K, Dighiero G. Basic biology of autoimmune phenomena in chronic lymphocytic leukemia. Semin Oncol 1998; 25(1):34–41.

29. Delves PJ, Roitt IM. The immune system. First of two parts. N Engl J Med 2000; 343(1):37–49.

30. Boes M. Role of natural and immune IgM antibodies in immune responses. Mol Immunol 2000; 37(18):1141–1149.

31. Chiorazzi N. CLL: at the intersection of autoimmunity, innate and adaptive immunity, and malignancy. Leuk Lymphoma 2007; 48(suppl 1):S5–S6.

32. Rai KR, Sawitsky A, Cronkite EP, et al. Clinical staging of chronic lymphocytic leukemia. Blood 1975; 46(2):219–234.

33. Binet JL, Auquier A, Dighiero G, et al. A new prognostic classification of chronic lymphocytic leukemia derived from a multivariate survival analysis. Cancer 1981; 48(1):198–206.

34. Cheson BD, Bennett JM, Grever M, et al. National Cancer Institute-sponsored Working Group guidelines for chronic lymphocytic leukemia: revised guidelines for diagnosis and treatment. Blood 1996; 87(12):4990–4997.

35. Eichhorst B, Hallek M. Revision of the guidelines for diagnosis and therapy of chronic lymphocytic leukemia (CLL). Best Pract Res Clin Haematol 2007; 20(3):469–477.

36. Diehl LF, Ketchum LH. Autoimmune disease and chronic lymphocytic leukemia: autoimmune hemolytic anemia, pure red cell aplasia, and autoimmune thrombocytopenia. Semin Oncol 1998; 25(1):80–97.

37. Engelfriet CP, Overbeeke MA, von dem Borne AE. Autoimmune hemolytic anemia. Semin Hematol 1992; 29(1):3–12.

38. Kyasa MJ, Parrish RS, Schichman SA, et al. Autoimmune cytopenia does not predict poor prognosis in chronic lymphocytic leukemia/small lymphocytic lymphoma. Am J Hematol 2003; 74(1):1–8.
39. Sthoeger ZM, Sthoeger D, Shtalrid M, et al. Mechanism of autoimmune hemolytic anemia in chronic lymphocytic leukemia. Am J Hematol 1993; 43(4):259–264.
40. Barcellini W, Capalbo S, Agostinelli RM, et al. Relationship between autoimmune phenomena and disease stage and therapy in B-cell chronic lymphocytic leukemia. Haematologica 2006; 91(12):1689–1692.
41. Mauro FR, Foa R, Cerretti R, et al. Autoimmune hemolytic anemia in chronic lymphocytic leukemia: clinical, therapeutic, and prognostic features. Blood 2000; 95(9):2786–2792.
42. Catovsky D, Richards S. Incidence of hemolytic anemia after chemotherapy in the CLL4 trial. A possible protective role for fludarabine plus cyclophosphamide. ASH Annual Meeting Abstracts 2004; 104(11):480.
43. Eichhorst BF, Busch R, Hopfinger G, et al. Fludarabine plus cyclophosphamide versus fludarabine alone in first-line therapy of younger patients with chronic lymphocytic leukemia. Blood 2006; 107(3):885–891.
44. Keating MJ, O'Brien S, Albitar M, et al. Early results of a chemoimmunotherapy regimen of fludarabine, cyclophosphamide, and rituximab as initial therapy for chronic lymphocytic leukemia. J Clin Oncol 2005; 23(18):4079–4088.
45. Sokol RJ, Hewitt S, Booker DJ, et al. An enzyme-linked direct antiglobulin test for assessing erythrocyte bound immunoglobulins. J Immunol Methods 1988; 106(1):31–35.
46. Hall AM, Vickers MA, McLeod E, et al. Rh autoantigen presentation to helper T cells in chronic lymphocytic leukemia by malignant B cells. Blood 2005; 105(5):2007–2015.
47. Barcellini W, Montesano R, Clerici G, et al. In vitro production of anti-RBC antibodies and cytokines in chronic lymphocytic leukemia. Am J Hematol 2002; 71(3):177–183.
48. Duhrsen U, Augener W, Zwingers T, et al. Spectrum and frequency of autoimmune derangements in lymphoproliferative disorders: analysis of 637 cases and comparison with myeloproliferative diseases. Br J Haematol 1987; 67(2):235–239.
49. Chikkappa G, Zarrabi MH, Tsan MF. Pure red-cell aplasia in patients with chronic lymphocytic leukemia. Medicine (Baltimore) 1986; 65(5):339–351.
50. Fisch P, Handgretinger R, Schaefer HE. Pure red cell aplasia. Br J Haematol 2000; 111(4): 1010–1022.
51. Mangan KF, Chikkappa G, Bieler LZ, et al. Regulation of human blood erythroid burst-forming unit (BFU-E) proliferation by T-lymphocyte subpopulations defined by Fc receptors and monoclonal antibodies. Blood 1982; 59(5):990–996.
52. Elson CJ, Barker RN, Thompson SJ, et al. Immunologically ignorant autoreactive T cells, epitope spreading and repertoire limitation. Immunol Today 1995; 16(2):71–76.
53. Barker RN, Elson CJ. Multiple self epitopes on the Rhesus polypeptides stimulate immunologically ignorant human T cells in vitro. Eur J Immunol 1994; 24(7):1578–1582.
54. Sakaguchi S. Naturally arising CD4+ regulatory t cells for immunologic self-tolerance and negative control of immune responses. Annu Rev Immunol 2004; 22:531–562.
55. O'Garra A, Vieira P. Regulatory T cells and mechanisms of immune system control. Nat Med 2004; 10(8):801–805.
56. Davidson A, Diamond B. Autoimmune diseases. N Engl J Med 2001; 345(5):340–350.
57. Barker RN, Hall AM, Standen GR, et al. Identification of T-cell epitopes on the Rhesus polypeptides in autoimmune hemolytic anemia. Blood 1997; 90(7):2701–2715.
58. Hall AM, Ward FJ, Vickers MA, et al. Interleukin-10-mediated regulatory T-cell responses to epitopes on a human red blood cell autoantigen. Blood 2002; 100(13):4529–4536.
59. Dazzi F, D'Andrea E, Biasi G, et al. Failure of B cells of chronic lymphocytic leukemia in presenting soluble and alloantigens. Clin Immunol Immunopathol 1995; 75(1):26–32.
60. Mittal S, Blaylock MG, Culligan DJ, et al. A high rate of CLL phenotype lymphocytes in autoimmune hemolytic anemia and immune thrombocytopenic purpura. Haematologica 2008; 93(1):151–152.

61. Eris JM, Basten A, Brink R, et al. Anergic self-reactive B cells present self antigen and respond normally to CD40-dependent T-cell signals but are defective in antigen-receptor-mediated functions. Proc Natl Acad Sci U S A 1994; 91(10):4392–4396.

62. Ranheim EA, Kipps TJ. Activated T cells induce expression of B7/BB1 on normal or leukemic B cells through a CD40-dependent signal. J Exp Med 1993; 177(4):925–935.

63. Wierda WG, Cantwell MJ, Woods SJ, et al. CD40-ligand (CD154) gene therapy for chronic lymphocytic leukemia. Blood 2000; 96(9):2917–2924.

64. Schattner EJ, Mascarenhas J, Reyfman I, et al. Chronic lymphocytic leukemia B cells can express CD40 ligand and demonstrate T-cell type costimulatory capacity. Blood 1998; 91(8): 2689–2697.

65. Viglianti GA, Lau CM, Hanley TM, et al. Activation of autoreactive B cells by CpG dsDNA. Immunity 2003; 19(6):837–847.

66. Caligaris-Cappio F. Biology of chronic lymphocytic leukemia. Rev Clin Exp Hematol 2000; 4(1):5–21.

67. Sneller MC, Wang J, Dale JK, et al. Clincal, immunologic, and genetic features of an autoimmune lymphoproliferative syndrome associated with abnormal lymphocyte apoptosis. Blood 1997; 89(4):1341–1348.

68. Greaney P, Nahimana A, Lagopoulos L, et al. A Fas agonist induces high levels of apoptosis in haematological malignancies. Leuk Res 2006; 30(4):415–426.

69. Panayiotidis P, Ganeshaguru K, Foroni L, et al. Expression and function of the FAS antigen in B chronic lymphocytic leukemia and hairy cell leukemia. Leukemia 1995; 9(7):1227–1232.

70. Kay NE, Han L, Bone N, et al. Interleukin 4 content in chronic lymphocytic leukaemia (CLL) B cells and blood CD8+ T cells from B-CLL patients: impact on clonal B-cell apoptosis. Br J Haematol 2001; 112(3):760–767.

71. Cantwell M, Hua T, Pappas J, et al. Acquired CD40-ligand deficiency in chronic lymphocytic leukemia. Nat Med 1997; 3(9):984–989.

72. Scrivener S, Goddard RV, Kaminski ER, et al. Abnormal T-cell function in B-cell chronic lymphocytic leukaemia. Leuk Lymphoma 2003; 44(3):383–389.

73. Beyer M, Kochanek M, Darabi K, et al. Reduced frequencies and suppressive function of CD4+CD25hi regulatory T cells in patients with chronic lymphocytic leukemia after therapy with fludarabine. Blood 2005; 106(6):2018–2025.

74. Shevach EM. Regulatory T cells in autoimmmunity*. Annu Rev Immunol 2000; 18:423–449.

75. Viglietta V, Baecher-Allan C, Weiner HL, et al. Loss of functional suppression by CD4+CD25+ regulatory T cells in patients with multiple sclerosis. J Exp Med 2004; 199(7): 971–979.

76. Crispin JC, Martinez A, Alcocer-Varela J. Quantification of regulatory T cells in patients with systemic lupus erythematosus. J Autoimmun 2003; 21(3):273–276.

77. Ichihara F, Kono K, Takahashi A, et al. Increased populations of regulatory T cells in peripheral blood and tumor-infiltrating lymphocytes in patients with gastric and esophageal cancers. Clin Cancer Res 2003; 9(12):4404–4408.

78. Woo EY, Yeh H, Chu CS, et al. Cutting edge: Regulatory T cells from lung cancer patients directly inhibit autologous T cell proliferation. J Immunol 2002; 168(9):4272–4276.

79. Wolf AM, Wolf D, Steurer M, et al. Increase of regulatory T cells in the peripheral blood of cancer patients. Clin Cancer Res 2003; 9(2):606–612.

80. Thornton AM, Shevach EM. CD4+CD25+ immunoregulatory T cells suppress polyclonal T cell activation in vitro by inhibiting interleukin 2 production. J Exp Med 1998; 188(2): 287–296.

81. Fallarino F, Fields PE, Gajewski TF. B7-1 engagement of cytotoxic T lymphocyte antigen 4 inhibits T cell activation in the absence of CD28. J Exp Med 1998; 188(1):205–210.

82. Pavkovic M, Georgievski B, Cevreska L, et al. CTLA-4 exon 1 polymorphism in patients with autoimmune blood disorders. Am J Hematol 2003; 72(2):147–149.

83. Hamblin TJ, Orchard JA, Myint H, et al. Fludarabine and hemolytic anemia in chronic lymphocytic leukemia. J Clin Oncol 1998; 16(9):3209–3210.

84. Gonzalez H, Leblond V, Azar N, et al. Severe autoimmune hemolytic anemia in eight patients treated with fludarabine. Hematol Cell Ther 1998; 40(3):113–118.
85. Weiss RB, Freiman J, Kweder SL, et al. Hemolytic anemia after fludarabine therapy for chronic lymphocytic leukemia. J Clin Oncol 1998; 16(5):1885–1889.
86. Myint H, Copplestone JA, Orchard J, et al. Fludarabine-related autoimmune haemolytic anaemia in patients with chronic lymphocytic leukaemia. Br J Haematol 1995; 91(2):341–344.
87. Catovsky D, Richards S, Matutes E, et al. Assessment of fludarabine plus cyclophosphamide for patients with chronic lymphocytic leukaemia (the LRF CLL4 Trial): a randomised controlled trial. Lancet 2007; 370(9583):230–239.
88. Leporrier M, Reman O, Troussard X. Pure red-cell aplasia with fludarabine for chronic lymphocytic leukaemia. Lancet 1993; 342(8870):555.
89. Di Raimondo F, Giustolisi R, Cacciola E, et al. Autoimmune hemolytic anemia in chronic lymphocytic leukemia patients treated with fludarabine. Leuk Lymphoma 1993; 11(1–2):63–68.
90. Robak T, Blasinska-Morawiec M, Krykowski E, et al. Autoimmune haemolytic anaemia in patients with chronic lymphocytic leukaemia treated with 2-chlorodeoxyadenosine (cladribine). Eur J Haematol 1997; 58(2):109–113.
91. Chasty RC, Myint H, Oscier DG, et al. Autoimmune haemolysis in patients with B-CLL treated with chlorodeoxyadenosine (CDA). Leuk Lymphoma 1998; 29(3–4):391–398.
92. Byrd JC, Hertler AA, Weiss RB, et al. Fatal recurrence of autoimmune hemolytic anemia following pentostatin therapy in a patient with a history of fludarabine-associated hemolytic anemia. Ann Oncol 1995; 6(3):300–301.
93. Lewis FB, Schwartz RS, Dameshek W. X-radiation and alkylating agents as possible "trigger" mechanisms in the autoimmune complications of malignant lymphophroliferative disease. Clin Exp Immunol 1966; 1(1):3–11.
94. Dearden C, Wade R, Else M, et al. The prognostic significance of a positive direct antiglobulin test in chronic lymphocytic leukemia: a beneficial effect of the combination of fludarabine and cyclophosphamide on the incidence of hemolytic anemia. Blood 2008; 111(4):1820–1826.
95. Flinn IW, Neuberg DS, Grever MR, et al. Phase III trial of fludarabine plus cyclophosphamide compared with fludarabine for patients with previously untreated chronic lymphocytic leukemia: US Intergroup Trial E2997. J Clin Oncol 2007; 25(7):793–798.
96. Borthakur G, O'Brien S, Wierda WG, et al. Immune anaemias in patients with chronic lymphocytic leukaemia treated with fludarabine, cyclophosphamide and rituximab–incidence and predictors. Br J Haematol 2007; 136(6):800–805.
97. Eberl G, Renggli J, Men Y, et al. Extracellular processing and presentation of a 69-mer synthetic polypetide to MHC class I-restricted T cells. Mol Immunol 1999; 36(2):103–112.
98. Zanotti R, Ambrosetti A, Andreoli A, et al. ZAP-70 expression in B-CLL is associated with increased risk of autoimmune cytopenias. Haematologica 2006; 91(s1):104.
99. Foon KA, Rai KR, Gale RP. Chronic lymphocytic leukemia: new insights into biology and therapy. Ann Intern Med 1990; 113(7):525–539.
100. Anhalt GJ, Kim SC, Stanley JR, et al. Paraneoplastic pemphigus. An autoimmune mucocutaneous disease associated with neoplasia. N Engl J Med 1990; 323(25):1729–1735.
101. Goodnough LT, Muir WA. Bullous pemphigoid as a manifestation of chronic lymphocytic leukemia. Arch Intern Med 1980; 140(11):1526–1527.
102. Hill PA, Firkin F, Dwyer KM, et al. Membranoproliferative glomerulonephritis in association with chronic lymphocytic leukaemia: a report of three cases. Pathology 2002; 34(2):138–143.
103. Macheta MP, Parapia LA, Gouldesbrough DR. Renal failure in a patient with chronic lymphocytic leukaemia treated with fludarabine. J Clin Pathol 1995; 48(2):181–182.
104. Tisler A, Pierratos A, Lipton JH. Crescentic glomerulonephritis associated with p-ANCA positivity in fludarabine-treated chronic lymphocytic leukaemia. Nephrol Dial Transplant 1996; 11(11):2306–2308.
105. Lipscombe TK, Orton DI, Bird AG, et al. Acquired C1-esterase inhibitor deficiency: three case reports and commentary on the syndrome. Australas J Dermatol 1996; 37(3):145–148.
106. Chevailler A, Arlaud G, Ponard D, et al. C-1-inhibitor binding monoclonal immunoglobins in three patients with acquired angioneurotic edema. J Allergy Clin Immunol 1996; 97(4):998–1008.

107. Michiels JJ, Budde U, van der Planken M, et al. Acquired von Willebrand syndromes: clinical features, aetiology, pathophysiology, classification and management. Best Pract Res Clin Haematol 2001; 14(2):401–436.

108. Mateo J, Martino R, Borrell M, et al. Acquired factor VIII inhibitor preceding chronic lymphocytic leukemia. Ann Hematol 1993; 67(6):309–311.

109. Mahipal A, Bilgrami S. Acquired hemophilia in chronic lymphocytic leukemia. Leuk Lymphoma 2007; 48(5):1026–1028.

110. Goodrick MJ, Prentice AG, Copplestone JA, et al. Acquired factor XI inhibitor in chronic lymphocytic leukaemia. J Clin Pathol 1992; 45(4):352–353.

111. Dameshek W, Komninos ZD. The present status of treatment of autoimmune hemolytic anemia with ACTH and cortisone. Blood 1956; 11(7):648–664.

112. Flores G, Cunningham-Rundles C, Newland AC, et al. Efficacy of intravenous immunoglobulin in the treatment of autoimmune hemolytic anemia: results in 73 patients. Am J Hematol 1993; 44(4):237–242.

113. Besa EC. Rapid transient reversal of anemia and long-term effects of maintenance intravenous immunoglobulin for autoimmune hemolytic anemia in patients with lymphoproliferative disorders. Am J Med 1988; 84(4):691–698.

114. Cortes J, O'Brien S, Loscertales J, et al. Cyclosporin A for the treatment of cytopenia associated with chronic lymphocytic leukemia. Cancer 2001; 92(8): 2016–2022.

115. Seymour JF, Cusack JD, Lerner SA, et al. Case/control study of the role of splenectomy in chronic lymphocytic leukemia. J Clin Oncol 1997; 15(1):52–60.

116. Dacie JV. Autoimmune hemolytic anemia. Arch Intern Med 1975; 135(10):1293–1300.

117. McMillan R. Therapy for adults with refractory chronic immune thrombocytopenic purpura. Ann Intern Med 1997; 126(4):307–314.

118. Guiney MJ, Liew KH, Quong GG, et al. A study of splenic irradiation in chronic lymphocytic leukemia. Int J Radiat Oncol Biol Phys 1989; 16(1):225–229.

119. Shaw T, Quan J, Totoritis MC. B cell therapy for rheumatoid arthritis: the rituximab (anti-CD20) experience. Ann Rheum Dis 2003; 62(suppl 2):ii55–ii59.

120. Tokunaga M, Fujii K, Saito K, et al. Down-regulation of CD40 and CD80 on B cells in patients with life-threatening systemic lupus erythematosus after successful treatment with rituximab. Rheumatology (Oxford) 2005; 44(2):176–182.

121. Stasi R, Brunetti M, Stipa E, et al. Selective B-cell depletion with rituximab for the treatment of patients with acquired hemophilia. Blood 2004; 103(12):4424–4428.

122. Dupuy A, Viguier M, Bedane C, et al. Treatment of refractory pemphigus vulgaris with rituximab (anti-CD20 monoclonal antibody). Arch Dermatol 2004; 140(1):91–96.

123. Sansonno D, De Re V, Lauletta G, et al. Monoclonal antibody treatment of mixed cryoglobulinemia resistant to interferon alpha with an anti-CD20. Blood 2003; 101(10): 3818–3826.

124. Pestronk A, Florence J, Miller T, et al. Treatment of IgM antibody associated polyneuropathies using rituximab. J Neurol Neurosurg Psychiatry 2003; 74(4):485–489.

125. Shanafelt TD, Madueme HL, Wolf RC, et al. Rituximab for immune cytopenia in adults: idiopathic thrombocytopenic purpura, autoimmune hemolytic anemia, and Evans syndrome. Mayo Clin Proc 2003; 78(11):1340–1346.

126. Zaja F, Vianelli N, Sperotto A, et al. Anti-CD20 therapy for chronic lymphocytic leukemia-associated autoimmune diseases. Leuk Lymphoma 2003; 44(11): 1951–1955.

127. Narat S, Gandla J, Hoffbrand AV, et al. Rituximab in the treatment of refractory autoimmune cytopenias in adults. Haematologica 2005; 90(9):1273–1274.

128. Gupta N, Kavuru S, Patel D, et al. Rituximab-based chemotherapy for steroid-refractory autoimmune hemolytic anemia of chronic lymphocytic leukemia. Leukemia 2002; 16(10): 2092–2095.

129. Ghazal H. Successful treatment of pure red cell aplasia with rituximab in patients with chronic lymphocytic leukemia. Blood 2002; 99(3):1092–1094.

130. Lundin J, Porwit-MacDonald A, Rossmann ED, et al. Cellular immune reconstitution after subcutaneous alemtuzumab (anti-CD52 monoclonal antibody, CAMPATH-1H) treatment as first-line therapy for B-cell chronic lymphocytic leukaemia. Leukemia 2004; 18(3):484–490.

131. Karlsson C, Hansson L, Celsing F, et al. Treatment of severe refractory autoimmune hemolytic anemia in B-cell chronic lymphocytic leukemia with alemtuzumab (humanized CD52 monoclonal antibody). Leukemia 2007; 21(3):511–514.

132. Rodon P, Breton P, Courouble G. Treatment of pure red cell aplasia and autoimmune haemolytic anaemia in chronic lymphocytic leukaemia with Campath-1H. Eur J Haematol 2003; 70(5):319–321.

133. Hillmen P, Skotnicki AB, Robak T, et al. Alemtuzumab compared with chlorambucil as first-line therapy for chronic lymphocytic leukemia. J Clin Oncol 2007; 25(35):5616–5623.

134. Orchard J, Bolam S, Myint H, et al. In patients with lymphoid tumours recovering from the autoimmune complications of fludarabine, relapse may be triggered by conventional chemotherapy. Br J Haematol 1998; 102(4):1112–1113.

135. Lortholary P, Boiron M, Ripault P, et al. Chronic lymphoid leukemia secondarily associated with a malignant reticulopathy richter's syndrome. Nouv Rev Fr Hematol 1964; 78:621–644.

136. Richter MN. Generalized reticular cell sarcoma of lymph nodes associated with lymphocytic leukemia. Am J Pathol 1928; 4:285–292.

137. Enno A, Catovsky D, O'Brien M, et al. 'Prolymphocytoid' transformation of chronic lymphocytic leukaemia. Br J Haematol 1979; 41:9–18.

138. Melo JV, Wardle J, Chetty M, et al. The relationship between chronic lymphocytic leukaemia and prolymphocytic leukaemia. III. Evaluation of cell size by morphology and volume measurements. Br J Haematol 1986; 64:469–478.

139. Gutteridge CN, Newland AC. Chronic lymphocytic leukaemia complicating null cell acute lymphoblastic leukaemia. Clin Lab Haematol 1986; 8:77–79.

140. Brouet JC, Fermand JP, Laurent G, et al. The association of chronic lymphocytic leukaemia and multiple myeloma: a study of eleven patients. Br J Haematol 1985; 59:55–66.

141. Morrison VA, Rai KR, Peterson BL, et al. Transformation to Richter's syndrome or prolymphocytic leukemia (PLL), and other second malignancies in patients with chronic lymphocytic leukemia (CLL): an Intrgroup Study (CALGB 9011). Blood 1999; 94(suppl.): 539a (abstract).

142. Tsimberidou AM, O'Brien S, Kantarjian HM, et al. Hodgkin transformation of chronic lymphocytic leukemia: the M. D. Anderson Cancer Center experience. Cancer 2006; 107:1294–1302.

143. Tsimberidou AM, O'Brien S, Khouri I, et al. Clinical outcomes and prognostic factors in patients with Richter's syndrome treated with chemotherapy or chemoimmunotherapy with or without stem-cell transplantation. J Clin Oncol 2006; 24:2343–2351.

144. Robak T, Blonski JZ, Gora-Tybor J, et al. Second malignancies and Richter's syndrome in patients with chronic lymphocytic leukaemia treated with cladribine. Eur J Cancer 2004; 40:383–389.

145. Armitage JO, Dick FR, Corder MP. Diffuse histiocytic lymphoma complicating chronic lymphocytic leukemia. Cancer 1978; 41:422–427.

146. Foucar K, Rydell RE. Richter's syndrome in chronic lymphocytic leukemia. Cancer 1980; 46:118–134.

147. Harousseau JL, Flandrin G, Tricot G, et al. Malignant lymphoma supervening in chronic lymphocytic leukemia and related disorders. Richter's syndrome: a study of 25 cases. Cancer 1981; 48:1302–1308.

148. Jelic S, Jovanovic V, Milanovic N, et al. Richter syndrome with emphasis on large-cell non-Hodgkin lymphoma in previously unrecognized subclinical chronic lymphocytic leukemia. Neoplasma 1997; 44:63–68.

149. Trump DL, Mann RB, Phelps R, et al. Richter's syndrome: diffuse histiocytic lymphoma in patients with chronic lymphocytic leukemia. A report of five cases and review of the literature. Am J Med 1980; 68:539–548.

150. Robertson LE, Pugh W, O'Brien S, et al. Richter's syndrome: a report on 39 patients. J Clin Oncol 1993; 11:1985–1989.

151. Long JC, Aisenberg AC. Richter's syndrome. A terminal complication of chronic lymphocytic leukemia with distinct clinicopathologic features. Am J Clin Pathol 1975; 63:786–795.

152. Mao Z, Quintanilla-Martinez L, Raffeld M, et al. IgVH mutational status and clonality analysis of Richter's transformation: diffuse large B-cell lymphoma and Hodgkin lymphoma in association with B-cell chronic lymphocytic leukemia (B-CLL) represent 2 different pathways of disease evolution. Am J Surg Pathol 2007; 31:1605–1614.

153. Ma Y, Mansour A, Bekele BN, et al. The clinical significance of large cells in bone marrow in patients with chronic lymphocytic leukemia. Cancer 2004; 100:2167–2175.

154. Tohda S, Morio T, Suzuki T, et al. Richter syndrome with two B cell clones possessing different surface immunoglobulins and immunoglobulin gene rearrangements. Am J Hematol 1990; 35:32–36.

155. Martinez-Lostao L, Briones J, Forne I, et al. Role of the STAT1 pathway in apoptosis induced by fludarabine and JAK kinase inhibitors in B-cell chronic lymphocytic leukemia. Leuk Lymphoma 2005; 46:435–442.

156. van Endert PM, Mechtersheimer G, Moller P, et al. Discordant differentiation antigen pattern in a case of Richter's syndrome with monoclonal idiotype expression and immunoglobulin gene rearrangement. Br J Cancer 1990; 62:248–252.

157. Robak E, Robak T. Skin lesions in chronic lymphocytic leukemia. Leuk Lymphoma 2007; 48:855–865.

158. Jimenez C, Ribera JM, Junca J, et al. Richter syndrome with exclusively cutaneous involvement. Sangre (Barc) 1993; 38:67–69.

159. Bayliss KM, Kueck BD, Hanson CA, et al. Richter's syndrome presenting as primary central nervous system lymphoma. Transformation of an identical clone. Am J Clin Pathol 1990; 93:117–123.

160. Lane PK, Townsend RM, Beckstead JH, et al. Central nervous system involvement in a patient with chronic lymphocytic leukemia and non-Hodgkin's lymphoma (Richter's syndrome), with concordant cell surface immunoglobulin isotypic and immunophenotypic markers. Am J Clin Pathol 1988; 89:254–259.

161. O'Neill BP, Habermann TM, Banks PM, et al. Primary central nervous system lymphoma as a variant of Richter's syndrome in two patients with chronic lymphocytic leukemia. Cancer 1989; 64:1296–1300.

162. Bagic A, Lupu VD, Kessler CM, et al. Isolated Richter's transformation of the brain. J Neurooncol 2007; 83:325–328.

163. Lazarevic V, Wahlin A, Hultdin M, et al. Chronic lymphocytic leukemia with osteolytic Richter's syndrome mimicking myeloma bone disease shows no over-expression of DKK1. Leuk Lymphoma 2006; 47:1987–1988.

164. Beaudreuil J, Lortholary O, Martin A, et al. Hypercalcemia may indicate Richter's syndrome: report of four cases and review. Cancer 1997; 79:1211–1215.

165. Ott MM, Ott G, Roblick U, et al. Localized gastric non-Hodgkin's lymphoma of high-grade malignancy in patients with pre-existing chronic lymphocytic leukemia or immunocytoma. Leukemia 1995; 9:609–614.

166. Noel P, Kyle RA. Monoclonal proteins in chronic lymphocytic leukemia. Am J Clin Pathol 1987; 87:385–388.

167. Briones J, Cervantes F, Montserrat E, et al. Hypercalcemia in a patient with chronic lymphocytic leukemia evolving into Richter's syndrome. Leuk Lymphoma 1996; 21:521–523.

168. Seymour JF, Khouri IF, Champlin RE, et al. Refractory chronic lymphocytic leukemia complicated by hypercalcemia treated with allogeneic bone marrow transplantation. Case report and review. Am J Clin Oncol 1994; 17:360–368.

169. Seymour JF, Gagel RF. Calcitriol: the major humoral mediator of hypercalcemia in Hodgkin's disease and non-Hodgkin's lymphomas. Blood 1993; 82:1383–1394.

170. Partyka S, O'Brien S, Podoloff D, et al. The usefulness of high dose (7-10mci) gallium (67Ga) scanning to diagnose Richter's transformation. Leuk Lymphoma 1999; 36:151–155.

171. Bruzzi JF, Macapinlac H, Tsimberidou AM, et al. Detection of Richter's transformation of chronic lymphocytic leukemia by PET/CT. J Nucl Med 2006; 47:1267–1273.
172. Travis LB, Curtis RE, Hankey BF, et al. Second cancers in patients with chronic lymphocytic leukemia. J Natl Cancer Inst 1992; 84:1422–1427.
173. Juneja S, Carney D, Ellis D, et al. Hodgkin's disease type Richter's syndrome in chronic lymphocytic leukemia. Leukemia 1999; 13:826–827.
174. Petrella T, Yaziji N, Collin F, et al. Implication of the Epstein-Barr virus in the progression of chronic lymphocytic leukaemia/small lymphocytic lymphoma to Hodgkin-like lymphomas. Anticancer Res 1997; 17:3907–3913.
175. Fayad L, Robertson LE, O'Brien S, et al. Hodgkin's disease variant of Richter's syndrome: experience at a single institution. Leuk Lymphoma 1996; 23:333–337.
176. Weisenberg E, Anastasi J, Adeyanju M, et al. Hodgkin's disease associated with chronic lymphocytic leukemia. Eight additional cases, including two of the nodular lymphocyte predominant type. Am J Clin Pathol 1995; 103:479–484.
177. Brecher M, Banks PM. Hodgkin's disease variant of Richter's syndrome. Report of eight cases. Am J Clin Pathol 1990; 93:333–339.
178. Fong D, Kaiser A, Spizzo G, et al. Hodgkin's disease variant of Richter's syndrome in chronic lymphocytic leukaemia patients previously treated with fludarabine. Br J Haematol 2005; 129:199–205.
179. Harland CC, Whittaker SJ, Ng YL, et al. Coexistent cutaneous T-cell lymphoma and B-cell chronic lymphocytic leukaemia. Br J Dermatol 1992; 127:519–523.
180. Strickler JG, Amsden TW, Kurtin PJ. Small B-cell lymphoid neoplasms with coexisting T-cell lymphomas. Am J Clin Pathol 1992; 98:424–429.
181. Lee A, Skelly ME, Kingma DW, et al. B-cell chronic lymphocytic leukemia followed by high grade T-cell lymphoma. An unusual variant of Richter's syndrome. Am J Clin Pathol 1995; 103:348–352.
182. Milkowski DA, Worley BD, Morris MJ. Richter's transformation presenting as an obstructing endobronchial lesion. Chest 1999; 116:832–835.
183. Ansell SM, Li CY, Lloyd RV, et al. Epstein-Barr virus infection in Richter's transformation. Am J Hematol 1999; 60:99–104.
184. Nakamura N, Abe M. Richter syndrome in B-cell chronic lymphocytic leukemia. Pathol Int 2003; 53:195–203.
185. Bessudo A, Kipps TJ. Origin of high-grade lymphomas in Richter syndrome. Leuk Lymphoma 1995; 18:367–372.
186. Miyamura K, Osada H, Yamauchi T, et al. Single clonal origin of neoplastic B-cells with different immunoglobulin light chains in a patient with Richter's syndrome. Cancer 1990; 66:140–144.
187. Sun T, Susin M, Desner M, et al. The clonal origin of two cell populations in Richter's syndrome. Hum Pathol 1990; 21:722–728.
188. Matolcsy A, Schattner EJ, Knowles DM, et al. Clonal evolution of B cells in transformation from low- to high-grade lymphoma. Eur J Immunol 1999; 29:1253–1264.
189. van Dongen JJ, Hooijkaas H, Michiels JJ, et al. Richter's syndrome with different immunoglobulin light chains and different heavy chain gene rearrangements. Blood 1984; 64:571–575.
190. Ohno T, Smir BN, Weisenburger DD, et al. Origin of the Hodgkin/Reed-Sternberg cells in chronic lymphocytic leukemia with "Hodgkin's transformation". Blood 1998; 91:1757–1761.
191. Momose H, Jaffe ES, Shin SS, et al. Chronic lymphocytic leukemia/small lymphocytic lymphoma with Reed-Sternberg-like cells and possible transformation to Hodgkin's disease. Mediation by Epstein-Barr virus. Am J Surg Pathol 1992; 16:859–867.
192. Williams J, Schned A, Cotelingam JD, et al. Chronic lymphocytic leukemia with coexistent Hodgkin's disease. Implications for the origin of the Reed-Sternberg cell. Am J Surg Pathol 1991; 15:33–42.
193. Choi H, Keller RH. Coexistence of chronic lymphocytic leukemia and Hodgkin's disease. Cancer 1981; 48:48–57.

194. Matolcsy A, Casali P, Knowles DM. Different clonal origin of B-cell populations of chronic lymphocytic leukemia and large-cell lymphoma in Richter's syndrome. Ann N Y Acad Sci 1995; 764:496–503.

195. Matolcsy A, Inghirami G, Knowles DM. Molecular genetic demonstration of the diverse evolution of Richter's syndrome (chronic lymphocytic leukemia and subsequent large cell lymphoma). Blood 1994; 83:1363–1372.

196. Timar B, Fulop Z, Csernus B, et al. Relationship between the mutational status of VH genes and pathogenesis of diffuse large B-cell lymphoma in Richter's syndrome. Leukemia 2004; 18:326–330.

197. Nakamura N, Kuze T, Hashimoto Y, et al. Analysis of the immunoglobulin heavy chain gene of secondary diffuse large B-cell lymphoma that subsequently developed in four cases with B-cell chronic lymphocytic leukemia or lymphoplasmacytoid lymphoma (Richter syndrome). Pathol Int 2000; 50:636–643.

198. Smit LA, van Maldegem F, Langerak AW, et al. Antigen receptors and somatic hypermutation in B-cell chronic lymphocytic leukemia with Richter's transformation. Haematologica 2006; 91:903–911.

199. de Leval L, Vivario M, De Prijck B, et al. Distinct clonal origin in two cases of Hodgkin's lymphoma variant of Richter's syndrome associated With EBV infection. Am J Surg Pathol 2004; 28:679–686.

200. Belsito VP, Iaccarino S, Liguon L, et al. Chronic lymphocytic leukemia in Richter's transformation: our experience. Blood 1999; 94(suppl.):295b (abstract).

201. Kipps TJ. Immunobiology of chronic lymphocytic leukemia. Curr Opin Hematol 2003; 10:312–318.

202. Tabuteau S, Fernandes J, Garidi R, et al. Richter's syndrome in B-CLL: Report of 37 cases. Blood 1999; 94(suppl.):306b (abstract).

203. Rossi D, Capello D, Cerri M, et al. Molecular, phenotypic and clinical predictors of Richter syndrome (RS) in chronic lymphocytic leukemia (CLL). Blood. 2007; 110:XX (abstract).

204. Thornton PD, Bellas C, Santon A, et al. Richter's transformation of chronic lymphocytic leukemia. The possible role of fludarabine and the Epstein-Barr virus in its pathogenesis. Leuk Res 2005; 29:389–395.

205. Damle RN, Wasil T, Fais F, et al. Ig V gene mutation status and CD38 expression as novel prognostic indicators in chronic lymphocytic leukemia. Blood 1999; 94:1840–1847.

206. Hamblin TJ, Davis Z, Gardiner A, et al. Unmutated Ig V(H) genes are associated with a more aggressive form of chronic lymphocytic leukemia. Blood 1999; 94:1848–1854.

207. Aoki H, Takishita M, Kosaka M, et al. Frequent somatic mutations in D and/or JH segments of Ig gene in Waldenstrom's macroglobulinemia and chronic lymphocytic leukemia (CLL) with Richter's syndrome but not in common CLL. Blood 1995; 85:1913–1919.

208. Hamblin TJ. Richter's syndrome–the downside of fludarabine? Leuk Res 2005; 29:1103–1104.

209. Traweek ST, Liu J, Johnson RM, et al. High-grade transformation of chronic lymphocytic leukemia and low-grade non-Hodgkin's lymphoma. Genotypic confirmation of clonal identity. Am J Clin Pathol 1993; 100:519–526.

210. Kantarjian HM, O'Brien S, Smith TL, et al. Results of treatment with hyper-CVAD, a dose-intensive regimen, in adult acute lymphocytic leukemia. J Clin Oncol 2000; 18:547–561.

211. Dabaja BS, O'Brien SM, Kantarjian HM, et al. Fractionated cyclophosphamide, vincristine, liposomal daunorubicin (daunoXome), and dexamethasone (hyperCVXD) regimen in Richter's syndrome. Leuk Lymphoma 2001; 42:329–337.

212. Tsimberidou AM, Kantarjian HM, Cortes J, et al. Fractionated cyclophosphamide, vincristine, liposomal daunorubicin, and dexamethasone plus rituximab and granulocyte-macrophage-colony stimulating factor (GM-CSF) alternating with methotrexate and cytarabine plus rituximab and GM-CSF in patients with Richter syndrome or fludarabine-refractory chronic lymphocytic leukemia. Cancer 2003; 97:1711–1720.

213. Giles FJ, O'Brien SM, Santini V, et al. Sequential cis-platinum and fludarabine with or without arabinosyl cytosine in patients failing prior fludarabine therapy for chronic lymphocytic leukemia: a phase II study. Leuk Lymphoma 1999; 36:57–65.

214. Tsimberidou AM, O'Brien SM, Cortes JE, et al. Phase II study of fludarabine, cytarabine (Ara-C), cyclophosphamide, cisplatin and GM-CSF (FACPGM) in patients with Richter's syndrome or refractory lymphoproliferative disorders. Leuk Lymphoma 2002; 43:767–772.
215. Tsimberidou AM, Wierda WG, Plunkett W, et al. Phase I-II study of oxaliplatin, fludarabine, cytarabine, and rituximab combination therapy in patients with richter's syndrome or fludarabine-refractory chronic lymphocytic leukemia. J Clin Oncol 2008; 26:196–203.
216. Rodriguez J, Keating MJ, O'Brien S, Champlin RE, Khouri IF. Allogeneic haematopoietic transplantation for Richter's syndrome. Br J Haematol 2000; 110:897–899.
217. Espanol I, Buchler T, Ferra C, et al. Richter's syndrome after allogeneic stem cell transplantation for chronic lymphocytic leukaemia successfully treated by withdrawal of immunosuppression, and donor lymphocyte infusion. Bone Marrow Transplant 2003; 31:215–218.
218. Milojkovic D, Aldouri M, Pagliuca A, et al. Prolonged remission in a case of Richter's transformation of B-cell chronic lymphocytic leukaemia following adoptive immunotherapy. Bone Marrow Transplant 2006; 38:461–462.
219. Russell NH, Byrne JL, Faulkner RD, et al. Donor lymphocyte infusions can result in sustained remissions in patients with residual or relapsed lymphoid malignancy following allogeneic haemopoietic stem cell transplantation. Bone Marrow Transplant 2005; 36:437–441.
220. van Besien K, Ha CS, Murphy S, et al. Risk factors, treatment, and outcome of central nervous system recurrence in adults with intermediate-grade and immunoblastic lymphoma. Blood 1998; 91:1178–1184.
221. Kapatai G, Murray P. Contribution of the Epstein Barr virus to the molecular pathogenesis of Hodgkin lymphoma. J Clin Pathol 2007; 60:1342–1349.
222. Kanzler H, Kuppers R, Helmes S, et al. Hodgkin and Reed-Sternberg-like cells in B-cell chronic lymphocytic leukemia represent the outgrowth of single germinal-center B-cell-derived clones: potential precursors of Hodgkin and Reed-Sternberg cells in Hodgkin's disease. Blood 2000; 95:1023–1031.
223. Rubin D, Hudnall SD, Aisenberg A, et al. Richter's transformation of chronic lymphocytic leukemia with Hodgkin's-like cells is associated with Epstein-Barr virus infection. Mod Pathol 1994; 7:91–98.
224. Yee KW, O'Brien SM, Giles FJ. Richter's syndrome: biology and therapy. Cancer J 2005; 11:161–174.
225. Bea S, Lopez-Guillermo A, Ribas M, et al. Genetic imbalances in progressed B-cell chronic lymphocytic leukemia and transformed large-cell lymphoma (Richter's syndrome). Am J Pathol 2002; 161:957–968.
226. Bentley G, Palutke M, Mohamed AN. Variant t(14; 18) in malignant lymphoma: a report of seven cases. Cancer Genet Cytogenet 2005; 157:12–17.
227. Gaidano G, Ballerini P, Gong JZ, et al. p53 mutations in human lymphoid malignancies: association with Burkitt lymphoma and chronic lymphocytic leukemia. Proc Natl Acad Sci U S A 1991; 88:5413–5417.
228. Cobo F, Martinez A, Pinyol M, et al. Multiple cell cycle regulator alterations in Richter's transformation of chronic lymphocytic leukemia. Leukemia 2002; 16:1028–1034.

15

Infectious Complications in Patients with Chronic Lymphocytic Leukemia

Elias Anaissie
Myeloma Institute for Research and Therapy, University of Arkansas for Medical Sciences, Little Rock, Arkansas, U.S.A.

INTRODUCTION

Infections constitute a significant challenge during the management of chronic lymphocytic leukemia (CLL). Indeed, more than 50% of patients with CLL suffer recurrent infections, and infection accounts for up to 60% to 80% of deaths from CLL (1–7). This increased risk for infectious complications is the result of the interplay between the immune defects inherent in CLL and the therapies given to control it. The introduction of purine analogs (fludarabine, cladribine, and pentostatin) (8) and monoclonal antibodies such as alemtuzumab (9) has led to significant progress in the treatment of CLL. Purine analogs interfere with DNA synthesis through inhibition of DNA polymerases and ribonucleotide reductase, leading to programmed cell death of malignant lymphoid cells, but with a similar effect on the normal resting lymphocytes (10). This results in prolonged lymphopenia, especially in the CD4 subset of T cells, which predisposes to opportunistic infections (1–3,6,7).

A number of monoclonal antibodies such as rituximab and alemtuzumab have been effectively used to treat CLL (9). These antibodies are directed against cell surface antigens expressed on the neoplastic cells and as such are associated with a limited toxicity profile. However, infections have been frequently reported when alemtuzumab is used in previously treated patients with advanced CLL or as consolidation therapy following induction with fludarabine-based regimens (11).

The efficacy of purine analogs as single agents and their limited extramedullary toxicity have led to their use in combination with alkylating agents (12,13) and, more recently, with monoclonal antibodies (14,15) in an attempt to improve response rates and survival. These combination therapies may further increase the predisposition to infections.

In this manuscript, the infectious complications of therapy of CLL are reviewed and the possible underlying factors discussed, including the immune defects inherent to the underlying disease and those that develop as a result of antileukemic therapy.

DISEASE-RELATED FACTORS

A number of factors predispose patients with CLL to infections. These include defects in humoral and cell-mediated immunity (CMI), quantitative and qualitative phagocytic cell defects, abnormalities of complement, and others (Table 1).

CLL is associated with a high incidence of hypogammaglobulinemia, which may be severe and correlates with disease duration and stage, i.e., more pronounced with increasing disease duration (16–20,24). An association between low IgG levels and increasing infections (and possibly shorter survival) is well described (Table 2). The etiology of this hypogammaglobulinemia is not clear; a number of factors, such as functional abnormalities of T cells resulting in dysregulation of nonclonal CD5$^-$ B cells, may be responsible (22,23). In vitro, CLL cells inhibit the interaction of activated T lymphocytes and normal B lymphocytes (27) and suppress the CD40 ligand-mediated helper signal necessary for normal lymphocyte differentiation (29). Transforming growth factor-beta (TGF-β), a potent inhibitor of B-cell proliferation, is also secreted by CLL lymphocytes (30). Furthermore, these cells produce high levels of circulating interleukin-2 (IL-2) receptor, which can remove endogenous IL-2 and downregulate T-helper cell function (31). These disorders of T-cell/B-cell interaction are likely to contribute to the various immune deficiencies of patients with CLL, including humoral defects (27).

IgA deficiency, the most common Ig class deficiency in CLL (25), is also strongly associated with higher risk for severe infections, and in one study, IgA deficiency was the only risk factor that was independent of clinical stage (26). This IgA deficiency may be responsible for the high incidence of sinopulmonary infections. Although hypogamma-globulinemia appears to predispose patients with CLL to infections (16–21), it is important to keep in mind that patients with a normal serum Ig level may also suffer from recurrent infections, whereas those with marked hypogammaglobulinemia may remain infection free (21,26,62).

Additional humoral risk factors for infections include the reductions in serum levels of the IgG subclasses (IgG 1–4) (26,28) and the deficiency of secondary IgG antibody response to common antigens, including *Escherichia coli* and *Streptococcus pneumoniae* (21).

Conflicting data exist regarding the role of the mutation of Ig VH gene on humoral immunity and risk for infections in CLL. In one report, no significant differences in Ig levels, mannan-binding lectin, and immune responses to *Hemophilus influenzae* type B vaccination or rate of infection were found between two groups of patients that differed in the mutational status of the B-cell clone (32), while another study of 280 patients concluded that an unmutated Ig VH gene status was independently associated with significantly shorter time to first infection and higher infection-related mortality as compared with mutated Ig VH gene status, despite comparable Ig levels between the two groups (33). Additional risk factors for shorter time to first infection included older age, clinical stage B or C disease, type of initial therapy, the presence of genetic abnormalities, and a positive CD38 status. However, unmutated gene status had no impact on the incidence of recurrent infections (33).

Quantitative and qualitative abnormalities of T cells have been reported in patients with CLL (Table 1) (34–39,43–52,63–65) and translated into impaired CMI as demonstrated by lack of response to recall antigens on skin testing, prolonged skin graft survival (53), diminished response to skin testing for tuberculin, mumps, and *Candida* (54), and anergy to recall skin testing (55). Patients with CLL may also have suppressed natural killer (NK) cell activity (25) and lymphocyte-activated killer (LAK) cell functions (57) and functional defects of the dendritic cell compartment with an inability to stimulate an effective CMI response (58) (Table 1).

Table 1 Inherent Immune Defects in Patients with Chronic Lymphocytic Leukemia

Immune Defects	Etiology	Risk for infection
Humoral immunity		
Hypogammaglobulinemia (16–20,30)	Possibly due to functional abnormalities of T cells resulting in dysregulation of nonclonal CD5$^-$ B cells (22,23)	IgG deficiency associated with ↑ infections and ↓ survival. (16–21)
↓IgA (most common Ig deficiency) (28)	*CLL cells*	IgA deficiency associated with ↑ infections, particularly sinopulmonary (29)
↓ IgG2, IgG4 (29)	-Inhibit the interaction of activated T lymphocytes and normal B lymphocytes (24)	↑Infections in patients with ↓ IgG2 and IgG4 (29,32)
↓IgG3, IgG4 (only moderate ↓ IgG1, IgG2) (30)	-Suppress the CD40 ligand-mediated helper signal necessary for normal lymphocyte differentiation (25)	↓ Antipneumococcal antibodies not directly associated with hypogammaglobulinemia. However, most patients with severe or multiple infections had ↓ both IgG and pneumococcal antibodies (30)
Deficiencies in secondary antibody response to common antigens, such as low IgG titers to *E. coli* and *S. pneumoniae*	-Secrete TGF-β, a potent inhibitor of B-cell proliferation (26)	No association with infection
Significant ↓ in mucosal (salivary) IgM (23)	-Produce high levels of circulating IL-2 receptor, which remove endogenous IL-2 and downregulate T-helper cell function (27)	No differences in Ig or MBL levels, immune responses to *H. influenzae* B vaccination or rate of infection between mutated and unmutated status (33)
Mutational status of the immunoglobulin VH gene (33,34)		Shorter time to first infection in patients with unmutated status (34)

(*Continued*)

Table 1 Inherent Immune Defects in Patients with Chronic Lymphocytic Leukemia (*Continued*)

Immune Defects	Etiology	Risk for infection
Cell-mediated immunity *Quantitative* (35–40) Imbalance in the T-cell subsets:	Mechanisms unclear; possibly related to the differential sensitivity of CD4 and CD8 T lymphocytes to the Fas-expressing CLL cells.	↑Risk for various infections associated with defects in cell-mediated immunity (1–3, 6–8, 64–66)
-↓ CD4/CD8 ratio especially in advanced stages (18,41,42) -↑ CD8 subpopulations (NK, suppressors and CTLs) (43,44) -Both ↑ and ↓ numbers of suppressor-inducer phenotype (CD45Ra) reported (43–46)		
Qualitative Suppression of helper T-cell function and excessive T-suppressor function -Variable CD8 cell function (reported to be normal, ↑ or ↓). (42,49)	Likely related to soluble factors released by CLL cells (52) CLL-derived T-helper cells may be normal but the predominance of neoplastic B cells as accessory cells alters T-cell function (53).	
-↓ T-cell response to PHA (37); normal response to PHA but ↑ response by IL-1 or IL-2 ↓ compared to normal T cells (51) -↓ Antibody-dependent cytotoxicity -↓ Delayed hypersensitivity responses (54–56)		
Natural killer and dendritic cells -↓ Function of NK (28) and LAK cells (28,57,58) -Functional and maturation defects of dendritic cells (59)		

Innate immunity

Neutrophils and monocytes

Qualitative: ↓β-glucuronidase, lysozyme, myeloperoxidase with ↓ phagocytic, bactericidal activity, chemotaxis	Marrow infiltration by CLL, suppression of neutrophil progenitors by CLL-related humoral and cellular factors	↑ Risk for various infections (66)
Quantitative: ↓ absolute neutrophil counts and monocytes counts		

Complement system

Suppression of classical and alternate pathways		May ↑ risk for various infections, though no association between complement deficiencies and infections in CLL
↓ Complement component levels		
Defects in complement activation and binding		

Splenomegaly

Sequestration of red cells, platelets, and white cells (60–62)	Splenic infiltration by CLL	Cytopenias and ↑ risk for various infections

Aging

↑ Immune dysfunction. Ability to mount primary immune responses against new antigens ↓ significantly	All of the above	May ↑ risk for various infections; ↓ efficacy of vaccination

Advanced disease

Immune incompetence associated with CLL is linked to disease duration and eventually develops in all patients[a]	All of the above	May ↑ risk for various infections; ↓ efficacy of vaccination

[a]Immune incompetence is partly secondary to hypogammaglobulinemia and impaired CMI to recall antigens.

Abbreviations: Lymph, lymphocyte; Ig, immunoglobulin; CLL, chronic lymphocytic leukemia; CTL, cytotoxic lymphocyte; LAK, lymphocyte-activated killer; NK, natural killer; MBL, Mannan-binding lectin; TGF-β, transforming growth factor-beta; PHA, phytohemagglutinin; IL, interleukin; IFN-γ, interferon-gamma.

Table 2 Association Between Hypogammaglobulinemia and Infection Rate in CLL

References	Total	IgG level (mg/dL)	Patients	Severe infection (%)	p value
20	52	<600	20	11[a]	<0.001
		>600	32	1[a]	
30[b]	59	<600	32	15	<0.001
		>600	27	3	

[a]Patients dying from severe infections, p value calculated for survival.
[b]Low levels of pneumococcal antibodies were strongly associated with severe or multiple infections ($p < 0.00001$)

Neutrophil and monocyte dysfunction also occur in patients with CLL, and neutropenia is commonly seen in patients with extensive marrow infiltration relapsing after multiple therapies. Neutropenia, however, is not a common feature of earlier-stage disease and as such does not contribute to the infection risk except in the setting of myelosuppressive therapy (1–3).

Splenomegaly may contribute to the cytopenias seen in advanced CLL because an enlarged spleen causes sequestration and destruction of large numbers of red cells, platelets, and white cells, including immune effector cells, and hence contributes to cytopenias (55,58–61).

The clinical influence of these immune defects, particularly in older patients and those with advanced disease stages, on the risk of infections during therapy for CLL has not been fully elucidated, partly because of the constant interplay between these defects and the immunosuppressive effects of antileukemic therapy.

THERAPY-RELATED FACTORS

Treatment-related factors further contribute to the immune incompetence seen in patients with CLL and to their risk for infections.

Corticosteroids

Corticosteroids are mainly indicated in the management of antibody-mediated (auto-immune) anemia and thrombocytopenia and are usually given for three to six months for this indication (2,3). Such prolonged used of corticosteroids, especially when given at doses greater than or equal to 60 mg prednisone equivalent per day for longer than two weeks, significantly increases the risk of opportunistic infections (OIs). This risk is compounded when steroids are used concomitantly with purine analogs (40–42).

Alkylating Agents

Chlorambucil

Until recently, chlorambucil, given alone or with corticosteroids, was the mainstay of therapy for patients with CLL (1–5,7,8). With this treatment, infections are common, although serious (grade 3–4) infections occur in only 7% to 17% of patients. Most infections involve the respiratory tract (sinusitis, bronchitis, and pneumonia) and are caused by common organisms such as *Staphylococcus aureus*, *S. pneumoniae*, *H. influenzae*, *E. coli*, *Klebsiella pneumoniae*, and *Pseudomonas aeruginosa* (Table 3).

Table 3 Infections in Patients with CLL: Treatment-Related Risk Factors, Spectrum, Monitoring, and Prevention

Risk factor	Effect on the immune system	Spectrum of infection	Monitoring and prevention
Disease and therapy related			
Active disease and receipt of any therapy (Table 1)	*Active CLL*: Hypogammaglobulinemia, other	*Active CLL*:	Prophylaxis against encapsulated bacteria with a fluoroquinolone
	Therapy related: see below	Encapsulated bacteria (*S. Pneumoniae*, others). Also, *S. aureus*, *E. coli*, *Klebsiella* spp. others	IVIG if IgG <500 mg/dL and recurrent serious infections despite prophylactic antibiotics
		Most commonly respiratory tract infections but also bacteremia, UTI, others	Vaccinate close contacts against the influenza virus and *H. influenzae*
		Therapy related: see below	
Chlorambucil (1–5,7,8)	Neutropenia, mild	Same as above. Fungal and viral infections rare unless after/in advanced-stage disease.	Same as with active disease
	↓ CMI, mild		
Purine analogs (1–8,10,69–71)	Same as with active CLL *plus* ↓ CMI: profound ↓ CD4$^+$ cells, rapid, persistent for several months after therapy	Bacteria (same as above) plus *L. monocytogenes*, *Nocardia*, *Legionella*, other	*For high-risk patients (Table 6)*
		Viruses: HSV, VZV, respiratory viruses, CMV	1. Screen patients for CMV, hepatitis B surface antigen and core antibody, HIV
		Fungi: *Candida*, *Cryptococcus*, *Aspergillus*, PCP	2. Obtain relevant history and serology in patients living in areas of endemicity for infections (fungal infections, tuberculosis, *stronguiloidis stercoralis*, meliodosis, scabies, other)
		Rarely: mycobacteria (tuberculosis and atypical), parasitic and endemic infections	3. Provide prophylaxis against: fungi, PCP, *Candida* species, influenza viruses, herpes viruses (HSV, VZV), and against infections likely to reactivate in a patient with history of infection (e.g., hepatitis B, tuberculosis, other)

(Continued)

Table 3 Infections in Patients with CLL: Treatment-Related Risk Factors, Spectrum, Monitoring, and Prevention (*Continued*)

Risk factor	Effect on the immune system	Spectrum of infection	Monitoring and prevention
			4. Transfuse CMV-seronegative blood or use filter if patient is CMV-seronegative 5. Monitor for CMV infection (PCR or antigenemia) and for aspergillosis[a]
Alemtuzumab (1–5,7,8,121–124)	Severe lymphopenia; rapid and persistent ↓ B and T cells in all patients: CD4+, CD8+, NK, NK-T, and $CD19^+5^-$	Same as with purine analogs	Same as with purine analogs
		CMV infection and disease problematic in high-risk patients and alemtuzumab consolidation	Particular attention to CMV monitoring
Rituximab (117–119)	↓ PBL, recover over 9–12 mo. Mild ↓ Ig (~ 15% patients), mild ↓ ANC	No ↑ infections or change in spectrum even when higher doses used	No special monitoring or prophylaxis
Corticosteroids (66)	↓ CMI, severe if high-dose steroids used	Same as in purine analogs if patient receiving high-dose steroids (≥60 mg/day equivalent for >2 wk)	Same as with active disease *plus* strict control of glycemia *plus*
	Effects of hyperglycemia		
Autologous stem cell transplant (ASCT) (142–144)	*Preengraftment*	*Preengraftment*: bacterial: staph, strep, enterococci; enterobacteriaceae, *P. aeruginosa;*	*Preengraftment*: same as with purine analogs and alemtuzumab *plus*
	Neutropenia, severe	Bacteremia, pneumonia, colitis (*C. difficile*)	High stem cell dose (>5 × 10^6 $CD34^+$ cells/kg)
	Mucositis, moderate severe	Fungal: *Candida, Aspergillus*	For mucositis: oral hygiene, cryotherapy. KGF if using TBI-conditioning regimens
		After engraftment: HSV, VZV, CMV, PCP	Monitor for CMV infection (PCR or antigenemia) and for aspergillosis[a]
	After engraftment: ↓ CMI		*After engraftment*: Monitor for CMV; Give PCP[b] and viral prophylaxis

Allogeneic stem cell transplant (142–144)	*Preengraftment*: same as ASCT.	*Preengraftment*: same as ASCT.	*Preengraftment*: same as ASCT.
	After engraftment: Very severe ↓ CMI with severe GVHD	*After engraftment*: same as ASCT plus ↑ aspergillosis with severe GVHD.	*After engraftment*: same as ASCT. If severe GVHD, continue fluconazole until day +100 And monitor for CMV infection (PCR or antigenemia) and for aspergillosis[a]
Renal failure (66)	↓ neutrophil function, ↓CMI ↓ expression of TLR-4	Various infections. Renal failure is a risk factor for infection	Adjust dose of purine analogs Avoid and immediately treat conditions that may cause/worsen renal failure[c]
Iron overload (66)	↓ function (phagocytes, NK cells)	Various infections	ESA instead of transfusions, iron chelation if iron overload is clinically severe
Splenectomy	Hyposplenism	Bacteremia/shock, with encapsulated bacteria	Same as with active disease
Exposure to pathogens			
History of infection (66)	Various infections including PCP and CMV		Targeted prophylaxis (e.g., TMP-SMX if history of PCP)
Exposure to pathogens in hospital and/or community (66)	Transmission from health care workers, equipment, and contaminated solutions		Patient education and appropriate infection control practices
	Respiratory viruses, waterborne or food-borne pathogens, others		Immunization of household contacts (e.g., influenza virus)
	Occupational, recreational, and geographical risks		Avoidance of high-risk activities during severe immunosuppression

The risk of infection persists after end of therapy in patients with extensive prior therapy (particularly with purine analogs and/or alemtuzumab) and with advanced/refractory disease. Prophylaxis should reflect the presence and duration of high-risk factors for infection.

[a]Monitor for aspergillosis with serum Aspergillus galactomannan antigen.

[b]PCP prophylaxis: trimethoprim-sulfamethoxazole.

[c]Sepsis, hypovolemia, drugs (NSAIDs, others) tumor lysis, obstruction.

Abbreviations: CMI, cell-mediated immunity; PCP, Pneumocystis carinii pneumonia; ANC, absolute neutrophil count; NA, not applicable; PBL, peripheral blood lymphocyte; IgG, immunoglobulin G; viral prophylaxis, acyclovir, valacyclovir, or famciclovir; TMP-SMX, trimethoprim-sulfamethoxazole; FQ, fluoroquinolone; IVIG, intravenous immunoglobulin; TLR, toll-like receptor; NSAID, nonsteroid anti-inflammatory; CMV, cytomegalovirus; HSV, herpes simplex virus; VZV, varicella-zoster virus; PCR, polymerase chain reaction; NK, natural killer; G-CSF, granulocyte colony-stimulating factor; TBI, total body irradiation; GVHD, graft versus host disease; ESA, erythropoietin-stimulating agents; KGF, keratinocyte growth factor; HIV, human immunodeficiency virus.

Fungal and viral infections such as herpes simplex virus (HSV) and varicella zoster virus (VZV) are less common except in the setting of therapy-related neutropenia in patients with advanced stage disease.

Bendamustine

Bendamustine is an alkylating agent that has been extensively used in Germany and was recently approved for use in the United States. A randomized comparative trial (RCT) evaluated bendamustine (139 patients) versus chlorambucil (125 patients) as initial therapy of patients with CLL aged 75 years or younger. Both drugs were administered for six cycles, with additional therapy given according to response. Overall, bendamustine-treated patients had superior overall and progression-free survival (PFS) but suffered higher rates of grades 3 to 4 myelosuppression (including 43% neutropenia) and infection (27% vs. 13%). However, the incidence of severe infections did not significantly differ among patients treated with bendamustine or chlorambucil (3% and 7%, respectively) (79). Another trial evaluated bendamustine plus rituximab in 81 patients with relapsed or refractory CLL. The bendamustine dose was reduced by 30% from the usual frontline dose (70 mg/m^2 instead of 100 mg/m^2 on days 1 and 2), and rituximab was given at 375 mg/m^2 in cycle one and at higher doses for subsequent cycles. A 65% overall response rate was observed, and the regimen was well tolerated with only six severe infections (80).

Cyclophosphamide

Cyclophosphamide is not typically used as a single agent for therapy of CLL but in combination with purine analogs (discussed under section "Purine Analogs").

Purine analogs   These are fludarabine, 2-chlorodeoxyadenosine (2CDA, cladribine), and 2′-deoxycoformycin (DCF, pentostatin).

Therapy with purine analogs in patients with CLL lead to a marked immunosuppression (6,10,66–68), including the following:

- A profound lymphopenia with decrease in CD3-positive T-lymphocytes and a fall in both CD4 and CD8 counts. A pronounced reduction in the various T-cell subpopulations occurs during and after therapy with fludarabine; T-cell lymphopenia, particularly CD4 cells, is universal, develops rapidly (within 2–3 months) after therapy, and may persist for more than two years after discontinuation of therapy (66–68). By contrast, CD8 and NK cell numbers normalize from elevated pretherapy levels. This T-cell lymphopenia aggravates the T-cell-mediated dysfunction associated with advanced-stage CLL, particularly in patients who have received prior therapy. Similar CD4 and CD8 lymphocyte count reductions occur in patients with CLL treated with cladribine and pentostatin. These immune defects appear to be more severe in patients with lymphoid malignancies compared with solid tumors, suggesting that the nature of the immune defects partially relates to the underlying disease.
- Neutropenia in 15% to 75% of patients, especially in previously treated patients.
- Decrease in monocyte counts and in B cells. The effect on immunoglobulin levels is variable.

Notably, therapy of patients with CLL with any of the purine analogs exerts similarly potent immunosuppressive effects (type, depth, and duration) and risk for and spectrum of OIs.

The spectrum of infections in patients with CLL treated with purine analogs differs from that seen with traditional alkylating agents. In addition to infections with common pathogens (such as neutropenia-associated bacteria, HSV, and candidal mucositis), therapy with purine analogs increases the risk of atypical infections by various organisms (1–3,6–8,40–42,81–83). These include bacteria (*Listeria monocytogenes, Nocardia spp*, and others), fungi (*Cryptococcus neoformans, Aspergillus spp, and Pneumocystis carinii* (reclassified as a fungus and renamed *Pneumocystis jiroveci*), and viruses, particularly cytomegalovirus (CMV) and, rarely, reactivation of adenovirus, hepatitis viruses, and Epstein–Barr virus (EBV) infections. Infections caused by *P. carinii* pneumonia (PCP) and *L. monocytogenes* have been observed when purine analogs are administered concomitantly with steroids (40–42). Rarely, these patients develop infections by parasites (*Toxoplasma gondii, Cryptosporidium parvum,* and *Balantidium coli*) and mycobacteria, most commonly pulmonary tuberculosis but also extrapulmonary infections, such as bloodstream, soft tissue, and bone and joint infections caused by atypical mycobacteria (42).

These atypical infections that develop after therapy with purine analogs reflect the severe CMI defects associated with these agents.

The timing of the infectious complications in patients receiving purine analogs varies according to extent of prior therapy (Table 4) (1–3,6–8,40–42,67,81–83). Most infections occur early, usually during the first six weeks of therapy, and a significant

Table 4 Infection in Patients with CLL Receiving Antileukemic Therapy: Spectrum According to Stage of Therapy (Early in the Course of the Disease or Late After Repeated Cycles of Therapy) (1–3,6–8,66,72)

Infection	Early	Late (same infections as in early stage, plus the following)
Bacterial	Encapsulated bacteria	*Listeria monocytogenes, Nocardia* spp, *Legionella* spp, others
	During neutropenia: streptococci, staphylococci, enterobacteriaceae, *Pseudomonas Aeruginosa*	
Viral	HSV (mucosal infection) Respiratory viral infections	HSV, VZV, rarely disseminated.
		CMV reactivation and disease
		Rarely reactivation of hepatitis viruses, adenovirus, Epstein–Barr virus
Fungal	Mucosal candidiasis	Disseminated candidiasis
		Invasive mould infections (Aspergillosis, others)
		Cryptococcus neoformans meningitis, pneumonia
		Pneumocystis carinii pneumonia
Mycobacterial	None	Pulmonary tuberculosis, various infections with atypical mycobacteria
Parasitic	None	*Toxoplasma gondii, cryptosporidium parvum, balantidium coli*

The risk of infection persists after end of therapy in patients with extensive prior therapy (particularly with purine analogs and/or alemtuzumab) and with advanced/refractory disease. Early infections are associated with neutropenia while late infections are caused by neutropenia and severe lymphopenia with defects in cell-mediated immunity. *Abbreviations*: HSV, herpes simplex virus; VZV, varicella zoster virus; CMV, cytomegalovirus.

Table 5 The Incidence of Severe Infections (Grades 3 and 4) After Purine Analog Therapy is Markedly Decreased with Prophylaxis

	Severe infections[a]	
Therapy	No prophylaxis	Prophylaxis[b]
Single agent		
Treatment-naïve (1–3,64,66,72,75–85)	35%	<10%
Previously treated (1–3,64,65,70,71,81,97)	50%	<10%
Combination		
Treatment naïve (100,105,108)	45%	<10%
Previously treated (101,103,106,109–112)	60%	<10%

[a]Approximate rate of severe infections based on a review of the largest studies.
[b]Trimethoprim-sulfamethoxazole plus acyclovir or similar antiviral agent. Colony-stimulating factor.
Other prophylaxis as in Table 7. Monitoring for CMV reactivation and early preemptive CMV therapy.

proportion of severe infections are caused by neutropenia-related opportunistic pathogens. At this stage, infections are caused by encapsulated bacteria (e.g., *S. pneumonia* and *H. influenzae*) and the common opportunistic bacterial infections and HSV and candidal mucosal disease (1,42,81). Late infections (particularly after repeated cycles of purine analog therapy) include opportunistic pathogens associated with depressed CMI (1–3,6–8,40–42,83).

Although pneumonia is the most frequent respiratory tract infection, upper respiratory tract infections such as sinusitis and tracheobronchitis are also common. Other manifestations of bacterial infection in these patients include bloodstream infection and urinary tract and skin and soft tissue infections. A small number of patients may experience overwhelming polymicrobial infections (42).

The frequency of severe infections associated with purine analog therapy varies according to whether these agents are used as frontline therapy ($\sim 35\%$ rate of infection) (1–3,6–8,41,42,81,84–95) or in previously treated patients ($\sim 50\%$, i.e., $\sim 15\%$ increase in risk) (1–3,6–8,40–42,65,67,83,90–94,96–107) and whether they are used alone ($\sim 30\%$) (68,81–94,96–107) or in combination with other agents ($\sim 40\%$) (1–3,6–8,40–42,108–122) (Table 5). Antimicrobial prophylaxis with acyclovir (or similar antiviral agent) and with trimethoprim sulfamethoxazole (TMP-SMX) markedly decreases the risk of severe infections in these patients (from 30–50% to <10%) (113,115,117). Response to purine analog therapy also appears to be associated with decreasing risk for infection (41). On the other hand, the use of corticosteroids concomitantly, prior to or after purine analog therapy, predisposes patients to atypical infections (40–42). Furthermore, patients refractory to purine analogs are at a very high risk for infections, which are common causes of morbidity and death in such a setting (123–126).

Treatment—naïve versus previously treated patients A review of over 400 patients with CLL who received fludarabine with or without prednisone indicated that a higher incidence of infections occurred in previously treated (58%) compared with untreated (34%) patients ($p < 0.001$) (41). Infections with *L. monocytogenes* or *P. carinii* occurred in 7% of 170 previously treated patients who received fludarabine plus prednisone, none of 78 previously treated patients who received fludarabine alone, and 1% of 154 previously untreated patients who received the combination ($p = 0.003$). Independent risk factors for major infection included Rai stages III and IV, prior therapy, and elevated serum creatinine. A baseline granulocyte count greater than 1×10^9/L was protective. Five (26%) of nineteen patients with CD4 counts less than 50 cells/µL developed dermatomal zoster, as compared with 9 (6%) of 139 patients with a CD4 count greater than 50 cells/µL ($p = 0.01$) (41). A similar association was made between CD4 counts less than 50 cells/µL and risk for PCP (67).

Analysis of the infectious complications following therapy with chlorambucil, fludarabine, or the combination of both drugs in 534 previously untreated patients with CLL was performed (81). A total of 1107 infections, including 241 major infections, occurred in 518 patients. The combination therapy arm of the study was closed early because of toxicity, predominantly myelosuppression, and infections. When comparing the single agent fludarabine and chlorambucil arms, fludarabine recipients had significantly higher incidence of infections (overall and severe infections). The majority of viral infections were herpes virus infections (including varicella zoster) and were more likely to occur not only in the combination arm ($p < 0.0001$) but also in fludarabine recipients compared with chlorambucil-treated patients ($p = 0.0006$). Overall, most of these viral infections were minor, not requiring hospitalization or parenteral therapy. Similarly, fungal infections were uncommon with the majority of infections being caused by *Candida* species in patients treated with fludarabine either alone or in combination. Three patients developed mycobacterial infections, and only one case of legionella infection was reported in a patient treated with the combination (81).

Older age, advanced Rai stage, and declining creatinine clearance were associated with risk for major infections in the combination arm only. Patients with a low IgG value at study initiation (<500 mg/dL) were at greater risk of infections compared with those with higher values (81).

Purine analog therapy in older patients   Although two studies suggested that purine analogs are well tolerated in older patients (93,122), a recent large RCT raised concerns about poorer outcome in this patient population (89). This study enrolled patients with CLL who were 65 years or older. Patients were randomized to receive fludarabine 25 mg/m^2/day for five days every 28 days (101 patients) or chlorambucil 0.4 mg/kg with planned dose escalation to 0.8 mg/kg every 15 days (105 patients). Overall and complete remission (CR) rates with fludarabine were significantly higher than those seen with chlorambucil. However, the PFS rate was not significantly different between the two arms, and although no significant difference was seen in overall survival (OS), the median OS time was substantially shorter with fludarabine versus chlorambucil (89). Although more myelotoxicity was observed among fludarabine recipients, no significant differences were seen in the incidences of grade 3 to 4 anemia, thrombocytopenia, or infection. The shorter OS time with fludarabine (89) contrasts with the nearly identical OS and PFS rates observed in younger patients (84–87), including in a study conducted by the same group (88), raising concerns that fludarabine may not be optimal frontline therapy for older patients.

Purine analog-based combinations   Several purine-based combinations have been used to treat patients with CLL (108–122). Fludarabine has been combined with the alkylating agent cyclophosphamide (FC) (109–112), with cyclophosphamide and the monoclonal antibody rituximab (FCR) (113–116), and, more recently, as a combination of FCR with the monoclonal antibody alemtuzumab (CFAR) (117). Similarly, cladribine has been combined with chlorambucil and/or prednisone (118,119), while pentostatin was given together with chlorambucil and/or prednisone (120) and with cyclophosphamide and rituximab (PCR) (15,121,122). When pentostatin was combined with chlorambucil and prednisone in previously untreated patients, a 31% rate of severe infections was observed (120), while the rate of such infections with the PCR combination was 10% in treatment naïve (121) compared with 28% in pretreated patients (122). These combination therapies increase severity of myelosuppression and the risk for OIs. However, antimicrobial and growth factor prophylaxis significantly reduce the rate of these complications even when these combinations included monoclonal antibodies such as in FCR (113,115) and more recently in CFAR (117). The latter study compared 26 patients treated with CFAR with historical FCR data (119 patients). Patients in both groups were younger than 70 years and had a serum β2-microglobulin (β2M) level greater than twice the upper limit normal. Both populations were well matched on key prognostic variables, including β2M, absolute lymphocyte count, platelet count, and Rai stage of disease at treatment initiation. Six 28-day courses were planned in the CFAR regimen and a median of five courses completed. The overall response rate was comparable between regimens. Neutropenia grade 3 to 4 was less common in CFAR (68% vs. 86%); however, 6 mg of Pegfilgastrim was given routinely to CFAR patients one day after the last alemtuzumab dose, while growth factor use was limited in the historical FCR control population. No difference in rates of infection was observed between groups for fever of unknown origin (FUO) (35% vs. 26%), major infections (8% vs. 15%), minor infections (23% vs. 18%), and HSV reactivation (4% vs. 3%) for CFAR and FCR, respectively. Most CFAR patients received valganciclovir prophylaxis; two of the seven who could not receive valganciclovir and received only valacyclovir had CMV reactivation compared with none of the 19 valganciclovir recipients (117). Although these results are encouraging, the small number of CFAR patients treated so far does not allow definitive conclusions regarding the safety of this regimen.

Finally, the addition of oblimersen (Bcl-2 antisense) to fludarabine plus cyclophosphamide in an RCT significantly increased the rate and duration of response in patients with relapsed or refractory CLL without increasing the incidence of OIs (109).

Refractoriness to purine analogs　Patients refractory to purine analogs are at a particularly high risk for serious infections, which are common causes of morbidity and death (123–125). Infections may involve any organ and typically occur at a median of four to six months from onset of the refractory state. Although infections with gram-positive organisms are most common, infections with gram-negative bacilli, invasive moulds, *P. carinii*, and other atypical organisms are not uncommon and can be particularly severe. Lack of response to salvage therapy is associated with increasing risk of infection (123–125).

Flavopiridol

Flavopiridol is a synthetic flavone that has been shown to be effective in heavily pretreated patients with CLL and appears to be well tolerated with manageable infectious complications (126).

Monoclonal Antibodies

Rituximab

Treatment with standard dose rituximab results in a significant reduction (by ∼90%) in the peripheral B-lymphocyte count within three days, followed by a slow recovery over 9 to 12 months (73,75). A mild decrease in serum Ig levels occurs in up to 20% of patients. Transient reductions in the white blood cell count to less than 3000/μL and in the absolute neutrophil count (ANC) to less than 1500/μL may be seen with spontaneous recovery. Isolated but reversible neutropenia of unclear etiology has also been reported after therapy with rituximab (74).

Significant myelosuppression and infection are uncommon, even in studies using higher doses of rituximab in patients with CLL (75,127). In fact, the incidence and severity of infections does not appear to be different from those in patients with CLL not receiving rituximab. Rituximab has also been administered in combination with other antileukemic agents in patients with large disease burden and/or prior extensive therapies without apparent effect on the incidence or severity of infections (although higher rates of grade 3 or 4 neutropenia may be seen) (15,113–117,121,122). In a recent RCT of 104 previously untreated patients with CLL, rituximab was used concurrently or sequentially with fludarabine (14). The rate of severe infections was 20%, and OIs were slightly higher among patients receiving sequential therapy (26% vs. 16% with concurrent therapy), although most were caused by localized herpes virus infections with only two cases of PCP (14).

Alemtuzumab

Therapy with alemtuzumab in patients with CLL leads to marked immunosuppression (69–72), which includes the following:

- Severe lymphopenia with a marked decrease in all peripheral blood lymphocytes (B and T cells) in all patients with median end-of-treatment counts for $CD4^+$, $CD8^+$, $CD3-56^+$ (NK), $CD3^+56^+$ (NK-T), and $CD19^+5^-$ (normal B) cells of 43, 20, 4, 1, and 8 cells/µL, respectively. This decrease is rapid and persists for several months after end of therapy (EOT) with the median cell count of all lymphoid subpopulations remaining at less than 25% of baseline values for greater than nine months posttreatment. Thereafter, cell numbers increase more rapidly except for normal B cells, which remain at a low level at 18 months. At four months after completion of therapy, $CD4^+$ and $CD8^+$ levels in the blood had reached greater than 100/µL in more than 50% of patients.
- Mild granulocytopenia and monocytopenia. Granulocytes return to baseline levels early during the follow-up.

No correlation appears to exist between alemtuzumab cumulative dose and route of administration (IV or subcutaneous) and immunosuppression. This long-lasting lymphopenia exacerbates the preexisting immune deficiencies in patients with CLL, particularly among those pretreated with purine analogs, resulting in increased risk for severe infections.

Treatment naïve patients With optimal antimicrobial prophylaxis, the incidence of infections with alemtuzumab therapy is low in previously untreated patients (70,71), even when alemtuzumab is used in combination with fludarabine, cyclophosphamide, and rituximab as in CFAR (117). A recent RCT compared alemtuzumab (149 patients) to chlorambucil (148 patients) as first-line treatment for patients with CLL (71). Alemtuzumab-treated patients had a superior leukemia outcome with predictable and manageable toxicity. More CMV events occurred in the alemtuzumab arm, but without apparent impact on efficacy.

Previously treated patients Therapy with alemtuzumab increases the vulnerability of pretreated patients to OIs. Infections include those caused by bacteria (*L. monocytogenes*, others), viruses (particularly HSV/VZV and CMV, rarely adenovirus and the hepatitis viruses), fungi (*Aspergillus* spp., *Cryptococcus neoformans*, zygomycetes, and *P. carinii*), and, less commonly, by protozoa (*Toxoplasma gondii, Cryptosporidium parvum*, acanthamoeba, and others) and mycobacteria (72,128–133). The risk for and spectrum of OIs in pretreated patients is shown in a multicenter study of 93 fludarabine-refractory patients with CLL who were treated with alemtuzumab; 55% developed at least one infection, and severe infections occurred in 27% of patients (72). Eleven patients with advanced disease developed OIs, including PCP, invasive fungal infections, viral infections, particularly CMV reactivation (7 patients) and *L. monocytogenes*, with some experiencing multiple episodes. Seven additional OIs occurred in the follow-up period. Risks for OIs included extensive prior therapy, advanced disease and possibly the addition of systemic corticosteroids (>5 days) (72). As with fludarabine, infections appear to be less common among patients responding to therapy than among nonresponders.

Reactivation of CMV infection occurs in 15% to 30% of patients treated with alemtuzumab (129–133) with low serum albumin identified as the only predictor of CMV reactivation (133).

Consolidation alemtuzumab   The efficacy and safety of alemtuzumab consolidation in patients with previously untreated CLL was examined in several trials (134–141). Patients included were those who responded to fludarabine-based induction chemotherapy but had residual disease. Alemtuzumab was given intravenously or subcutaneously two to –six months after completion of induction therapy, and antimicrobial prophylaxis (acyclovir or valacyclovir and TMP-SMX) was provided. Dosing of alemtuzumab varied from 10 to 30 mg, and duration of treatment was also different in the various studies.

Although effective at increasing response rates, alemtuzumab consolidation was associated with severe infections (0–64%), but the incidence varied markedly between studies. These infections included OI such as *L. monocytogenes*, aspergillosis, tuberculosis, and others (134–141). Viral infections were common, particularly CMV reactivation. Two studies were terminated early because of the occurrence of severe infections (139,140). Notably, in both studies with the high rates of infection, the interval between chemotherapy and alemtuzumab treatment was short, at only two months.

In the only randomized study, 21 patients with CLL in first remission received alemtuzumab, 30 mg IV three times weekly for 12 weeks (11 patients), or were observed (10 patients) (139). Patients were randomized two months after fludarabine-based therapy. The study was terminated early because of the occurrence of severe infections in 7 of 11 patients who received a median of four weeks of alemtuzumab. These infections included CMV reactivations (3), pulmonary aspergillosis, pulmonary tuberculosis, and herpes zoster (1 each), all of which were successfully treated; no deaths occurred. This compared to only one VZV infection and one episode of sinusitis in the observation arm. Hematologic toxicity with six grade 4 events developed in 4 of 11 alemtuzumab recipients (139). Another study included 51 patients who received induction therapy with fludarabine plus rituximab (140). Patients with stable/responsive disease following induction received consolidation therapy with subcutaneous alemtuzumab 30 mg three times weekly for six weeks, given two months after chemotherapy. The study was discontinued because of unacceptable toxicity after alemtuzumab consolidation. Infections were mostly seen in patients who received consolidation when in CR after induction compared with patients who were only in PR (47% and 26% rate of infections, respectively). Patients in CR had 50% lower baseline lymphocyte counts, although the median ANC was similar between the two patient populations. Seven patients died after alemtuzumab therapy, five deaths occurred after EOT. This included two deaths in PR patients (EBV hepatitis and transfusion-associated graft vs. host disease, 1 and 8 months after end of therapy (EOT), respectively) and five deaths in CR patients; two during alemtuzumab therapy (Listeria meningitis and CMV glomerulonephropathy, 1 patient each) and three after EOT (*Legionella* pneumonia, sepsis, and viral meningitis, 1 case each, 1, 5, and 7 months after EOT, respectively) (140).

In contrast to the data reported above, two single arm trials used alemtuzumab as consolidation after fludarabine-based therapy, but in both of these trials, the interval between chemotherapy and alemtuzumab was four to –six months. In the Italian trial where alemtuzumab was given at 10 mg subcutaneously three times a week for six weeks to 34 patients, no bacterial or fungal infections were seen. CMV reactivation was detected on the basis of screening in 53% of patients, but no cases of CMV disease occurred. In a larger trial of 58 patients who received alemtuzumab 30 mg intravenously three times a week for four weeks, there were only three bacterial infections noted and no fungal infections. Symptomatic CMV reactivation occurred in 20% of patients. Thus, although these trials had different doses and different routes of administration, the common feature that may be associated with lower risk of infection is a longer interval between the chemotherapy and the initiation of alemtuzumab consolidation.

A recent publication (in abstract form) provided a comparative analysis of the infectious complications of treatment naïve patients with CLL treated in three sequential trials: fludarabine followed by alemtuzumab, single-agent fludarabine, and a randomized comparison of fludarabine with rituximab, either concurrent or sequential (141). Significantly higher rates of infection occurred with the alemtuzumab regimen (38%) compared with fludarabine alone (23%) or fludarabine plus rituximab (20%). Most infections were due to CMV reactivation, which occurred more commonly in the alemtuzumab study (14% vs. <1% in the other 2 studies). The incidence of PCP in all three studies was very low because most patients received PCP prophylaxis (141). Known risk factors for infection in CLL, including age, renal function, serum albumin levels, and others, were not evaluated in this preliminary report.

Denileukin Diftitox

The diphtheria fusion protein DAB (389) IL-2 (denileukin diftitox) is directed at the human IL-2) receptor, which is expressed on cells from some patients with CLL. After binding, the diphtheria toxin moiety is internalized and results in apoptosis or lysis. Eighteen patients with fludarabine-refractory CLL received denileukin diftitox without clinical evidence of immunosuppression or CMV reactivation (142). However, CMV status and peripheral blood lymphocytes counts were not monitored. Four severe infections occurred but without clear association with treatment with denileukin diftitox.

Splenectomy

Patients with CLL may develop splenomegaly and profound cytopenia, often responsive to chemotherapy, at least initially (95,143). However, marked splenomegaly may be present in some patients, especially those with advanced disease, and they may have cytopenias refractory to treatment with corticosteroids and/or chemotherapeutic agents. Splenic irradiation has been occasionally used in managing these patients, although splenectomy remains the preferred approach (95,143). The resulting asplenia significantly increases the risk for infection not only by encapsulated bacteria, particularly *S. pneumoniae*, but also infections due to *H. influenzae*, *Neisseria* spp, *Capnocytophaga canimorsus*, intraerythrocytic parasites (e.g., *Babesia microti*), group B streptococci, *S. aureus*, enterobacteriaceae, and *L. monocytogenes* (144).

Radiation Therapy

Radiation therapy is rarely indicated in CLL, except as a palliative measure, when bulky and symptomatic lymphoid masses or massive splenomegaly are present, in a patient unresponsive to chemotherapy. Radiation is typically delivered to these lymphoid masses and/or spleen and may provide temporary relief (143). The risk of severe infections because of radiation to these sites is likely to be limited.

Hematopoietic Stem Cell Transplantation

Autologous and allogeneic hematopoietic stem cell transplantation (HSCT) is increasingly being used in younger patients. The spectrum of infections associated with HSCT has been recently reviewed (76–78) and is briefly summarized in Table 3.

RISK FACTORS FOR INFECTIONS AND PERIOD AT RISK

The High-risk Patient

A number of factors place CLL patients at high risk for severe infections when receiving antileukemic therapy (Table 6). These include factors related to the host, the underlying process, and the therapy given. Recognition of these factors in individual patients is critical to formulate a risk-based preventive strategy.

Table 6 Risk Factors for Infection in Patients with CLL Receiving Antileukemic Therapy

Host related
   Older age (72,80,81)
   Renal dysfunction (64,72)
   Low serum albumin (64,146)
Therapy related
   Extensive prior therapy (64)
   Type of therapy: higher risk with
      Purine analogs and alemtuzumab (1–3,6,7,64)
      Concurrent high-dose corticosteroid therapy[a] (63,64)
      Combination of agents (1–3,6,7,64)
   Pretreatment granulocyte count $<1000/\mu L$ (64) and/or $CD4^+$ <50 cells/μL (64,70)
   Dose density and intensity (higher than recommended doses and/or aggressive schedule of
      therapy)
   Lack of dose reduction for prior treatment-related toxicities and unfavorable host-related factors
      (as above)
Disease related
   Advanced stage (Rai III and IV) (64,72)
   Refractoriness to purine analogs (113–115)
   Poor, slow, or no response to therapy (64)
   Hypogammaglobulinemia (16–20)
   Unmutated status of immunoglobulin Vh gene (34)
   FISH-detectable genetic abnormalities (such as p53) (34)
   Presence of $CD\text{-}38^+$ cells (34)
Factors related to microbial exposure
   No antimicrobial prophylaxis (66,107,146)
   History of severe infection or significant exposure to potential pathogen and secondary
      antimicrobial prophylaxis is not given (66)

The risk of infection persists after end of therapy in patients with extensive prior therapy (particularly with purine analogs and/or alemtuzumab) and those with advanced/refractory disease.

Text in Bold refers to the most important risk factors.

[a]High-dose corticosteroid therapy refers to treatment with ≥ 60 mg/day of prednisone equivalent for ≥ 2 wk.

The Period at Risk

In addition to identifying high-risk patients, the period of risk for infection should also be determined so that preventive strategies are applied throughout that period. Therapy with purine analogs and/or alemtuzumab is associated with profound defects in CMI, which may persist for longer than a year after EOT and with severe OIs posttherapy. In such patients, the period of risk extends for at least six months after discontinuation of purine analogs or alemtuzumab. When additional high-risk features for infection are present (Table 6), the period at risk should be extended beyond six months and until these additional risk features have resolved. Monitoring CD4 counts in such patients may be useful with CD4 counts less than or equal to 50 cells/μL, indicating persistence of severe immunosuppression, i.e., risk for OIs.

PREVENTION OF INFECTION: A RISK-BASED STRATEGY

Prevention of infection in patients with CLL requires a multifaceted effort, which includes the following:

1. Understanding the immune defects (both inherent to CLL and therapy related). Particular attention should be paid to the profound and persistent T-cell immunosuppression that follows therapy with purine analogs and alemtuzumab, especially when high-dose corticosteroids are added (Table 3).
2. Identifying patients at high-risk for infection (Table 6) and the period of risk.
3. Developing strategies aimed at preventing serious infections in these patients (Tables 3, 7, 8).

The following strategies can be applied to reduce the risk of infections in patients with CLL (Table 8)

Judicious Utilization of Antineoplastic Therapy

Treatment Indications

Indications for therapy include advanced disease, high tumor burden, severe CLL-related "B" symptoms, or repeated infections (severe hypogammaglobulinemia and indolent CLL are not).

Types of Therapy

- In patients younger than 65 years and with favorable host factors (Table 6), frontline therapy with purine analogs should be considered because of the high response rate and manageable toxicity (e.g., opportunistic infections, auto-immune cytopenias). However, longer follow-up of the comparative trials is necessary before final recommendations can be made.
- Treating older patients (65 years and older) with chlorambucil-based regimens or investigational agents because they do not tolerate purine analogs.
- Limiting the concomitant use of corticosteroids to their established indications.

Dose Density and Intensity

- Reducing the dose density and intensity of cycles of purine analog therapy.
- Early discontinuation of purine analog therapy in poorly responsive patients.

Table 7 Antimicrobial Prophylaxis During and After Therapy of CLL

Prophylaxis	Chlorambucil	Purine analog	Alemtuzumab	Steroids[a]	Duration of prophylaxis
Fluoroquinolone[b]	+	+	+	NA	During neutropenia ($<$100 cell/μL)
Antifungal azole[c]	+	+	+	+	During neutropenia ($<$100 cell/μL)
TMP-SMX[d]	—	($\pm$)[e]	+	+	$\geq$4–6 mo after stopping fludarabine or alemtuzumab[f]
Antiviral agent active against HSV/VZV[g]	($\pm$)	+	+	+	2 wk after last chlorambucil dose $\geq$4–6 mo after stopping fludarabine or alemtuzumab[f]
Neuraminidase inhibitor[h]	—	+	+	+	During the influenza virus season $\geq$4–6 mo after stopping fludarabine or alemtuzumab[f]

The risk of infection persists after end of therapy in patients with extensive prior therapy (particularly with purine analogs and/or alemtuzumab) and with advanced/refractory disease. Prophylaxis should reflect the presence and duration of high-risk factors for infection.

[a]High-dose corticosteroids: i.e., more than 2 wk of $\geq$60 mg/day of prednisone equivalent.

[b]Fluoroquinolone: e.g., levofloxacin 500 mg orally per day.

[c]Antifungal azole: e.g., fluconazole, 200 mg orally per day.

[d]TMP-SMX: Trimethoprim-sulfamethoxazole 1 tablet single or double strength orally per day; TMP-SMX prevents *P. carinii* pneumonia, listeriosis, nocardiosis, legionellosis, and other more common bacterial infections.

[e]TMP-SMX prophylaxis not recommended in patients treated with purine analogs unless they are also receiving corticosteroids or have other high-risk features for infection (Table 6).

[f]Acyclovir, famciclovir, or valacyclovir for patients who are seropositive for herpes simplex or herpes zoster or with history of previous herpetic infections.

[g]Continue prophylaxis in patients whose CD4 counts are or expected to drop below 50 cells/μL.

[h]Neuraminidase inhibitor: oseltamivir (Tamiflu) at 75 mg orally once daily during the influenza season.

Abbreviations: NA, not applicable; HSV, herpes simplex virus; VZV, varicella zoster virus.

- Reducing chemotherapy doses in high-risk patients (Table 6), particularly older patients (65 years and older) and those with renal dysfunction or a history of serious treatment-related toxicities during prior cycles of therapy.

Antimicrobial Prophylaxis/Preemptive Therapy

Prophylaxis should include antibacterial agents such as a fluoroquinolone, an antiviral agent active against HSV/VZV, an antifungal agent targeting candidal infections and TMP-SMX (Table 7).

A fluoroquinolone (e.g., levofloxacin, ciprofloxacin, or comparable agent) and an antifungal azole (e.g., fluconazole) should be given to patients with persistent ($>$10 days) severe neutropenia ($<$100 cells/μL).

Table 8 Prevention of Infections in Patients with CLL: Efficacy of Various Strategies

Preventive strategy	Efficacy
During therapy	
Judicious use of antileukemic therapy	+++
Antimicrobial prophylaxis	+++
Vaccination of caregivers and household contacts	++
Reducing exposure to pathogens	+
Growth factors (G-CSF, GM-CSF)	+
Intravenous immunoglobulin (IVIG) replacement	±
Vaccination of patient	±
After *end of therapy*[a]	
Antimicrobial prophylaxis	+++
Preemptive, patient self-administered antibiotic therapy	++
Reducing exposure to pathogens	+

+++: highly efficacious, strongly recommended.
++: efficacious and recommended.
+: likely efficacious.
±: limited efficacy.
Both G-CSF and GM-CSF shorten the duration of neutropenia and may reduce the risk of infection. IVIG is only indicated in patients with recurrent severe infections (pneumonia, bacteremia) despite prophylactic antibiotics and with serum IgG level <500 mg/dL.
[a]Applies to high-risk patients (Table 6), particularly those treated with alemtuzumab or purine analogs and high-dose corticosteroids.
Abbreviations: G-CSF, granulocyte colony–stimulating factor; GM-CSF, granulocyte macrophage CSF.

In patients at risk for invasive mould infections, prophylaxis with a mould-active antifungal triazole (itraconazole, voriconazole, or Posaconazole) may be used (78). Alternatively, serial monitoring for circulating *Aspergillus* galactomannan antigen can be performed and diagnostic-based therapy applied with the mould-active triazoles or an amphotericin B product (78). Because of the high rate of HSV and VZV infections with the use of purine analogs and alemtuzumab, and because of the morbidity associated with VZV-related post-herpetic neuralgia, especially in older patients, antiviral prophylaxis is recommended using acyclovir (400 mg po b.i.d.), famciclovir, or valacyclovir (500 mg po once daily). Prophylaxis should be given to all patients at risk for HSV/VZV infections (positive herpes serology or previous herpetic infections and patients with unknown serostatus), particularly when CD4 counts are or expected to be less than 50 CD4$^+$ cells/µL. Maintenance therapy is justified in patients with persistently depressed CD4 counts because of the correlation between very low CD4 counts after fludarabine therapy and VZV infection.

Reactivation of CMV infection occurs in 15% to 30% of patients receiving alemtuzumab-containing regimens and peaks between weeks 3 and 6 of therapy at the time of nadir T-cell count. Patients can be monitored for evidence of CMV reactivation with weekly CMV antigenemia or quantitative CMV PCR; alternatively, febrile patients can be evaluated for CMV at the time of symptoms and anti-CMV therapy (IV ganciclovir or oral valganciclovir) given to prevent progression to CMV disease (146). Induction therapy can be given with ganciclovir IV (5 mg/kg twice daily) or valganciclovir (900 mg orally twice daily) with dosage adjustment for renal dysfunction for both agents. Once CMV infection is brought under control, maintenance therapy with either agent can be commenced at half the induction dose.

An alternative strategy is prophylaxis with valganciclovir in CMV seropositive patients receiving an alemtuzumab-containing regimen as supported by the results of an

RCT that compared prophylaxis (145) with either valacyclovir 500 mg orally daily or valganciclovir 450 mg orally twice daily. The study enrolled 29 patients with CLL and 11 with related disorders who were receiving various alemtuzumab-containing regimens. The study was terminated early because stopping rules were met; CMV reactivation was prevented among the 20 patients randomized to valganciclovir compared to a 35% rate of reactivation among the 20 valacyclovir recipients ($p = 0.004$) (145).

CMV seronegative patients should only receive transfusions with CMV seronegative or filtered blood.

In high-risk patients, TMP-SMX should be started after hematologic recovery (platelets $\geq$ 75.000/µL) at a dose of one double-strength or single-strength tablet per day. Prophylaxis for PCP is not necessary in younger patients, particularly in absence of concomitant corticosteroids. Because PCP has been reported in CLL patients allergic to TMP-SMX, alternative prophylactic strategies, including dapsone (100 mg orally per day, or 5 days a week, after G6PD screen), atovaquone (750 mg of suspension orally twice per day, with food), or aerosolized pentamidine (AP), 300 mg per month, should be considered (76). Unlike TMP-SMX, however, none of these agents protect against listeriosis, nocardiosis, legionellosis, and other common bacterial infections; atovaquone and AP are expensive, and the latter associated with the rare risk of extrapulmonary pneumocystosis. Desensitization should therefore be seriously considered in patients with allergy to TMP-SMX (78).

Preventing influenza virus infections is important and is best accomplished by vaccinating health care workers, caregivers, and household members, and providing patients with neuraminidase inhibitor prophylaxis such as oseltamivir (Tamiflu) at 75 mg orally once daily during the influenza season (78).

Patients with CLL may have a coinfection with hepatitis viruses, which may reactivate following immunosuppressive therapies. Prevention of reactivation of hepatitis B infection can be achieved by lamivudine 150 mg once daily. Lamivudine should be started as early as possible and continued for several months after the EOT. Close monitoring of liver function tests is needed, particularly after EOT when immune reconstitution begins, because of the risk of liver dysfunction following resolution of immunosuppression. Prophylaxis against hepatitis C reactivation is not recommended given the narrow therapeutic index of hepatitis C-active agents.

Finally, a careful history should be obtained focused on history on latent infections, particularly in areas of endemicity for some infections (e.g., tuberculosis, endemic fungal infections such as histoplasmosis, blastomycosis, coccidioidomycosis, paracoccidioidomycosis, and others).

The appropriate duration of antimicrobial prophylaxis in patients with CLL receiving antileukemic therapy is unclear. However, because patients who achieve a significant response to treatment have a lower risk for major infection, prophylaxis could be discontinued after the completion of purine analog therapy in responding patients, particularly if they do not display any high-risk features (Table 6). By contrast, patients at high risk for major infections should continue to receive prophylaxis as long as these risk factors persist, for a minimum of six months after last dose of therapy. CD4 counts should be monitored in such patients and prophylaxis continued until CD4 counts reaches greater than or equal to 200 cells/µL for two consecutive months (78).

Secondary Prophylaxis

Patients who have suffered a severe infection such as PCP, HSV/VZV, aspergillosis, and tuberculosis are likely to experience relapse with continued therapy. Targeted secondary prophylaxis should be given to all such patients.

Growth Factors

Prophylactic growth factors (such as G-CSF 5 µg/kg, subcutaneously starting one day after the last dose of chemotherapy) reduce the duration of myelosuppression and appear to decrease the risk of infections following therapy with purine analogs and alemtuzumab (98,117).

Antimicrobials and Other Measures Following Completion of Therapy

Because patients receiving immunosuppressive agents (purine analogs and/or alemtuzumab) may develop severe infections long after their last dose of therapy, it is recommended that PCP and HSV/VZV prophylaxis be continued in such patients until the high-risk features have resolved and for a minimum of six months after EOT (42). When antimicrobial prophylaxis is stopped, these patients should also be provided with a supply of antimicrobial agents for self-administration (42). An agent active against encapsulated organisms (e.g., a fluoroquinolone or amoxicillin-clavulanate) should be started at the first onset of signs and symptoms suggestive of infection (e.g., fever and chills); early antibiotics can lessen the severity of bacterial infections associated with encapsulated bacteria such as *S. pneumoniae*, particularly in asplenic patients. Similarly, it is recommended that such patients be provided with a supply of acyclovir, valacyclovir, or famciclovir to commence if mucocutaneous lesions develop; early antiviral therapy may abort or shorten the course of HSV/VZV infections and may decrease the risk of dissemination and the severity of postherapeutic neuralgia.

All patients receiving therapy, particularly those at high risk for major infections, should be educated about the need to avoid activities, which may increase their risk for infection (42). This includes avoidance of occupational and recreational activities known to be associated with risk for infection and minimizing exposure to individuals with signs and symptoms of respiratory infections. Because waterborne or food-borne pathogens may cause serious infections in severely immunosuppressed patients, it is recommended that high-risk patients be educated about drinking sterile water only and avoiding foods likely to contain *L. monocytogenes* (e.g., unpasteurized milk, raw vegetables, under-cooked poultry or meat) during the high-risk period (95,40–42).

INTRAVENOUS IMMUNOGLOBULIN (IVIG) REPLACEMENT

In patients with CLL treated with chlorambucil, prophylactic IVIG replacement (400 mg/kg, every 3 weeks for 1 year) decreases the risk of mild and moderate bacterial infections (147–150). Lower doses (250 mg/kg, every 4 weeks or 10 grams every 3 weeks; given for 1 year or for 6 months) appear equally effective (151–154). Even so, the cost of IVIG and the availability of less expensive and more effective antibiotics limit the role of IVIG in CLL patients. IVIG can however be recommended in patients with IgG levels less than or equal to 500 mg/dL who continue to suffer recurrent sinopulmonary infections and/or bacteremias despite antibiotic prophylaxis. In such patients, the trough serum IgG should be kept greater than 500 mg/dL (2,42).

The role of IVIG replacement in the setting of therapy with purine analogs and monoclonal antibodies has not been extensively evaluated.

Vaccination

Vaccination of patients with CLL may be effective in decreasing the incidence of *H. influenzae* type b (Hib) and pneumococcal infections and infections caused by influenza virus in a subset of patients (155–164). However, antibody response to vaccine antigens is highly variable in patients with CLL and always lower compared with controls. In general, response to vaccination against influenza viruses A and B, *S. pneumoniae*, Hib, and tetanus toxoid ranges from 5% to 50%, with a modest increase in protective antibodies against influenza viruses following booster vaccination (155–164).

Predictors of a significant vaccination response include younger age, early-stage disease, elevated serum levels of IgM, IgA, and total IgG (>700 mg/dL) and of IgG subclasses 1, 2, and 4, suggesting that vaccination should be given at diagnosis, prior to initiation of chemotherapy and the worsening of hypogammaglobulinemia. However, response to vaccination may not be sustained, and booster vaccination should be considered on the basis of the levels of protective antibodies. Patients with advanced disease and those with extensive prior therapy are unlikely to develop adequate responses to vaccination, even if given before chemotherapy.

A more effective strategy is to vaccinate household members against influenza virus and Hib, because it is likely to decrease the risk of infection among high-risk patients (42). These high-risk patients are not expected to respond to vaccination, particularly after therapy with purine analogs and/or alemtuzumab (Table 5).

Interleukin-2

IL-2 was given as a specific CD 4^+ T-cell activator in an attempt to reverse fludarabine-induced immunosuppression. In a study of 19 patients, IL-2 led to a less profound $CD4^+$ decline. However, no data exist to support a role for IL-2 in the clinical setting (165).

CONCLUSION

Infectious complications continue to play a significant role in the management of patients with CLL, particularly with the advent of newer and more effective therapies. Several risk factors for infection have been identified in various subsets of patients, perhaps the most important of which is lack of application of antimicrobial prophylaxis. Indeed, the availability of safe and highly effective antimicrobial agents for the prevention of infections in these patients, coupled with powerful monitoring tools, has significantly reduced the incidence and severity of infectious complications even among heavily pretreated patients.

REFERENCES

1. Morrison VA. Management of infectious complications in patients with chronic lymphocytic leukemia. Hematology Am Soc Hematol Educ Program 2007; 2007:332–338.
2. Ravandi F, Anaissie EJ, O'Brien S. Infections in chronic leukemias and other hematological malignancies. In: Wingard JR, Bowden RA, eds. Management of Infections in Oncology Patients. London and New York: Martin Dunitz, 2003:105–128.
3. O'Brien SN, Blijlevens NM, Mahfouz TH, et al. Infections in patients with hematological cancer: recent developments. Hematology Am Soc Hematol Educ Program 2003:438–472.
4. Twomey JJ. Infections complicating multiple myeloma and chronic lymphocytic leukemia. Arch Intern Med 1973; 132:562–565.
5. Molica S. Infections in chronic lymphocytic leukemia: risk factors, and impact on survival, and treatment. Leuk Lymphoma 1994; 13:203–214.

6. Cheson BD. Infectious and immunosuppressive complications of purine analog therapy. J Clin Oncol 1995; 13:2431–2448.
7. Samonis G, Kontoyiannis DP. Infectious complications of purine analog therapy. Curr Opin Infect Dis 2001; 14:409–413.
8. Ferrajoli A, O'Brien SM. Treatment of chronic lymphocytic leukemia. Semin Oncol 2004; 31:60–65.
9. Mavromatis B, Cheson BD. Monoclonal antibody therapy of chronic lymphocytic leukemia. J Clin Oncol 2003; 21:1874–1881.
10. Dighiero G. Adverse and beneficial immunological effects of purine nucleoside analogues. Hematol Cell Ther 1996; 38(suppl 2):S75–S81.
11. Keating MJ, Flinn I, Jain V, et al. Therapeutic role of alemtuzumab (Campath-1H) in patients who have failed fludarabine: results of a large international study. Blood 2002; 99:3554–3561.
12. O'Brien SM, Kantarjian HM, Cortes J, et al. Results of the fludarabine and cyclophosphamide combination regimen in chronic lymphocytic leukemia. J Clin Oncol 2001; 19:1414–1420.
13. Weiss MA, Maslak PG, Jurcic JG, et al. Pentostatin and cyclophosphamide: an effective new regimen in previously treated patients with chronic lymphocytic leukemia. J Clin Oncol 2003; 21:1278–1284.
14. Byrd JC, Peterson BL, Morrison VA, et al. Randomized phase 2 study of fludarabine with concurrent versus sequential treatment with rituximab in symptomatic, untreated patients with B-cell chronic lymphocytic leukemia: results from Cancer and Leukemia Group B 9712 (CALGB 9712). Blood 2003; 101:6–14.
15. Weiss MA, Nicole L, Jurcic JG, et al. Pentostatin, Cyclophosphamide, and Rituximab (PCR therapy): A new active regimen for previously treated patients with Chronic Lymphocytic Leukemia (CLL). Blood 2003; 102.
16. Fairley GH, Scott RB. Hypogammaglobulinemia in chronic lymphocytic leukemia. Br Med J 1961; 2:920.
17. Rozman C, Montserrat E, Vinolas N. Serum immunoglobulins in B-chronic lymphocytic leukemia. Natural history and prognostic significance. Cancer 1988; 61:279–283.
18. Foa R, Catovsky D, Brozovic M, et al. Clinical staging and immunological findings in chronic lymphocytic leukemia. Cancer 1979; 44:483–487.
19. Itala M, Helenius H, Nikoskelainen J, et al. Infections and serum IgG levels in patients with chronic lymphocytic leukemia. Eur J Haematol 1992; 48:266–270.
20. Fiddes P, Penny R, Wells JV, et al. Clinical correlations with immunoglobulin levels in chronic lymphatic leukaemia. Aust N Z J Med 1972; 2:346–350.
21. Griffiths H, Lea J, Bunch C, et al. Predictors of infection in chronic lymphocytic leukaemia (CLL). Clin Exp Immunol 1992; 89:374–377.
22. Dighiero G. An attempt to explain disordered immunity and hypogammaglobulinemia in B-CLL. Nouv Rev Fr Hematol 1988; 30:283–288.
23. Dighiero G. Hypogammaglobulinemia and disordered immunity in CLL. In: Cheson DB, ed. Chronic Lymphocytic Leukemia: Scientific Advances and Clinical Developments. New York: Marcel Dekker, Inc.1993:147–166.
24. Whelan CA, Willoughby R, McCann SR. Relationship between immunoglobulin levels, lymphocyte subpopulations and Rai staging in patients with B-CLL. Acta Haematol 1983; 69:217–223.
25. Foa R. Pathogenesis of immunodeficiency in chronic lymphocytic leukemia. In: Cheson BD, ed. Chronic Lymphocytic Leukemia: Scientific Advances and Clinical Developments. New York: Marcel Dekker, Inc., 1993:147–166.
26. Aittoniemi J, Miettinen A, Laine S, et al. Opsonising immunoglobulins and mannan-binding lectin in chronic lymphocytic leukemia. Leuk Lymphoma 1999; 34:381–385.
27. Kneitz C, Goller M, Wilhelm M, et al. Inhibition of T cell/B cell interaction by B-CLL cells. Leukemia 1999; 13:98–104.
28. Copson ER, Ellis BA, Westwood NB, et al. IgG subclass levels in patients with B cell chronic lymphocytic leukaemia. Leuk Lymphoma 1994; 14:471–473.
29. Noelle RJ, Ledbetter JA, Aruffo A. CD40 and its ligand, an essential ligand-receptor pair for thymus-dependent B-cell activation. Immunol Today 1992; 13:431–433.

30. Lotz M, Ranheim E, Kipps TJ. Transforming growth factor beta as endogenous growth inhibitor of chronic lymphocytic leukemia B cells. J Exp Med 1994; 179:999–1004.
31. Semenzato G, Foa R, Agostini C, et al. High serum levels of soluble interleukin 2 receptor in patients with B chronic lymphocytic leukemia. Blood 1987; 70:396–400.
32. Sinisalo M, Aittoniemi J, Koski T, et al. Similar humoral immunity parameters in chronic lymphocytic leukemia patients independent of VH gene mutation status. Leuk Lymphoma 2004; 45:2451–2454.
33. Francis S, Karanth M, Pratt G, et al. The effect of immunoglobulin V(H) gene mutation status and other prognostic factors on the incidence of major infections in patients with chronic lymphocytic leukemia. Cancer 2006; 107:1023.
34. Rossi E, Matutes E, Morilla R, et al. Zeta chain and CD28 are poorly expressed on T lymphocytes from chronic lymphocytic leukemia. Leukemia 1996; 10:494–497.
35. Kunicka JE, Platsoucas CD. Defective helper function of purified T4 cells and excessive suppressor activity of purified T8 cells in patients with B-cell chronic lymphocytic leukemia. T4 suppressor effector cells are present in certain patients. Blood 1988; 71:1551–1560.
36. Prieto A, Garcia-Suarez J, Reyes E, et al. Diminished DNA synthesis in T cells from B chronic lymphocytic leukemia after phytohemagglutinin, anti-CD3, and phorbol myristate acetate mitogenic signals. Exp Hematol 1993; 21:1563–1569.
37. Dianzani U, Omede P, Marmont F, et al. Expansion of T cells expressing low CD4 or CD8 levels in B-cell chronic lymphocytic leukemia: correlation with disease status and neoplastic phenotype. Blood 1994; 83:2198–2205.
38. Semenzato G, Pezzutto A, Foa R, et al. T lymphocytes in B-cell chronic lymphocytic leukemia: characterization by monoclonal antibodies and correlation with Fc receptors. Clin Immunol Immunopathol 1983; 26:155–161.
39. Serrano D, Monteiro J, Allen SL, et al. Clonal expansion within the CD4+CD57+ and CD8+CD57+ T cell subsets in chronic lymphocytic leukemia. J Immunol 1997; 158:1482–1489.
40. Anaissie EJ, Kontoyiannis DP, O'Brien S, et al. Infections in patients with chronic lymphocytic leukemia treated with fludarabine. Ann Intern Med 1998; 129:559–566.
41. Anaissie E, Kontoyiannis DP, Kantarjian H, et al. Listeriosis in patients with chronic lymphocytic leukemia who were treated with fludarabine and prednisone. Ann Intern Med 1992; 117:466–469.
42. Anaissie Elias J. Overview of infectious complications following purine analog therapy. UpToDate 2008 http://www.utdol.com.
43. Platsoucas CD, Galinski M, Kempin S, et al. Abnormal T lymphocyte subpopulations in patients with B cell chronic lymphocytic leukemia: an analysis by monoclonal antibodies. J Immunol 1982; 129:2305–2312.
44. Kay NE. Abnormal T-cell subpopulation function in CLL: excessive suppressor (T gamma) and deficient helper (T mu) activity with respect to B-cell proliferation. Blood 1981; 57: 418–420.
45. Totterman TH, Carlsson M, Simonsson B, et al. T-cell activation and subset patterns are altered in B-CLL and correlate with the stage of the disease. Blood 1989; 74:786–792.
46. Peller S, Kaufman S. Decreased CD45RA T cells in B-cell chronic lymphatic leukemia patients: correlation with disease stage. Blood 1991; 78:1569–1573.
47. Vuillier F, Tortevoye P, Binet JL, et al. CD4, CD8 and NK subsets in B-CLL. Nouv Rev Fr Hematol 1988; 30:331–334.
48. Reyes E, Prieto A, Carrion F, et al. Morphological variants of leukemic cells in B chronic lymphocytic leukemia are associated with different T cell and NK cell abnormalities. Am J Hematol 1997; 55:175–182.
49. Burton JD, Weitz CH, Kay NE. Malignant chronic lymphocytic leukemia B cells elaborate soluble factors that down-regulate T cell and NK function. Am J Hematol 1989; 30:61–67.
50. Han T, Ozer H, Henderson ES, et al. Defective immunoregulatory T-cell function in chronic lymphocytic leukemia. Blood 1981; 58:1182–1189.
51. Decker T, Flohr T, Trautmann P, et al. Role of accessory cells in cytokine production by T cells in chronic B- cell lymphocytic leukemia. Blood 1995; 86:1115–1123.

52. Briggs PG, Kraft N, Atkins RC. T-lymphocyte response to cytokines in B-chronic lymphocytic leukemia. Leuk Res 1991; 15:859–865.
53. Miller D, Lizardo JG, Snyderman RK. Homologous and heterologous skin transplantation in patients with lymphomatous disease. J Natl Cancer Inst 1961; 26:569–579.
54. Miller D, Karnofsky DA. Immunologic factors and resistance to infection in chronic lymphocytic leukemia. Am J Med 1961; 31:748–757.
55. Chapel HM, Bunch C. Mechanisms of infection in chronic lymphocytic leukemia. Semin Hematol 1987; 24:291–296.
56. Foa R, Lauria F, Lusso P, et al. Discrepancy between phenotypic and functional features of natural killer T-lymphocytes in B-cell chronic lymphocytic leukaemia. Br J Haematol 1984; 58:509–516.
57. Foa R, Fierro MT, Raspadori D, et al. Lymphokine-activated killer (LAK) cell activity in B and T chronic lymphoid leukemia: defective LAK generation and reduced susceptibility of the leukemic cells to allogeneic and autologous LAK effectors. Blood 1990; 76:1349–1354.
58. Orsini E, Guarini A, Chiaretti S, et al. The circulating dendritic cell compartment in patients with chronic lymphocytic leukemia is severely defective and unable to stimulate an effective T-cell response. Cancer Res 2003; 63:4497–4506.
59. Donaldson GW, McArthur M, Macpherson AI, et al. Blood volume changes in splenomegaly. Br J Haematol 1970; 18:45–55.
60. Wright CS, Doan CA, Bouroncle BA, et al. Direct splenic arterial and venous blood studies in the hypersplenic syndromes before and after epinephrine. Blood 1951; 6:195–212.
61. Crosby WH. Hypersplenism. Annu Rev Med 1962; 13:127–146.
62. Rai KR, Montserrat E. Prognostic factors in chronic lymphocytic leukemia. Semin Hematol 1987; 24:252–256.
63. Lundin J, Porwit-MacDonald A, Rossmann ED, et al. Cellular immune reconstitution after subcutaneous alemtuzumab (anti-CD52 monoclonal antibody, CAMPATH-1H) treatment as first-line therapy for B-cell chronic lymphocytic leukaemia. Leukemia 2004; 18:484–490.
64. Tinhofer I, Marschitz I, Kos M, et al. Differential sensitivity of CD4+ and CD8+ T lymphocytes to the killing efficacy of Fas (Apo-1/CD95) ligand+ tumor cells in B chronic lymphocytic leukemia. Blood 1998; 91:4273–4281.
65. Lauria F, Foa R, Mantovani V, et al. T-cell functional abnormality in B-chronic lymphocytic leukaemia: evidence of a defect of the T-helper subset. Br J Haematol 1983; 54:277–283.
66. Wijermans PW, Gerrits WB, Haak HL. Severe immunodeficiency in patients treated with fludarabine monophosphate. Eur J Haematol 1993; 50:292–296.
67. Fenchel K, Bergmann L, Wijermans P, et al. Clinical experience with fludarabine and its immunosuppressive effects in pretreated chronic lymphocytic leukemias and low-grade lymphomas. Leuk Lymphoma 1995; 18:485–492.
68. Bergmann L, Fenchel K, Jahn B, et al. Immunosuppressive effects and clinical response of fludarabine in refractory chronic lymphocytic leukemia. Ann Oncol 1993; 4:371–375.
69. Osterborg A, Werner A, Halapi E, et al. Clonal CD8+ and CD52- T cells are induced in responding B cell lymphoma patients treated with Campath-1H (anti-CD52). Eur J Haematol 1997; 58:5–13.
70. Lundin J, Kimby E, Bjorkholm M, et al. Phase II trial of subcutaneous anti-CD52 monoclonal antibody alemtuzumab (Campath-1H) as first-line treatment for patients with B- cell chronic lymphocytic leukemia (B-CLL). Blood 2002; 100:768–773.
71. Hillmen P, Skotnicki AB, Robak T, et al. Alemtuzumab compared with chlorambucil as first-line therapy for chronic lymphocytic leukemia. J Clin Oncol 2007; 25(35):5616–5623. [Epub 2007, Nov 5].
72. Osterborg A, Dyer MJ, Bunjes D, et al. Phase II multicenter study of human CD52 antibody in previously treated chronic lymphocytic leukemia. European Study Group of CAMPATH-1H Treatment in Chronic Lymphocytic Leukemia. J Clin Oncol 1997; 15:1567–1574.
73. Onrust SV, Lamb HM, Balfour JA. Rituximab. Drugs 1999; 58:79–88; (discussion 89–90).
74. Voog E, Morschhauser F, Solal-Celigny P. Neutropenia in patients treated with rituximab. N Engl J Med 2003; 348:2691–2694; (discussion 2691–4).

75. O'Brien SM, Kantarjian H, Thomas DA, et al. Rituximab dose-escalation trial in chronic lymphocytic leukemia. J Clin Oncol 2001; 19:2165–2170.
76. Anaissie Elias J. Overview of infections following hematopoietic cell transplantation. UpToDate 2008. Available at: http://www.utdol.com.
77. Anaissie Elias J. Evaluation for infection before hematopoietic cell transplantation. UpToDate 2008. Available at: http://www.utdol.com.
78. Anaissie Elias J. Prophylaxis of infections in hematopoietic cell transplant recipients. UpToDate 2008. Available at: http://www.utdol.com.
79. Knauf WU, Lissichkov T, Aldaoud A, et al. Bendamustine versus chlorambucil in treatment-naive patients with B-cell chronic lymphocytic leukemia (B-CLL): results of an International Phase III Study. Program and abstracts of the 49th Annual Meeting of the American Society of Hematology, Atlanta, Georgia 2007, December 8-11 (abstr 2043).
80. Fischer K, Stilgenbauer S, Schweighofer C, et al. Bendamustine in combination with rituximab (BR) for patients with relapsed chronic lymphocytic leukemia (CLL): a multicentre phase II trial of the German CLL Study Group (GCLLSG). Program and abstracts of the 49th Annual Meeting of the American Society of Hematology, Atlanta, Georgia 2007, December 8–11 (abstr 3106).
81. Morrison VA, Rai KR, Peterson BL, et al. Impact of therapy with chlorambucil, fludarabine, or fludarabine plus chlorambucil on infections in patients with chronic lymphocytic leukemia: Intergroup Study Cancer and Leukemia Group B 9011. J Clin Oncol 2001; 19:3611–3621.
82. Van Den Neste E, Delannoy A, Vandercam B, et al. Infectious complications after 2-chlorodeoxyadenosine therapy. Eur J Haematol 1996; 56:235–240.
83. Byrd JC, Hargis JB, Kester KE, et al. Opportunistic pulmonary infections with fludarabine in previously treated patients with low-grade lymphoid malignancies: a role for Pneumocystis carinii pneumonia prophylaxis. Am J Hematol 1995; 49:135–142.
84. Keating MJ, Kantarjian H, O'Brien S, et al. Fludarabine: a new agent with marked cytoreductive activity in untreated chronic lymphocytic leukemia. J Clin Oncol 1991; 9:44–49.
85. Saven A, Lemon RH, Kosty M, et al. 2-Chlorodeoxyadenosine activity in patients with untreated chronic lymphocytic leukemia. J Clin Oncol 1995; 13:570–574.
86. Leporrier M, Chevret S, Cazin B, et al. Randomized comparison of fludarabine, CAP, and ChOP in 938 previously untreated stage B and C chronic lymphocytic leukemia patients. Blood 2001; 98:2319–2325.
87. Rai KR, Peterson BL, Appelbaum FR, et al. Fludarabine compared with chlorambucil as primary therapy for chronic lymphocytic leukemia. N Engl J Med 2000; 343:1750–1757.
88. Eichhorst BF, Busch R, Schweighofer C, et al. German CLL Study Group (GCLLSG). Due to low infection rates no routine anti-infective prophylaxis is required in younger patients with chronic lymphocytic leukaemia during fludarabine-based first line therapy. Br J Haematol 2007; 136(1):63–72.
89. Eichhorst BF, Busch R, Stauch M, et al. No significant clinical benefit of first line therapy with fludarabine (F) in comparison to chlorambucil (Clb) in elderly patients (pts) with advanced chronic lymphocytic leukemia (CLL): results of a phase III study of the German CLL Study Group (GCLLSG). Program and abstracts of the 49th Annual Meeting of the American Society of Hematology, 2007, December 8–11, Atlanta, Georgia (abstr 629).
90. O'Brien S, Kantarjian H, Beran M, et al. Results of fludarabine and prednisone therapy in 264 patients with chronic lymphocytic leukemia with multivariate analysis-derived prognostic model for response to treatment [see comments]. Blood 1993; 82:1695–1700.
91. Keating MJ, O'Brien S, Kantarjian H, et al. Long-term follow-up of patients with chronic lymphocytic leukemia treated with fludarabine as a single agent. Blood 1993; 81:2878–2884.
92. Robak T, Blonski JZ, Urbanska-Rys H, et al. 2-Chlorodeoxyadenosine (Cladribine) in the treatment of patients with chronic lymphocytic leukemia 55 years old and younger. Leukemia 1999; 13:518–523.
93. Robak T, Blasinska-Morawiec M, Blonski JZ, et al. 2-Chlorodeoxyadenosine (cladribine) in the treatment of elderly patients with B-cell chronic lymphocytic leukemia. Leuk Lymphoma 1999; 34:151–157.

94. Dillman RO, Mick R, McIntyre OR. Pentostatin in chronic lymphocytic leukemia: a phase II trial of Cancer and Leukemia group B. J Clin Oncol 1989; 7:433–438.

95. Ravandi F, Keating M, O'Brien S. Supportive care in chronic lymphocytic leukemia. In: Cheson BD, ed. Chronic Lymphoid Leukemias. New York, Basel: Marcel Dekker, Inc., 2000:485–504.

96. Molteni A, Nosari A, Montillo M, et al. Multiple lines of chemotherapy are the main risk factor for severe infections in patients with chronic lymphocytic leukemia with febrile episodes. Haematologica 2005; 90(8):1145–1147.

97. Perkins JG, Flynn JM, Howard RS, et al. Frequency and type of serious infections in fludarabine-refractory B- cell chronic lymphocytic leukemia and small lymphocytic lymphoma: implications for clinical trials in this patient population. Cancer 2002; 94:2033–2039.

98. O'Brien S, Kantarjian H, Beran M, et al. Fludarabine and granulocyte colony-stimulating factor (G-CSF) in patients with chronic lymphocytic leukemia. Leukemia 1997; 11:1631–1635.

99. Juliusson G, Liliemark J. High complete remission rate from 2-chloro-2′-deoxyadenosine in previously treated patients with B-cell chronic lymphocytic leukemia: response predicted by rapid decrease of blood lymphocyte count. J Clin Oncol 1993; 11:679–689.

100. Tallman MS, Hakimian D, Zanzig C, et al. Cladribine in the treatment of relapsed or refractory chronic lymphocytic leukemia. J Clin Oncol 1995; 13:983–988.

101. Keating MJ, Kantarjian H, Talpaz M, et al. Fludarabine: a new agent with major activity against chronic lymphocytic leukemia. Blood 1989; 74:19–25.

102. Johnson S, Smith AG, Loffler H, et al. Multicentre prospective randomised trial of fludarabine versus cyclophosphamide, doxorubicin, and prednisone (CAP) for treatment of advanced-stage chronic lymphocytic leukaemia. The French Cooperative Group on CLL. Lancet 1996; 347:1432–1438.

103. Juliusson G, Liliemark J. Long-term survival following cladribine (2-chlorodeoxyadenosine) therapy in previously treated patients with chronic lymphocytic leukemia. Ann Oncol 1996; 7:373–379.

104. Ho AD, Thaler J, Stryckmans P, et al. Pentostatin in refractory chronic lymphocytic leukemia: a phase II trial of the European Organization for Research and Treatment of Cancer. J Natl Cancer Inst 1990; 82:1416–1420.

105. Fenchel K, Bergmann L, Wijermans P, et al. Clinical experience with fludarabine and its immunosuppressive effects in pretreated chronic lymphocytic leukemias and low-grade lymphomas. Leuk Lymphoma 1995; 18:485–492.

106. Zinzani PL, Lauria F, Rondelli D, et al. Fludarabine in patients with advanced and/or resistant B-chronic lymphocytic leukemia. Eur J Haematol 1993; 51:93–97.

107. Montserrat E, Lopez-Lorenzo JL, Manso F, et al. Fludarabine in resistant or relapsing B-cell chronic lymphocytic leukemia: the Spanish Group experience. Leuk Lymphoma 1996; 21:467–472.

108. Johnston JB, Verburg L, Shore T, et al. Combination therapy with nucleoside analogs and alkylating agents. Leukemia 1994; 8(suppl 1):S140–S143.

109. O'Brien S, Moore JO, Boyd TE, et al. Randomized phase III trial of fludarabine plus cyclophosphamide with or without oblimersen sodium (Bcl-2 antisense) in patients with relapsed or refractory chronic lymphocytic leukemia. J Clin Oncol 2007; 25(9): 1114–1120.

110. Kowal M, Dmoszynska A, Lewandowski K, et al. Efficacy and safety of fludarabine and cyclophosphamide combined therapy in patients with refractory/recurrent B-cell chronic lymphocytic leukaemia (B-CLL)-Polish multicentre study. Leuk Lymphoma 2004; 45(6): 1159–1165.

111. Hallek M, Schmitt B, Wilhelm M, et al. Fludarabine plus cyclophosphamide is an efficient treatment for advanced chronic lymphocytic leukaemia (CLL): results of a phase II study of the German CLL Study Group. Br J Haematol 2001; 114(2): 342–348.

112. Flinn IW, Neuberg DS, Grever MR, et al. Phase III trial of fludarabine plus cyclophosphamide compared with fludarabine for patients with previously untreated chronic lymphocytic leukemia: US Intergroup Trial E2997. J Clin Oncol 2007; 25(7):793–798.

113. Wierda W, O'Brien S, Faderl S, et al. Improved survival in patients with relapsed refractory Chronic Lymphocytic Leukemia (CLL) treated with Fludarabine, Cyclophosphamide, and Rituximab (FCR) combination. Blood 2003; 102.

114. Schulz H, Klein SK, Rehwald U, et al. Phase 2 study of a combined immunochemotherapy using rituximab and fludarabine in patients with chronic lymphocytic leukemia. Blood 2002; 100:3115–3120.

115. Keating M.J., O'Brien S, Albitar M, et al. Early results of a chemoimmunotherapy regimen of fludarabine, cyclophosphamide, and rituximab as initial therapy for chronic lymphocytic leukemia. J Clin Oncol 2005; 23(18):4079–4088. [Epub 2005, Mar 14].

116. Wierda W, O'Brien S, Wen S et al. Chemoimmunotherapy with fludarabine, cyclophosphamide, and rituximab for relapsed and refractory chronic lymphocytic leukemia. J Clin Oncol 2005; 23(18):4070–4078.

117. Wierda WG, O'Brien S, Ferrajoli A, et al. Combined cyclophosphamide, fludarabine, alemtuzumab, and rituximab (CFAR), an active frontline regimen for high-risk patients with CLL. Program and abstracts of the 49th Annual Meeting of the American Society of Hematology, 2007 December 8–11, Atlanta, Georgia (abstr 628).

118. Robak T, Blonski JZ, Kasznicki M, et al. Cladribine with prednisone versus chlorambucil with prednisone as first-line therapy in chronic lymphocytic leukemia: report of a prospective, randomized, multicenter trial. Blood 2000; 96:2723–2729.

119. Robak T, Blonski J.Z, Kasznicki M, et al. Cladribine with or without prednisone in the treatment of previously treated and untreated B-cell chronic lymphocytic leukaemia - updated results of the multicentre study of 378 patients. Br J Haematol 2000; 108(2):357–368.

120. Oken MM, Lee S, Kay NE, et al. Pentostatin, chlorambucil and prednisone therapy for B-chronic lymphocytic leukemia: a phase I/II study by the Eastern Cooperative Oncology Group study E1488. Leuk Lymphoma 2004; 45(1):79–84.

121. Lamanna N, Kalaycio M, Maslak P, et al. Pentostatin, cyclophosphamide, and rituximab is an active, well-tolerated regimen for patients with previously treated chronic lymphocytic leukemia. J Clin Oncol 2006; 24(10):1575–1581.

122. Shanafelt TD, Lin T, Geyer SM, et al. Pentostatin, cyclophosphamide, and rituximab regimen in older patients with chronic lymphocytic leukemia. Cancer 2007; 109(1):2291–2298.

123. Keating MJ, O'Brien S, Kontoyiannis D, et al. Results of first salvage therapy for patients refractory to a fludarabine regimen in chronic lymphocytic leukemia. Leuk Lymphoma 2002; 43:1755–1762.

124. Byrd JC, Peterson B, Piro L, et al. A phase II study of cladribine treatment for fludarabine refractory B cell chronic lymphocytic leukemia: results from CALGB Study 9211. Leukemia 2003; 17(2):323–327.

125. Juliusson G, Elmhorn-Rosenborg A, Liliemark J. Response to 2-chlorodeoxyadenosine in patients with B-cell chronic lymphocytic leukemia resistant to fludarabine. N Engl J Med 1992; 327:1056.

126. Byrd JC, Lin TS, Dalton JT, et al. Flavopiridol administered using a pharmacologically derived schedule is associated with marked clinical efficacy in refractory, genetically high-risk chronic lymphocytic leukemia. Blood 2007; 109:399.

127. Byrd JC, Murphy T, Howard RS, et al. Rituximab using a thrice weekly dosing schedule in B-cell chronic lymphocytic leukemia and small lymphocytic lymphoma demonstrates clinical activity and acceptable toxicity. J Clin Oncol 2001; 19:2153–2164.

128. Lundin J, Osterborg A, Brittinger G, et al. CAMPATH-1H monoclonal antibody in therapy for previously treated low- grade non-Hodgkin's lymphomas: a phase II multicenter study. European Study Group of CAMPATH-1H Treatment in Low-Grade Non-Hodgkin's Lymphoma. J Clin Oncol 1998; 16:3257–3263.

129. Rai KR, Freter CE, Mercier RJ, et al. Alemtuzumab in previously treated chronic lymphocytic leukemia patients who also had received fludarabine. J Clin Oncol 2002; 20:3891–3897.

130. Ferrajoli A, O'Brien SM, Cortes JE, et al. Phase II study of alemtuzumab in chronic lymphoproliferative disorders. Cancer 2003; 98:773–778.

131. Elter T, Borchmann P, Schulz H, et al. Results of a phase II trial of fludarabine with concomitant application of alemtuzumab in a four-weekly schedule (FluCam) in patients with relapsed CLL. Proceedings of ASCO 2004; 23:603.

132. Cao TM, Nguyen DD, Dugan k, et al. Incidence of cytomegalovirus (CMV) viremia during Campath-1H therapy for relapsed/refractory chronic lymphocytic leukemia (CLL). Blood 2001; 98:366a.

133. Borthakur G, Lin E, Faderl S, et al. Low serum albumin level is associated with cytomegalovirus reactivation in patients with chronic lymphoproliferative diseases treated with alemtuzumab(Campath-1H)-based therapies. Cancer 2007; 110(11):2478–2483.

134. O'Brien SM, Kantarjian HM, Thomas DA, et al. Alemtuzumab as treatment for residual disease after chemotherapy in patients with chronic lymphocytic leukemia. Cancer 2003; 98:2657–2663.

135. Montillo M, Cafro AM, Tedeschi A, et al. Safety and efficacy of subcutaneous Campath-1H for treating residual disease in patients with chronic lymphocytic leukemia responding to fludarabine. Haematologica 2002; 87:695–700; (discussion 700).

136. Rai K, Byrd J, Peterson BL, et al. A phase II trial of fludarabine followed by alemtuzumab (Campath-1H) in previously untreated chronic lymphocytic leukemia (CLL) patients with active disease: Cancer and Leukemia Group B (CALGB) study 19901. Blood 2002; 100:205a.

137. Rai KR, Byrd JC, Peterson B, et al. Subcutaneous alemtuzumab following fludarabine for previously untreated patients with chronic lymphocytic leukemia (CLL): CALGB Study 19901. Blood 2003; 102:676a.

138. Vitolo U, Orsucci L, di Celle PF, et al. Alemtuzumab (Campath, MabCampath) consolidation after fludarabine phosphate and cyclophosphamide second-Line chemotherapy for progressive chronic lymphocytic leukemia. Blood 2003; 102.

139. Wendtner CM, Ritgen M, Schweighofer CD, et al. Consolidation with alemtuzumab in patients with chronic lymphocytic leukemia (CLL) in first remission - Experience on safety and efficacy within a randomized multicenter phase III trial of the German CLL Study Group (GCLLSG). Blood 2003; 102:676a.

140. Lin TS, Donohue KA, Lucas MS. Consolidation therapy with subcutaneous (SC) alemtuzumab results in severe infectious toxicity in previously untreated CLL patients who achieve a complete response (CR) after fludarabine and rituximab (FR) induction therapy: interim safety analysis of the CALGB study 10101. Program and abstracts of the 49th Annual Meeting of the American Society of Hematology (ASH), 2007, December 8–11, Atlanta, Georgia (abstr) 755.

141. Morrison VA, Peterson BL, Rai KR, et al. Alemtuzumab increases serious infections in patients with previously untreated chronic lymphocytic leukemia (CLL) receiving fludarabine-based therapy: a comparative analysis of 3 cancer and leukemia group B studies (CALGB 9011, 9712, 19901). Program and abstracts of the 49th Annual Meeting of the American Society of Hematology, 2007, December 8–11, Atlanta, Georgia (abstr) 756.

142. Frankel AE, Fleming DR, Hall PD, et al. A phase II study of DT fusion protein denileukin diftitox in patients with fludarabine-refractory chronic lymphocytic leukemia. Clin Cancer Res 2003; 9:3555–3561.

143. Rai K, Keating M. Treatment of chronic lymphocytic leukemia. UpToDate 2008. Available at: http://www.utdol.com.

144. Pasternack MS. Clinical features, management, and prevention of sepsis in the splenectomized patient. UpToDate 2008. Available at: http://www.utdol.com.

145. O'Brien S, Ravandi F, Riehl T, et al. Valganciclovir prevents cytomegalovirus reactivation in patients receiving alemtuzumab-based therapy. Blood 2008; 111(4):1816–1819. [Epub 2007, Nov 26].

146. Keating M, Coutre S, Rai K, et al. Management guidelines for use of alemtuzumab in B-cell chronic lymphocytic leukemia. Clin Lymphoma 2004; 4:220–227.

147. Besa EC. Use of intravenous immunoglobulin in chronic lymphocytic leukemia. Am J Med 1984; 76:209–218.

148. Griffiths H, Brennan V, Lea J, et al. Crossover study of immunoglobulin replacement therapy in patients with low-grade B-cell tumors. Blood 1989; 73:366–368.

149. Bunch C, Chapel H, Raj K. Intravenous immunoglobulin reduces bacterial infections in chronic lymphocytic leukemia: a controlled, randomized clinical trial. Blood 1987; 70:224a.

150. Intravenous immunoglobulin for the prevention of infection in chronic lymphocytic leukemia. N Engl J Med 1988; 6:902–907.
151. Gamm H, Huber C, Chapel H, et al. Intravenous immune globulin in chronic lymphocytic leukaemia. Clin Exp Immunol 1994; 97(suppl 1):17–20.
152. Chapel H, Dicato M, Gamm H, et al. Immunoglobulin replacement in patients with chronic lymphocytic leukaemia: a comparison of two dose regimes. Br J Haematol 1994; 88:209–212.
153. Molica S, Musto P, Chiurazzi F, et al. Prophylaxis against infections with low-dose intravenous immunoglobulins (IVIG) in chronic lymphocytic leukemia. Results of a crossover study. Haematologica 1996; 81:121–126.
154. Jurlander J, Geisler CH, Hansen MM. Treatment of hypogammaglobulinaemia in chronic lymphocytic leukaemia by low-dose intravenous gammaglobulin. Eur J Haematol 1994; 53:114–118.
155. Gribabis DA, Panayiotidis P, Boussiotis VA, et al. Influenza virus vaccine in B-cell chronic lymphocytic leukaemia patients [see comments]. Acta Haematol 1994; 91:115–118.
156. Bucalossi A, Marotta G, Galieni P, et al. Immunological response to influenza virus vaccine in B-cell chronic lymphocytic leukaemia patients. Acta Haematol 1995; 93:56.
157. van der Velden AM, Mulder AH, Hartkamp A, et al. Influenza virus vaccination and booster in B-cell chronic lymphocytic leukaemia patients. Eur J Intern Med 2001; 12(5):420–424.
158. Sinisalo M, Aittoniemi J, Käyhty H, et al. Vaccination against infections in chronic lymphocytic leukemia. Leuk Lymphoma 2003; 44(4):649–652.
159. Sinisalo M, Aittoniemi J, Oivanen P, et al. Response to vaccination against different types of antigens in patients with chronic lymphocytic leukaemia. Br J Haematol 2001; 114(1):107–110.
160. Jurlander J, de Nully Brown P, Skov PS, et al. Improved vaccination response during ranitidine treatment, and increased plasma histamine concentrations, in patients with B cell chronic lymphocytic leukemia. Leukemia. 1995; 9(11):1902–1909.
161. Sinisalo M, Vilpo J, Itälä M, et al. Antibody response to 7-valent conjugated pneumococcal vaccine in patients with chronic lymphocytic leukaemia. Vaccine 2007; 26(1):82–87. [Epub 2007, Nov 12].
162. Sinsalo M, Aittoniemi J, Käyhty H, et al. *Haemophilus influenzae* type b (Hib) antibody concentrations and vaccination responses in patients with chronic lymphocytic leukaemia: predicting factors for response. Leuk Lymphoma 2002; 43(10):1967–1969.
163. Hartkamp A, Mulder AH, Rijkers GT, et al. Antibody responses to pneumococcal and haemophilus vaccinations in patients with B-cell chronic lymphocytic leukaemia. Vaccine 2001; 19(13–14):1671–1677.
164. Van der Velden AM, Van Velzen-Blad H, Claessen AM, et al. The effect of ranitidine on antibody responses to polysaccharide vaccines in patients with B-cell chronic lymphocytic leukaemia. Eur J Haematol 2007; 79(1):47–52. [Epub 2007, May 28].
165. Fenchel K, Atzpodien J, E.J. B, et al. Interleukin-2 is effective in reducing the fludarabine-induced CD4+ depletion. Blood 1997; 90.

Index

Absolute neutrophil count (ANC), 274
Acquired angioedema, 236
Actimid, 167
Acute lymphoblastic leukemia (ALL), 21
Acute myeloid leukemia (AML), 21
Acyclovir, 272
ADAM29 genes, 24
Adaptive immune-based treatment
    strategies, 202
Adeno-associated virus (AAV) vectors, 204
Adenovirus, 204
Adult T-cell lymphoma/leukemia (ATLL), 108
Agranulocytosis, 104
AIRC. *See* Associazione Italiana Ricerca sul
    Cancro (AIRC)
Alemtuzumab
    autoimmunity treatment, 237
    consolidation therapy, 154
    induction therapy, 151–154
        in fludarabine-refractory patients, 155–158
Alemtuzumab-based chemoimmunotherapy,
    130–131
Alkylating agents, 266–278
    bendamustine, 270
    chlorambucil, 266–270
    combination chemotherapies with, 126
    cyclophosphamide, 270–278
    monotherapy with, 123–124
    salvage therapy, 142, 143
ALL. *See* Acute lymphoblastic leukemia (ALL)
Allogenic stem cell transplantation, 186–188
    reduced-intensity conditioning (RIC),
        188–192
AML. *See* Acute myeloid leukemia (AML)
ANC. *See* Absolute neutrophil count (ANC)
Angioedema, acquired, 236

Animal models, monoclonal B lymphocytes
    (MBL) in, 72–74
Anthracycline, fludarabine with, 128
Anticipation phenomenon, 70
Antigen–presenting cells
    function of CLL as, 233–234
Antigens, CLL, 201–204
Antileukemic therapy, 261, 266
Antimicrobial prophylaxis, 280–282
Antimicrobials therapy, 283
Antineoplastic therapy, 279–280
Apoptosis dysregulation in CLL, 91–99
Associazione Italiana Ricerca sul Cancro
    (AIRC), 12
ATM mutation, 222
ATM or TP53 genes, 29
Autoimmune cytopenias, 232
Autoimmune hemolytic anemia (AIHA), 104
    prevalence, 232–233
    prognostic significance, 235–236
    risk factors, 235
    treatment, 237
Autoimmune thrombocytopenia, 104
Autoimmunity, 231–238
    pathogenesis, 233–236
    prevalence, 232–233
    prognostic significance, 235–236
    risk factors, 235
    treatment, 236–238
    treatment-related complications, 234–235
Autologous stem cell transplantation, 192–194,
    195–196

B-1a cells, 2
BAK, 97–98
BAX, 97–98

B-1b cells, 2
B-cells, 1, 2, 8, 21, 25, 262
  anergy, 56, 57
  subsets, 2, 4
B-cell maturation antigen (BCMA), 6
B-cell prolymphocytic leukemia (B-PLL),
    217–222
  cell morphology, 219
  clinical and laboratory features, 218–220
  cytogenetics, 220
  differential diagnosis, 220
  immunophenotyping, 219
  monoclonal antibodies therapy, 221
  pathogenesis, 217–218
  prognosis, 220–222
  purine analogue therapy in, 221
  splenectomy for, 221
  stem cell transplantation, 221–222
  treatment, 220–222
B-cell receptors (BCR)
  complex on CLL cells, 44–47
  coreceptors, 52–55
  costimulation, 55–56
  signaling, CLL cells, 51–52
  signaling in normal B cells, 47–50
  structure, 6–7
  and TLR engagement, in vitro, 4–5
B-1 cells, 2, 8
  vs B-2 cells, 7–8
B-2 cells, 2, 8
  vs B-1 cells, 7–8
B-cell subsets in animal and man, 7–9
  B-1 vs B-2 cells, 7–8
  IgM⁺IgD⁺CD27⁺Cells, 9
  MZ B Cells, 8–9
  transitional B cells, 9
B-cell variant of PLL (B-PLL), 108
Bcl-2 family–targeted therapies
  fludarabine-refractory patients, 158–159
BCL-2 proteins
  control of mitochondrial apoptosis in CLL,
      94–96
  intrinsic apoptosis pathway, CLL, 91–93
BCMA. See B-cell maturation antigen
    (BCMA)
BCR. See B-cell receptors (BCR)
BCR-antigen, 4
BCR-signaling pathway, 47
Bendamustine, 270
  monotherapy, 124–126
BFL-1 protein, 96
BH-3 mimetics, 178
BH3-only proteins, 97
BH3 profiling, 94–95

BIM protein, 94–95
Binet staging system, 109, 111
Biologic agents for the treatment of CLL,
    176–177
Biological risk factors
  Richter's syndrome, 244
Blood-borne microbial infection, 8
Blood cell specificity, autoimmunity, 234
B lymphocytes, 8
  BCR signaling in normal, 47–50
BLyS receptor 3 (BR3), 5
B2M. See B2-microglobulin (β2M)
B2-microglobulin (β2M), 111, 112, 274
BR3. See BLyS receptor 3 (BR3)
Burkitt lymphoma, 27

Calcium signaling, 49
CALGB 9712 protocol, 128
Caspase activation, 98–99
CD5, 3, 53–54
CD10, 3
CD19, 53
CD21, 53
CD22, 3, 54
CD23, 3, 111, 112
CD27, 3
CD38, 54–55
CD72, 54
CD80, 206
CD86, 206
CD154, 206–207
  clinical trials with, 209
CD79α expression, 46–47
CD5⁺ B cell, 25
CD27⁺ B cells, 25, 26, 28
CD79β expression, 46–47
CD5 cell, 25
CD38 cell, 22, 23
CD4 cells, 270
CD5⁺ cells, 10
CD40-ligand, 206–207
Cell-mediated immunity (CMI), 262
Cellular counterpart of CLL cells, 9–12
  M-CLL cells, 10–11
  U-CLL cells, 10
Cellular origin of CLL, 25–27
Cellular therapy, 210–211
CFAR. See Combination of FCR with the
    monoclonal antibody alemtuzumab
    (CFAR)
Chemokine receptors, 3
Chemotherapy, 276
Chimeric receptors, 210

Chlorambucil, 123–124, 127, 266–270
2-chlorodeoxyadenosine, 270
Chromosomal aberrations, in CLL, 35–37
Chronic lymphocytic leukemia (CLL),
    2, 19, 261
  adaptive immune-based treatment
    strategies, 202
  agents in early-stage clinical trials for
    treatment, 171, 172–175
  antigens, 201–204
  apoptosis dysregulation in, 91–99
  BCR complex on cells of, 44–47
  BCR signaling in cells of, 51–52
  biologic agents, 176–177
  biological association between MBL and,
    79–82
  cellular therapy, 210–211
  chromosomal aberrations in, 35–37
  clinical association between MBL and,
    82–83
  complications, 231–249
  consolidation therapy, 131–133
  control of mitochondrial apoptosis in BCL-2
    proteins, 94–96
  diagnosis, 103–104
    National Cancer Institute (NCI) guide-
      lines, 110
  differential diagnosis, 106–108
  etiology of, 69–71
  familial, 77–78
  frontline therapy, 123–131
    in patients with del(17p)/p53
      mutation, 133
  genomic aberrations and, 114–115
  histology, 105–106
  immune gene therapy, 204–209
  immune therapy, 201–204
  immunophenotyping, 106
  inherited susceptibility, 77–78
  miRNAs in pathogenesis of, 37
  morphology of lymphocytes in, 104–105
  physiology, 28–29
  prognosis, 110–116
  relapsed
    agents in phase I to II trial for treatment,
      166–171
    treatment of patients with, 141–159
  relation to mature B cell malignancies,
    27–28
  response assessment, 122–123, 142, 143
  silvestrol, 178–179
  staging for patients with, 109–110
  stem cell transplantation in, 185–196
  subsets, 3

[Chronic lymphocytic leukemia (CLL)]
  subtypes, 23–25
  targeted small molecules, 177–178
  transgenes, 205–207
  treatment
    decision, 121–122
    indications for salvage, 141–142
  tumor cells, 23, 27, 29
  ultraconsereved genes and, 41–42
  vaccine strategies, 210–211
Chronic lymphocytic leukemia (CLL) B cells,
    2, 3, 4, 5, 10, 262
  anatomic location and pattern, 3–4
  cellular counterpart of, 9–12
  characteristics, 3–7
    anatomic location and pattern, 3–4
    BCR structure, 6–7
    composite, 7
    gene expression, 6
    stimulation, 4–6
    surface membrane phenotype, 3
Cladribine (2-CdA), 148, 270
  with cyclophosphamide (CC), combination
    chemotherapy, 127
  monotherapy, 124
  salvage therapy in fludarabine-refractory
    patients, 155
X light chain gene, 24
CLL. *See* Chronic lymphocytic leukemia
    (CLL)
CLL antigen, potential, 203
CMI. *See* Cell-mediated immunity (CMI)
Combination chemotherapies
  with alkylating agents, 126
  with purine analogs, 126–128
Combination of FCR with the monoclonal
    antibody alemtuzumab (CFAR), 261,
    273, 275–277
  treatments, 275–276
Consolidation therapy
  alemtuzumab, 154
  CLL, 131–133
Coreceptors, BCR, 52–55
Corticosteroids, 266
Cyclophosphamide (FC), 123, 270–278, 273
  and fludarabin (FC), combination che-
    motherapy, 126
  and mitoxantrone, combination chemother-
    apy, 127
Cytogenetics
  B-cell PLL, 220
  Richter's syndrome, 248–249
  T-cell PLL, 223–224
Cytokine and chemokine influences, 5–6

Cytokine genes, 205–207
Cytometry, 24
Cytopenias, 266
   autoimmune, 232

Death-inducing signaling complex (DISC), 93
Del(17p)
   frontline therapy of CLL patients with, 133
Dendritic cell vaccines, 211
Denileukin diftitox, 277
2′-deoxycoformycin, 270
Diffuse large B-cell lymphoma (DLBCL), 21,
   239–241
   clonal relatedness, 243
   histological features of, 242
   Richter's syndrome, treatment options,
      245–247
Disease-related factors, 262–266
DLBCL. *See* Diffuse large B-cell lymphoma
   (DLBCL)
DNA, 4, 20
   microarrays, 20, 23
Donor lymphocyte infusion (DLI), response
   to, 187

Early-stage clinical trials, agents, 171,
   172–175
EBV, human Herpes virus, 248
Electroporation, 205
End of therapy (EOT), 275
EOT. *See* End of therapy (EOT)
Escherichia coli, 262
European Organization for Research and
   Treatment of Cases (EORTC)
   trial, 148
Extrinsic apoptotic pathway, CLL, 93
Ex vivo purging, of stem cells, 194

Familial CLL, 77–78
Family studies, 77–78
Fas-mediated apoptosis, latent sensitivity
   to, 207
FC. *See* Cyclophosphamide (FC)
FcγR engineered anti-CD20 antibodies, 176
FcγRIIb, 54
FCR. *See* Fludarabine/ cyclophosphamide plus
   rituximab (FCR)
Feinstein Institute for Medical Research, 12
Fever of unknown origin (FUO), 274
First-line treatment in CLL, 134
Flavopiridol, 169–171, 274

Fludarabine, 29, 261, 270
   monotherapy, 124
   plus anthracycline, combination chemother-
      apy, 128
   plus cyclophosphamide (FC), combination
      chemotherapy, 126
   salvage therapy, 144–147
Fludarabine cyclophosphamide, and rituximab
   (FCR), 148, 150, 273, 274–275
Fludarabine (purine analog)-sensitive patients,
   142, 143
Fludarabine-refractory patients, 154–155
   alemtuzumab therapy, 152
Fluorescence in situ hybridization (FISH)
   biological association between MBL and, 81–82
   genomic aberrations and CLL, 114, 115
18-F fluoro-deoxy-glucose (FDG) positron
   emission tomography (PET)
   Richter's syndrome detection, 240–241
FMC7, 3
Follicular lymphoma, 27
Frontline therapy, 123–131, 272
FUO. *See* Fever of unknown origin (FUO)

G3139. *See* Oblimersen sodium
GC. *See* Germinal centers (GC)
GC B cells, 6, 25, 28
Genasense. *See* Oblimersen sodium
Gene expression, 6
   profile analysis, 20–22
Gene therapy, immune, 204–209
   clinical trials of, 207–209
Genomic aberrations
   and CLL, 114–115
   VH mutation status and, 116
German CLL Study Group (GCLLSG) trial,
   148, 225, 235
Germinal centers (GC), 1, 22
Global gene expression profiling (GEP), 19
Graft *versus* leukemia (GVL) effect, 186, 187,
   191, 192
Gumprecht's phenomenon, 104

Hairy cell leukemia (HCL), 107
Hematopoietic stem cell transplantation
   (HSCT), 278
Hemophilus influenzae, 262
Herpes simplex virus (HSV), 205, 270
High-risk patient, 278
Histone deacetylase (HDAC) inhibitors, 178
Hodgkin lymphoma, 241–242
   clonal relatedness, 243
   histological features of, 242–243

[Hodgkin lymphoma]
  Richter's syndrome, treatment options, 247–248
Homogeneous gene expression profile of CLL, 22–23
Hospital outpatients
  detection of MBL in, 75–77
HS1, 48–49
HSCT. *See* Hematopoietic stem cell transplantation (HSCT)
HSP90 inhibitors, 177
HSV. *See* Herpes simplex virus (HSV)
Human Herpes virus, EBV, 248
Human marginal zone B cell, 11
HuMax CD20 (Ofatumumab), 166
HyperIgM syndrome, 5
Hypogammaglobulinemia, 262

IAP (Inhibitors of Apoptosis) proteins, 98–99
IDEC-152 (Lumiliximab), 166–167
IFN-γ induced monokine (Mig), 4
IFN-inducible protein 10 (IP-10), 4
Ig. *See* Immunoglobulin (Ig)
IgD-signaling pathways, 50
IgG levels, 262
IGHV gene
  usage in MBL, 80–81
Ig loci, 28
IgM antibodies, 1, 7, 10
IgM$^+$IgD$^+$CD27$^+$Cells, 9, 11
IgM-signaling pathways, 50
Ig VH gene, 262
IgV somatic hypermutation, 22, 24, 30
IL-2 family, 6
IL-15 family, 6
IL-21 family, 6
Immune effector cells, 266
Immune gene therapy, 204–209
  clinical trials of, 207–209
Immune system senescence
  MBL and, 78–79
Immune therapy, 201204
Immune thrombocytopenia (ITP)
  prevalence, 233
Immunoglobulin (Ig), 19, 270
Immunophenotypic analyses, 26
Immunophenotyping, 106
  B-cell PLL, 219
  T-cell PLL, 223
Immunoreceptor tyrosine-based inhibitory motif (ITIM), 53
Inhibitors of Apoptosis (IAP) proteins, 98–99
Inhibitory coreceptors, 53

Interferon consolidation therapy, 131–132
Interleukin-2, 205, 284
Interleukin-12, 205
Interleukin 21 (IL-21), 176
International Workshop Group on CLL (IWCLL), staging recommendations, 109
Intravenous immunoglobulin (IVIG), 283
Intrinsic apoptosis pathway, CLL, 91–93
In vivo purging of stem cells, 194
IP-10. *See* IFN-inducible protein 10 (IP-10)
Italian study
  MBL detection in hospital outpatients, 76–77
IVIG. *See* Intravenous immunoglobulin (IVIG)

Joseph Eletto Leukemia Research Fund, 12

LAK. *See* Lymphocyte-activated killer (LAK) cell
Large granular lymphocyte (LGL) leukemia, 108
Latent sensitivity to Fas-mediated apoptosis, 207
Lenalidomide, 167–169
Leukemia, 3
  hairy cell, 107
  large granular lymphocyte (LGL), 108
  prolymphocytic, 107–108, 217–226
Leukemic cells, 4
Leukemic clones, 3, 4
LPL genes, 24
Lumiliximab (IDEC-152), 166–167
Lymphocyte-activated killer (LAK) cell, 262
Lymphocytes, 21
Lymphoid malignancies, 21, 270
Lymphoid tissues, 4
Lymphopenia, 270
Lymphoplasmacytic lymphoma, 107
Lyn tyrosine kinase, 48

Mantle cell lymphoma, 107
MAPK pathway, 49–50
Marginal zone (MZ), 1
Mature B-cell malignancies, 27
M-CLL cells, 3, 5, 10–11
  IgM$^+$IgD$^+$CD27$^+$Cells and MZ B cells, 11
  murine B-2 cells, 10–11
MCL-1 protein, 97
Microarray profiling
  biological association between MBL and CLL, 79–80
Mig. *See* IFN-γ induced monokine (Mig)
HLL1 (milatuzumab), 177
Milatuzumab (hLL1), 177

miRNAs
   involved in CLL pathogenesis, 37–41
   as TCL1 interactors, 40
   as tumor suppressors, 37–40
miRnome, 30
Mitochondrial apoptosis in CLL
   BCL-2 family of proteins, control of, 94–96
Mitoxantrone
   with cyclophosphamide, combination che-
      motherapy, 127
   with cyclophosphamide and fludarabin (FC),
      combination chemotherapy, 126
Monoclonal antibodies, 261, 274–278
   alemtuzumab, 275–277
   consolidation therapy, CLL, 132–133
   rituximab, 274–275
   therapy for B-cell PLL, 221
Monoclonal B lymphocytes (MBL)
   in animal models, 72–74
   biological association between CLL and,
      79–82
   clinical association between CLL and, 82–83
   definition, 71–72
   detection in hospital outpatients, 75–77
   diagnostic criteria, 71–72
   IGHV gene usage in, 80–81
   immune system senescence and, 78–79
Monotherapy
   with alkylating agents, 123–124
   with purine analogs, 124
mRNA, 20, 24
Murine B-1 cell, 10
   subset, 10
Murine B-2 cells, 10–11
Mutated IgV genes, 23
P53 mutation
   frontline therapy of CLL patients with, 133
Myeloablative allogeneic transplantation, 186
Myelodysplasia (MDS), 195
Myelosuppressive therapy, 266
MZ. *See* Marginal zone (MZ)
MZ B cells, 4, 8–9, 10

National Cancer Institute, 12
National Cancer Institute - International
      Workshop on Chronic Lymphocytic
      Leukemia (NCI-IWCLL) guidelines, 71
National Cancer Institute (NCI) guidelines,
      diagnosis and assessment, 110
Natural killer (NK) cell, 262
NCI-IWCLL guidelines. *See* National Cancer
      Institute - International Workshop on
      Chronic Lymphocytic Leukemia (NCI-
      IWCLL) guidelines

Neoplastic cells, 261
Neutropenia, 266, 270
Neutrophil, 266
New Zealand black (NZB)
   mice, 74
   strain, 39
NF-AT transcription factors, 50
NF$_\kappa$B-inhibitory drug, 28
NF-kB/Rel transcription factors, 50
NF-$_\kappa$B target genes, 29
NK. *See* Natural killer (NK) cell
Non-Hodgkin lymphoma. *See* Diffuse large
      B-cell lymphoma (DLBCL)
Nonlymphoid cells, 5
North Shore University Hospital, 12
Nurse-like cells, 5

Oblimersen sodium, 158–159, 171
Ofatumumab (HuMax CD20), 166
Ohio State University (OSU) group study
   lenalidomide therapy, 168–169
Oncogenic transformation, 23
Oxidized autologous leukemia cell vaccine, 211

P. carinii pneumonia (PCP), 271
Paraneoplastic pemphigus, 236
PCP. *See P. carinii* pneumonia (PCP)
PCR. *See* Polymerase chain reaction (PCR)
Pentostatin, 148, 270
   salvage therapy in fludarabine-refractory
      patients, 155
Pentostatin with cyclophosphamide and ritux-
      imab (PCR), combination chemother-
      apy, 130
Peyer's patches, 1
PFS. *See* Progression-free survival (PFS)
Phagocytic cell, 262
Phosphatidylinositol 3-kinase pathway, 49
Phospholypase Cγ2, 49
PKCβ2, BCR signaling molecule, 52
Plasma cell, 5
PLL. *See* Prolymphocytic leukemia (PLL)
Polymerase chain reaction (PCR), 23
Positron emission tomographic (PET) scan-
      ning, 110
Precursor cells, 23
Preemptive therapy. *See* Antimicrobial pro-
      phylaxis
Prevention, of infection, 279–283
   antimicrobial prophylaxis, 280–282
   antineoplastic therapy, 279–280
   secondary prophylaxis, 282

Prognosis, 110–116

Prognostic factors
after development of Richter's syndrome, 245

Progression-free survival (PFS), 270
allogenic stem cell transplantation, 187–188

Prolymphocytic leukemia (PLL), 107–108, 217–226
B-cell, 217–222
clinical characteristics of, 218
laboratory characteristics of, 218
T-cell, 222–226

Prophylaxis, 272

Protein tyrosine kinase family, 23

Proximal BCR-signaling mediators, 48–49

Pseudoemperipolesis, 3

P53 target genes, 29

Pure red cell aplasia (PRCA), 233

Purine analogs, 270–274
combination chemotherapy with, 126–128
combinations, 273–274
monotherapy with, 124
salvage therapy, 144–148
fludarabine-refractory patients, 155, 156
treatments, 272–273

Purine analogue therapy
in B-cell PLL, 221
in older patients, 273

Radiation therapy, 277–278

Radiological assessment, 109–110

Raf kinase, 49–50

Rai staging system, 109, 111

Randomized comparative trial (RCT), 270

RCT. *See* Randomized comparative trial (RCT)

Reduced-intensity conditioning (RIC) allogenic stem cell transplantation, 188–191
risk factors for poor outcome after, 191–192

Relapsed CLL
investigational agents for, 166–171
treatment of patients with, 141–159

Respiratory tract infection, 272

Response assessment, CLL, 122–123, 142, 143

RIC. *See* Reduced-intensity conditioning (RIC)

Richter's syndrome, 238–249
clinical and laboratory features, 238–242
cytogenetics, 248–249
DLBCL, 245–247
epidemiology, 243–245
histological features of, 242–243
history, 238
Hodgkin lymphoma, 247–248
incidence, 243–245
molecular abnormalities, 248

[Richter's syndrome]
molecular features of, 248–249
pathogenesis, 248–249
radiological features, 238–242
risk factors, 243–245
scope, 238

Risk factors
for infections, 278–279
high-risk patient, 278
risk period, 279
Richter's syndrome, 243–245

Risk period, 29

Rituximab
autoimmunity treatment, 237
induction therapy, 148–151

Rituximab-based chemoimmunotherapy, 128–130

Rituximab induction therapy
in fludarabine-refractory patients, 155

RNA, 20

Salvage therapy
indications for, 141–142
therapeutic options for, 142–159

Secondary prophylaxis, 282

Second-line treatment in CLL, 134

Sezary syndrome, 108

Silvestrol, 178–179

Sinopulmonary infections, 283

Small lymphocytic lymphoma (SLL), 69, 103
diagnosis, 106

SmIgD, 4, 5

SmIgM, 4, 5

Splenectomy, 277
autoimmunity, 237
for B-cell PLL, 221

Splenic marginal zone lymphoma (SMZL)
with villous lymphocytes, 107

Splenomegaly, 266

SRC inhibitors, 178

Staging, CLL, 109–110

Stem cell transplantation, 185–196
allogeneic, 186–188
autologous, 192–194, 195–196
B-cell PLL, 221–222
late complications, 195
reduced-intensity conditioning (RIC), 188–192
T-cell PLL, 226

Stimulation, 4–6
BCR and TLR engagement, in vitro, 4–5
cytokine and chemokine influences, 5–6
T-cell dependence of CLL cell, 5

Streptococcus pneumoniae, 262
Stromal cells, 5
Subclinical organ-system dysfunction, population studies for, 74–77
Superfund sites
in United States, 74–75
Surface function-associated molecules, 205–206
Surface membrane phenotype, 3
Surrogate markers, VH mutation status, 112–114
Surveillance, Epidemiology, and End Results (SEER) Registry, United States, 69
Syk kinase, 48
Syk-ZAP-70, 23

TACI. *See* Transmembrane activator and CAML-interactor (TACI)
T-cell, 1, 4, 5, 23, 262
defects, autoimmunity, 234
dependence of CLL cell, 5
T-cell prolymphocytic leukemia (T-PLL), 108, 222–226
cell morphology, 223
clinical and laboratory features, 222–224
cytogenetics, 223–224
differential diagnosis, 224–225
immunophenotyping, 223
pathogenesis, 222
prognosis, 225–226
treatment, 225–226
T2 cells, 9
TCL1 interactors
miRNAs as, 40
Therapy-related factors, 266–278
alkylating agents, 266–278
corticosteroids, 266
Thrombocytopenia, autoimmune, 104
Thymidine kinase, 111–112
TI-2 antigens, 10
T-independent antigens, 26
TLR stimulation, 10
T-lymphocytes, 5, 270
TMP-SMX. *See* Trimethoprim sulfamethoxazole (TMP-SMX)
TNF. *See* Tumor necrosis factor (TNF) family
Toll-like receptors, 55–56
TP53 mutations, 220
TRAIL ligands, 93
Transcription factors
NF-AT family, 50
NF-kB/Rel family, 50

Transduction of CLL cells, 204–205
Transgenes, 205–207
Transitional B cells, 9, 10
Transmembrane activator and CAML-interactor (TACI), 6
Treatment
autoimmunity, 236–238
B-cell prolymphocytic leukemia (B-PLL), 220–222
T-cell PLL, 225–226
Treatment-naive CLL patients, trials, 124, 125
Treatment-related autoimmune complications, 234–235
Treatment-related risk factors
Richter's syndrome, 244–245
TRICOM, 206
Trimethoprim sulfamethoxazole (TMP-SMX), 272
Tru16, 176–177
Tumor-associated antigen (TAA), 202
Tumor cells, 23
Tumor necrosis factor (TNF) family, 5
Tumor-specific antigen (TSA), 202
Tumor suppressors
miRNAs as, 37–40
Type-2 antigens, 8

U-CLL cells, 3, 4, 5, 10
murine B-1 cell subset, 10
MZ B-cell, 10
transitional B cells, 10
U.K. study
MBL detection in hospital outpatients, 75–76
Ultraconsereved genes
and CLL, 41–42
United States
superfund sites in, 74–75
Unmutated IgV genes, 23

Vaccination, 283–284
Vaccine strategies, 210–211
Varicella zoster virus (VZV), 270
VDJ-junctional repertoire, 24
VDJ recombination, 28
$V_H DJ_H$ gene, 8
VH3-21-expressing CLL cases, 24
VH3-21 gene, 24

VH mutation status, 112
  genomic aberrations and, 116
  surrogate markers for, 112–114
Villous lymphocytes
  splenic marginal zone lymphoma (SMZL)
    with, 107
Virgin B cells, 6
VZV. *See* Varicella zoster virus (VZV)

Xcellerated T cells, 210

ZAP-70, 3, 4, 23, 24, 48, 112–114
  impact on outcome of RIC allogenic stem
    cell transplantation, 192